MW01205237

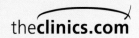

SLEEP MEDICINE CLINICS

Sleep in the Older Adult

Guest Editor
SONIA ANCOLI-ISRAEL, PhD

June 2006 • Volume 1 • Number 2

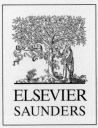

ELSEVIER
SAUNDERS

An imprint of Elsevier, Inc
PHILADELPHIA LONDON TORONTO MONTREAL SYDNEY TOKYO

W.B. SAUNDERS COMPANY
A Division of Elsevier Inc.

1600 John F. Kennedy Boulevard • Suite 1800 • Philadelphia, PA 19103-2899

http://www.sleep.theclinics.com

SLEEP MEDICINE CLINICS Volume 1, Number 2
June 2006 ISSN 1556-407X, ISBN 1-4160-3565-6

Editor: Sarah E. Barth

Copyright © 2006 Elsevier Inc. All rights reserved. No part of this publication may be reproduced or transmitted in any form or by any means, electronic or mechanical, including photocopy, recording, or any information storage and retrieval system, without written permission from the publisher.

Single photocopies of single articles may be made for personal use as allowed by national copyright laws. Permission of the publisher and payment of a fee is required for all other photocopying, including multiple or systematic copying, copying for advertising or promotional purposes, resale, and all forms of document delivery. Special rates are available for educational institutions that wish to make photocopies for non-profit educational classroom use. Permissions may be sought directly from Elsevier's Rights Department in Philadelphia, PA, USA; phone: (215) 239-3804, fax: (215) 239-3805, e-mail: healthpermissions@elsevier.com. Requests may also be completed on-line via the Elsevier homepage (http://www.elsevier.com/locate/permissions). In the USA, users may clear permissions and make payments through the Copyright Clearance Center, Inc., 222 Rosewood Drive,
Danvers, MA 01923, USA; phone: (978) 750-8400, fax: (978) 750-4744, and in the UK through the Copyright Licensing Agency Rapid Clearance Service (CLARCS), 90 Tottenham Court Road, London W1P 0LP, UK; phone: (+44) 171 436-5931; fax: (+44) 171 436 3986. Other countries may have a local reprographic rights agency for payments.

The ideas and opinions expressed in *Sleep Medicine Clinics* do not necessarily reflect those of the Publisher. The Publisher does not assume any responsibility for any injury and/or damage to persons or property arising out of or related to any use of the material contained in this periodical. The reader is advised to check the appropriate medical literature and the product information currently provided by the manufacturer of each drug to be administered to verify the dosage, the method and duration of administration, or contraindications. It is the responsibility of the treating physician or other health care professional, relying on independent experience and knowledge of the patient, to determine drug dosages and the best treatment for the patient. Mention of any product in this issue should not be construed as endorsement by the contributors, editors, or the Publisher of the product or manufacturers' claims.

Sleep Medicine Clinics (ISSN: 1556-407X) is published quarterly by W.B. Saunders Company, a division of Elsevier Inc., 360 Park Avenue South, New York, NY 10010-1710. Months of issue are March, June, September and December. Business and Editorial Offices: 1600 John F. Kennedy Blvd., Suite 1800, Philadelphia, PA 19103-2899. Accounting and Circulation offices: 6277 Sea Harbor Drive, Orlando, FL 32887-4800. Application to mail at periodicals postage rates is pending at New York, NY and additional mailing offices. **POSTMASTER**: Send address changes to *Sleep Medicine Clinics*, Elsevier Inc. Periodicals Department, 6277 Sea Harbor Drive, Orlando, FL 32887-4800.
Customer Service: 1-800-654-2452 (US). From outside of the United States,
call 1-407-345-4000. E-mail: hhspcs@wbsaunders.com.

Reprints: For copies of 100 or more, of articles in this publication, please contact the Commercial Reprints Department, Elsevier Inc., 360 Park Avenue South, New York, New York 10010-1710. Tel.: (212) 633-3813, Fax: (212) 462-1935, e-mail: reprints@elsevier.com

Printed in the United States of America.

GOAL STATEMENT

The goal of *Sleep Clinics of North America* is to keep practicing physicians up to date with current clinical practice in the diagnosis and treatment of sleep disorders by providing timely articles reviewing the state of the art in patient care.

ACCREDITATION

The *Sleep Clinics of North America* is planned and implemented in accordance with the Essential Areas and Policies of the Accreditation Council for Continuing Medical Education (ACCME) through the joint sponsorship of the University of Virginia School of Medicine and Elsevier. The University of Virginia School of Medicine is accredited by the ACCME to provide continuing medical education for physicians.

The University of Virginia School of Medicine designates this educational activity for a maximum of 15 AMA PRA Category 1 Credits™. Physicians should only claim credit commensurate with the extent of their participation in the activity.

The American Medical Association has determined that physicians not licensed in the US who participate in this CME activity are eligible for 15 AMA PRA Category 1 Credits™.

Category 1 credit can be earned by reading the text material, taking the CME examination online at *http://www. theclinics.com/home/cme*, and completing the evaluation. After taking the test, you will be required to review any and all incorrect answers. Following completion of the test and evaluation, your credit will be awarded and you may print your certificate.

FACULTY DISCLOSURE/CONFLICT OF INTEREST

The University of Virginia School of Medicine, as an ACCME accredited provider, endorses and strives to comply with the Accreditation Council for Continuing Medical Education (ACCME) Standards of Commercial Support, Commonwealth of Virginia statutes, University of Virginia policies and procedures, and associated federal and private regulations and guidelines on the need for disclosure and monitoring of proprietary and financial interests that may affect the scientific integrity and balance of content delivered in continuing medical education activities under our auspices.

The University of Virginia School of Medicine requires that all CME activities accredited through this institution be developed independently and be scientifically rigorous, balanced and objective in the presentation/discussion of its content, theories and practices.

All authors/editors participating in an accredited CME activity are expected to disclose to the readers relevant financial relationships with commercial entities occurring within the past 12 months (such as grants or research support, employee, consultant, stock holder, member of speakers bureau, etc.). The University of Virginia School of Medicine will employ appropriate mechanisms to resolve potential conflicts of interest to maintain the standards of fair and balanced education to the reader. Questions about specific strategies can be directed to the Office of Continuing Medical Education, University of Virginia School of Medicine, Charlottesville, Virginia.

The authors/editors listed below have identified no professional or financial affiliations for themselves or their spouse/partner:
Steven R. Barczi, MD; Amanda Schurle Bruce, MS; Lavinia Fiorentino, MS; Timothy M. Juergens, MD; Kathryn A. Lee, RN, PhD; Christine McCrae, PhD; Sidney D. Nau, PhD; Erik Naylor, PhD; Kristen L. Payne, MA; Susan Redline, M.D., M.P.H.; Kristen C. Stone, MS; Katie L. Stone, PhD; Michael V. Vitiello, PhD; and, Phyllis C. Zee, MD, PhD.

The authors/editors listed below identified the following professional or financial affiliations for themselves or their spouse/partner:
Mark S. Aloia, PhD is a consultant for Respironics.
Sonia Ancoli-Israel, PhD is a consultant and is on the advisory committee for Acadia, Cephalon, Inc, King Pharmaceuticals, Inc., Merck, Neurocrine Biosciences, Inc., Neurogen, Inc., Pfizer, Inc., Sanofi-Aventis, Sepracor, Inc., Somaxon, and Takeda Pharmaceuticals North America, Inc.; and, is on the speaker's bureau for Acadia, Cephalon, Inc, King Pharmaceuticals, Inc., Merck, Neurocrine Biosciences, Inc., Neurogen, Inc., Pfizer, Inc., Sanofi-Aventis, Sepracor, Inc., Somaxon, and Takeda Pharmaceuticals North America, Inc.
Alon Y. Avidan, MD, MPH is a consultant for Takeda Pharmaceutical; is on the speaker's bureau for Takeda Pharmaceutical, Sepracor, and GlaxoSmithKline; and, is on the advisory committee for Sepracor, Neurocrine, and GlaxoSmithKline.
Donald L. Bliwise, PhD is an independent contractor for GlaxoSmithKlime
Kenneth Lichstein, PhD is an independent contractor for Respironics, has stock in Sepracor, and is a consultant for Lilly.
Jennifer L. Martin, PhD is a consultant for Sepracor, Inc.

Disclosure of Discussion of non-FDA approved uses for pharmaceutical products and/or medical devices:
The University of Virginia School of Medicine, as an ACCME provider, requires that all faculty presenters identify and disclose any "off label" uses for pharmaceutical and medical device products. The University of Virginia School of Medicine recommends that each physician fully review all the available data on new products or procedures prior to instituting them with patients.

TO ENROLL

To enroll in the Sleep Clinics of North America Continuing Medical Education program, call customer service at 1-800-654-2452 or visit us online at www.theclinics.com/home/cme. The CME program is available to subscribers for an additional fee of $99.95.

THE CLINICS ARE NOW AVAILABLE ONLINE!

Access your subscription at:
www.theclinics.com

SLEEP IN THE OLDER ADULT

CONSULTING EDITOR

TEOFILO LEE-CHIONG, MD
National Jewish Medical and Research Center,
Denver, Colorado

GUEST EDITOR

SONIA ANCOLI-ISRAEL, PhD
Professor of Psychiatry, University of California San
Diego, La Jolla, California; Veterans Affairs San
Diego Healthcare System, San Diego, California

CONTRIBUTORS

MARK S. ALOIA, PhD
Assistant Professor, Department of Psychiatry and
Human Behavior, Brown Medical School,
Providence, Rhode Island

SONIA ANCOLI-ISRAEL, PhD
Professor of Psychiatry, University of California
San Diego, La Jolla, California; Veterans Affairs San
Diego Healthcare System, San Diego, California

ALON Y. AVIDAN, MD, MPH
Associate Professor and Associate Director, Sleep
Disorders Center UCLA, Department of
Neurology, Los Angeles, California

STEVEN R. BARCZI, MD
Associate Professor of Medicine, Section of
Geriatrics, University of Wisconsin School of
Medicine and Public Health, Madison, Wisconsin,
and Clinical Director, Madison VA Geriatrics,
Research, Education and Clinical Center,
Wm. S. Middleton Veterans Hospital, Madison,
Wisconsin

DONALD L. BLIWISE, PhD
Professor of Neurology and Director, Program in
Sleep, Aging and Chronobiology, Department of
Neurology, Emory University Medical School,
Atlanta, Georgia

AMANDA SCHURLE BRUCE, MS
Protocol Therapist, Department of Psychiatry and
Human Behavior, Brown Medical School,
Providence, Rhode Island

LAVINIA FIORENTINO, MS
Department of Psychiatry, University of California
San Diego, SDSU/UCSD Joint Doctoral Program
in Clinical Psychology, La Jolla, California;
Veterans Affairs San Diego Healthcare System, San
Diego, California

TIMOTHY M. JUERGENS, MD
Assistant Professor of Psychiatry, University of
Wisconsin School of Medicine and Public Health,
Madison, Wisconsin, and Director, Clinical Sleep
Laboratory, Geriatric Psychiatry, Wm. S. Middleton
Veterans Hospital, Madison, Wisconsin

KATHRYN A. LEE, PhD, RN, FAAN, CBSM
Professor of Nursing, James and Marjorie
Livingston Endowed Chair, Department of Family
Health Care Nursing, School of Nursing,
University of California, San Francisco, San
Francisco, California

KENNETH L. LICHSTEIN, PhD
Professor of Psychology, The University of
Alabama, Tuscaloosa, Alabama

JENNIFER L. MARTIN, PhD
Assistant Research Professor, Department of
Medicine, University of California, Los Angeles;
and Research Health Scientist, Geriatric Research,
Education and Clinical Center, VA Greater Los
Angeles Healthcare System, North Hills, California

CHRISTINA S. McCRAE, PhD
Assistant Professor of Psychology, University of
Florida, Gainesville, Florida

SIDNEY D. NAU, PhD
Research Scientist, Department of Psychology,
The University of Alabama, Tuscaloosa,
Alabama

ERIK NAYLOR, PhD
Postdoctoral Fellow, Department of Neurology,
Northwestern University Medical School, Chicago,
Illinois

KRISTEN L. PAYNE, MA
Graduate Student, Department of Psychology, The
University of Alabama, Tuscaloosa, Alabama

SUSAN REDLINE, MD
Professor of Pediatrics, Medicine, and
Epidemiology and Biostatistics, Case Western
Reserve University, Cleveland, Ohio

KATIE L. STONE, PhD
Scientist, San Francisco Coordinating Center/
California Pacific Medical Center Research
Institute, San Francisco, California

KRISTEN C. STONE, MS
Graduate Student, Department of Psychology,
University of Memphis, Memphis, Tennessee

MICHAEL V. VITIELLO, PhD
Professor, Department of Psychiatry and
Behavioral Sciences, University of Washington,
Seattle, Washington

PHYLLIS C. ZEE, MD, PhD
Professor, Department of Neurology,
Northwestern University Medical School, Chicago,
Illinois

SLEEP IN THE OLDER ADULT

Volume 1 • Number 2 • June 2006

Contents

The sleep of an older adult is not necessarily disturbed or of poor quality. Many high-functioning older adults are satisfied with their sleep, even though it is of objectively poorer quality compared with younger adults. When the various factors that can disrupt sleep are screened out, optimally or successfully aging adults can expect to undergo little change in their sleep, relative to those in the early to middle adult life span, and not be likely to experience excessive daytime sleep and the concomitant need to nap regularly during the day. Nevertheless, even successfully aging older adults can expect on average to be earlier to bed and to rise and to be less tolerant of circadian phase shifts than younger similarly healthy adults.

Research shows that napping and subjective daytime sleepiness are more common among older than among younger adults. This age-related increase in napping is likely caused by disruption in nighttime sleep, changes in circadian rhythms, lifestyle factors, and medical and psychiatric comorbidities. Some studies show that napping is associated with negative health outcomes, cognitive impairment, and increased mortality risk among older persons. Additional epidemiologic research is needed to describe more fully the timing and characteristics of daytime sleeping among older people, and further experimental research is needed to explore the mechanisms underlying the relationship between napping and health outcomes.

This article discusses the current knowledge and theory underlying circadian changes with age and their possible contribution to decreased sleep quality in this population. Sleep disturbances show higher prevalence with advanced age. Age-related circadian changes are seen at all levels; however, modifications in circadian rhythms alone do not fully explain common age-related difficulties. It is likely that changes in both circadian and sleep homeostatic processes, or the interaction between the two, are responsible for the impaired sleep of older adults. Advances in understanding of the circadian system and its interactions with sleep have resulted in some promising treatment options.

For midlife women, sleep disturbance is a major complaint associated with menopausal transition. Sleep during the menopausal years was reviewed using a biopsychosocial framework; cross-sectional and longitudinal study findings are compared. Biologic factors associated with sleep disturbance include diet and body mass index, inactivity, ovarian hormonal changes, and temperature fluctuations associated with hot flashes and night sweats. Psychologic factors include anxiety and depression. Sociocultural factors include race and ethnicity; income and education; and multiple role demands related to employment, relationships with family members, children leaving home, and caregiving for young children and elderly parents.

There has long been interest in the relationship between sleep and cognitive functioning. The literature demonstrating a negative effect of sleep abnormalities on cognitive functioning has developed rapidly over the past decade. This article addresses questions designed to summarize the existing literature and to theorize about the mechanisms behind the findings and their implications for future research. Addressed are questions of specificity, including which aspects of cognition are most affected by different types of sleep changes in the elderly. Also explored is functionality, asking how sleep might interfere with functional abilities.

Compared with other age groups, insomnia is more prevalent and more severe among older adults. Insomnia can signal the presence of other sleep disorders and is a health risk factor for depression, anxiety, substance abuse, and suicide. This article comprehensively examines older adults with insomnia, emphasizing a behavioral sleep medicine perspective.

As the field of medicine continues to advance, people are living longer with more comorbid medical and psychiatric conditions. This higher burden of illness and the numbers of medications used to treat these conditions plays an important role in the quality and quantity of sleep in older adults. In approaching sleep complaints in geriatric patients, it is essential that practitioners recognize the multidimensional mechanisms by which illness impacts sleep. Equally important, a balanced management approach that includes optimizing the underlying illness, adjusting medications, using cognitive-behavioral approaches, and using judicious hypnotic therapy seems justified based on the current evidence.

SLEEP
MEDICINE
CLINICS

Sleep Med Clin 1 (2006) xi–xiii

Preface
Sleep in the Older Adult

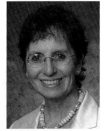

Sonia Ancoli-Israel, PhD
Professor of Psychiatry, Department of Psychiatry,
University of California San Diego,
9500 Gilman Drive #0603, La Jolla, CA 92093

E-mail address:
sancoliisrael@ucsd.edu

Sonia Ancoli-Israel, PhD
Guest Editor

"Aging seems to be the only available way to live a long life."
—Daniel Francois Esprit Auber

Yes, one has to age to live a long life, and if one is going to age, the key is to do it gracefully, to stay as healthy as possible, and to keep getting a good night's sleep.

Sleep changes over the life span. Young children sleep in multiple bouts throughout the day and night, whereas adults sleep in one or, at the most, two bouts (nighttime sleep and one "siesta"). Sleep stages change, with deeper levels of sleep decreasing with age. Sleep problems are very common in the older adult, often independent of the normal changes seen in sleep architecture. There has been much debate in the field of sleep medicine about whether older adults sleep less because their need for sleep decreases. Whether need for sleep decreases or not, it is clear that the ability to sleep does decrease with age, not because of aging per se, but because of all the other things that happen to us as we age. For example, poor sleep is associated with medical illness, psychiatric illness, medication use, and circadian rhythm changes. Poor sleep is also a result of specific sleep disorders, such as sleep-disordered breathing (SDB), restless legs syndrome (RLS), and periodic limb movements in sleep (PLMS). Dementia and being institutionalized also negatively affect sleep. This issue of the *Sleep Medicine Clinics* focuses on each of the different aspects of sleep disturbance in the older adult, and, as the reader will see, the topics of many of the articles intersect with each other.

In the first article, on sleep in normal aging, Vitiello describes some studies that recently have had great impact on what we understand about sleep in normal aging. For example, a recent meta-analysis found that the changes in sleep believed to be part of aging, such as decreased total sleep time and decreased slow-wave sleep, actually begin to decrease at an early age and remain stable in those aged 60 and over. Vitiello points out that there is no reason to assume that because an adult is older, sleep will necessarily be disturbed. He correctly states that many high-functioning, healthy older adults are very satisfied with their sleep and many have no sleep problems. He also points out that some high-functioning, healthy older adults have no complaints despite having objectively poorer quality sleep compared to younger adults. This brings up the question of which is more

1556-407X/06/$ – see front matter © 2006 Elsevier Inc. All rights reserved.
sleep.theclinics.com

doi:10.1016/j.jsmc.2006.04.012

important—the subjective perception of sleep or the objective measurement of sleep? This question remains unanswered within our field, and many believe that in fact, both are important.

In the second article, on napping, Martin and Ancoli-Israel review the research that confirms that napping is common in older adults, probably because of disruption of nighttime sleep, changes in circadian rhythms, lifestyle, and comorbidites (the effect of each of these factors on nighttime sleep are also covered separately in subsequent articles). The question of whether napping is beneficial or detrimental is quite controversial, and the authors review the evidence both for and against. Whereas brief naps may increase late afternoon and evening alertness, long naps may interfere with the ability to fall sleep. The authors also make the distinction between napping and daytime sleepiness. Daytime sleepiness is not synonymous with napping. Some older adults may be sleepy during the day without actually napping, and sleepiness and napping both may independently result in negative consequences. One of the negative consequences of napping is believed to be an increased risk of mortality. The authors review the evidence and summarize it in tabular form, allowing the reader to compare between the different studies. They conclude that the current literature does not allow for causal links between napping and negative health outcomes and that more research is needed to understand the potential mechanisms underlying the relationship between napping and increased mortality risk.

In the next article, on circadian rhythm alterations with aging, Naylor and Zee review the current knowledge and theories about changes in circadian rhythms as well as the contribution of these changes to decreased sleep quality in the older adult. Both the amplitude and the phase of the rhythm change with age, but this may be due in part to reductions in exposure to external entraining, *zeitgebers* (cues). The authors point out that age-related changes in the circadian system, on both the molecular and cellular level, and in the physiological, hormonal, and behavioral outputs of the circadian clock, do not fully explain the advanced sleep phase or the decrease in the amplitude of the sleep/wake activity cycle. Rather, it is most likely a combination of changes in the circadian and homeostatic processes that result in impaired sleep in this population.

Lee, in the article on sleep in midlife women, reviews the literature on the effect of menopause on sleep. In addition to the hormonal changes and hot flashes and sweats, many other factors also affect sleep in these women, including diet, weight, activity levels, and mood (particularly depression and anxiety). In addition, changes in lifestyle, such as children leaving home or needing to care for elderly parents, can also have an effect on sleep. This is important, because many clinicians assume that poor sleep in older women is just secondary to menopausal changes. Lee provides recommendations for the clinician on how to assess sleep problems in midlife women. Lee concludes that the extent to which menopausal symptoms influence sleep remains to be determined in larger longitudinal studies. But as importantly, more research is also needed to determine the extent to which other factors, such as obesity, depressed mood, sedentary lifestyle, or poor sleep behaviors may interact with menopause.

As part of normal aging, cognitive function begins to change, and poor sleep may contribute to further decrements in cognition. There is extensive literature on dementia and sleep, but Bruce and Aloia, in their article on sleep and cognition in older adults, review the literature on the relationship between sleep and cognition in cognitively intact, i.e., normal older adults. In addition, the authors theorize about the mechanisms that may underlie this relationship. Questions of which aspects of cognition are affected by sleep disruption are addressed, as are questions of how sleep disruption interferes with functional ability. Bruce and Aloia conclude by suggesting that research is needed to test whether improving sleep will also maximize functioning, i.e., whether improving sleep will improve cognition and whether improving cognition can also improve sleep.

The next article takes us away from normal aging, inasmuch as it is the first of a series of articles on sleep disorders. Lichstein et al., in their article on insomnia in the elderly, review the epidemiology, causes, consequences, and treatments of insomnia. As mentioned above, insomnia is most often comorbid with medical and psychiatric illnesses and the medications used to treat them. It may also be a symptom of other sleep disorders, such as SDB, RLS, PLMS, and circadian rhythm disorders. Not only can mood disorders result in insomnia, but as the authors describe, insomnia is a risk factor for depression, anxiety, substance abuse, and suicide. The National Institute on Health held a State-of-the-Science conference on insomnia in June of 2005 and concluded, among other things, that behavioral therapies for insomnia are the most efficacious and safe [1]. In this article, the authors emphasize a behavioral sleep medicine approach to the treatment of insomnia, but also give an unbiased overview of pharmacological treatments available for the older adult. As the authors conclude, clinicians must examine the efficacy, convenience, adherence, and safety of all treatment options when considering the clinical management of insomnia in older adults.

As mentioned in several articles, sleeping difficulties, and particularly insomnia, are most often comorbid with medical and psychiatric disorders as well as the medications used to treat those disorders. Barczi and Juergens, in their article on psychiatric, medical, medication, and substance use, review the comorbidities and how each affects sleep. They note that given the high prevalence of disease in older adults, it is highly likely that sleep disturbances will be seen in these patients. In addition, the more medical problems present, the worse the sleep. Barczi and Juergens conclude by reminding practitioners to look for and recognize the interaction between illness and sleep, and to adopt a balanced management approach that treats the underlying illness at the same time that the sleep disorder is treated, adjusts the medications, and uses behavioral therapy and, when needed, judicious hypnotic therapy.

Stone and Redline, in their article on SDB in the elderly, review the physiological and clinical features, epidemiology including risk factors, morbidity and mortality (in particular increased risk of cardiovascular and metabolic consequences, and cognitive impairment), and clinical assessment and treatment of SDB in the older adult. There is much discussion within the field of Sleep Medicine as to whether SDB in the older adult is equivalent to SDB in the younger adult. Stone and Redline review evidence on both sides of the argument, and conclude that whether it is the same or not, older adults who present with symptoms of SDB, or who exhibit comorbidities usually associated with SDB, need to be evaluated and considered for appropriate treatment.

In the next article, on PLMS and RLS, Bliwise reviews the epidemiology, characteristics, and treatment of these two related but independent conditions. Both conditions are very common in the older adult, and the risk factors for both are the same as those for younger adults, i.e., diabetes, neuropathy, renal insufficiency, and cardiovascular disease. The question of the clinical significance of periodic leg movements, without accompanying complaints of sleep disturbance, has not yet been answered; however, Bliwise presents evidence suggesting that PLMS with no symptoms is quite common in older adults and that these individuals may not need treatment. The same cannot be said for RLS, which can be a major problem for the older patient, and which clinicians should consider in every patient complaining of restlessness (or in dementia patients who pace).

Although neurological problems could have been covered in the article on comorbidities, there is sufficient research on sleep in these conditions, particularly dementia, to warrant a separate article. Avidan, in his article on sleep and neurological problems in the elderly, reviews the evidence on sleep in neurodegenerative diseases (e.g., Alzheimer's disease, Parkinson's disease, rapid eye movement behavior disorder, Lewy Body dementia, and multiple system atrophy, to name a few) and then describes the diagnostic approach to each. Inasmuch as these conditions often lead to institutionalization, it is crucial for the clinician to carefully examine the contribution of sleep disturbances to the symptoms of excessive sleepiness, wandering, and cognitive impairment, because these may be reversible with successful treatment of the sleep problem.

In the final article, on sleep disturbances in nursing home patients, Fiorentino and Ancoli-Israel review the sleep of the institutionalized, demented patient, as well as the effect of institutionalization on sleep. All of the sleep problems described in the previous articles also apply to the older adult in the nursing home. In addition, poor sleep at night in this population increases the risk of falls and affects overall concentration and recall. Often, environmental factors, such as poor light exposure and noise, contribute to poor sleep, yet these are contributing factors that can easily be remedied. Over two thirds of patients in nursing homes have sleep problems, but sleep disturbance and daytime sleeping are rarely documented in medical records. These patients should receive a complete sleep evaluation and, when needed, treatment for their sleep problems.

In closing, I would like to thank my colleagues who contributed to this issue and all my colleagues who study sleep in aging. It is a small group of very dedicated investigators who work on understanding sleep in the older adult. I am sure we all feel that there is no better way to honor older individuals than by trying to make their days more comfortable by filling their nights with good sleep.

Reference

[1] NIH State of the Science Conference Statement. Manifestations and management of chronic insomnia in adults. Sleep 2005;28(9):1049–57.

SLEEP
MEDICINE
CLINICS

Sleep Med Clin 1 (2006) 171–176

Sleep in Normal Aging

Michael V. Vitiello, PhD

- Sleep in normal aging
- Circadian rhythms in normal aging
- Napping and excessive daytime sleepiness in normal aging
- Causes of disturbed sleep in older adults
- Summary
- References

As of 2006 persons 65 years of age or older comprise approximately 12% of the United States population, but by 2030 the proportion of older adults will rise to 20%. This older portion of the national population is increasing twice as fast as other age groups, so that by 2030 the number of persons 65 year of age or older in the United States will effectively double to 72 million. In this rapidly expanding older portion of the national population, one of the major changes that commonly accompany the aging process is an often profound disruption of an individual's daily sleep-wake cycle. As many as 50% of older individuals complain about sleep problems, including disturbed or "light" sleep, frequent awakenings, early morning awakenings, and undesired daytime sleepiness [1–3]. Such disturbances can lead to impaired daytime function and seriously compromise quality of life.

The most striking change in sleep in older adults is the repeated and frequent interruption of sleep by long periods of wakefulness, possibly the result of an age-dependent intrinsic lightening of sleep homeostatic processes [4,5]. Further, older adults are more easily aroused from nighttime sleep by auditory stimuli suggesting that they may be more sensitive to environmental stimuli [6]. Both of these changes are indicative of impaired sleep maintenance and depth and contribute to the characterization of the sleep of older adults

as lighter, or more fragile, than that of younger adults.

These age-associated increases of nighttime wakefulness are mirrored by increases in daytime fatigue, excessive daytime sleepiness (EDS), and increased likelihood of napping or falling asleep during the day. Aging is also associated with a tendency to fall asleep and awaken earlier [7] (ie, a tendency for older individuals to be "larks" rather than "owls"). Older individuals also tend to be less tolerant of phase shifts in time of the sleep-wake schedule, such as those produced by jet lag and shift work [8,9]. These changes suggest an age-related breakdown of the normal adult circadian sleep-wake cycle.

It is important to note that even carefully screened older adults who do not complain of sleep disturbance and with minimal medical burdens show the changes described previously when compared with younger adults [10,11]. This suggests that at least some of the sleep disturbance seen in older adults is part of the aging process per se, apparently independent of any medical or psychiatric illnesses or primary sleep disorders, and often referred to as "age-related sleep change" [12,13]. A 60-year-old generally does not expect to be able to do all things as well as they did when they were 20. Similarly, their ability to sleep need not be the same. Just as an older individual can no longer

Supported by PHS grants AG025515, HP70139, AT002108, MH072736, and NR04101
Department of Psychiatry and Behavioral Sciences, University of Washington, Box 356560, 1959 NE Pacific Street, Room BB-1520D, Seattle, WA 98195–6560, USA
E-mail address: vitiello@u.washington.edu

run a 100-yd dash with the speed of their youth because of the physiologic changes that accompany the aging process, so too they can no longer sleep with the relatively undisturbed length and depth of the sleep of their younger years. As to whether this age-related decline in the ability to generate sleep equates with a decreased need for sleep in the later years of the human lifespan remains unclear. Nevertheless, the available scientific evidence suggests it is important to remember that, as one ages it might be best to modify the expectations about "inalienable rights" to life, liberty, and 8 hours of sound, uninterrupted sleep.

Sleep in normal aging

Sleep changes with advancing age, but the question remains, exactly when do these changes occur. Since the classic publication of Roffwarg and coworkers in 1966 [14], the accepted wisdom has been that the age-related sleep changes that characterize the sleep of older adults begin to appear in early adulthood and progress steadily across the full continuum of adult human lifespan, including the older adult years. Nearly 50 years of regular republication of Roffwarg and coworkers' [15] figure illustrating sleep change across the human life span, by the current author among many others, essentially reified this assumption.

Recent findings, however, call this assumption into serious question. The results of an extensive meta-analysis of objective sleep measures across the human lifespan by Ohayon and coworkers [15] demonstrated that the bulk of the changes seen in adult sleep patterns occur between early adulthood, beginning at age 19 through age 60, and that changes in sleep macroarchitecture effectively asymptote, declining only minimally from age 60 to age 102 [15].

The adult life span sleep changes reported by Ohayon and coworkers [15] are summarized in Table 1. These results are based on meta-analyses conducted on data from 2391 adults ages 19 to 102. When the full adult life span was examined, Ohayon and coworkers [15] confirmed the four consistently reported age-related changes in polysomnographic studies of sleep macroarchitecture: decreases in total sleep time, sleep efficiency, and slow wave sleep; and increases in wake after sleep onset. Ohayon and coworkers [15] also demonstrated that less consistently reported age-related sleep changes, increases in stage 1 and stage 2 sleep, and decreases in rapid eye movement sleep were all confirmed by their meta-analyses. Ohayon and coworkers [15] reported that age-related changes in either sleep latency or rapid eye movement latency were minimal.

Table 1: Summary of significant findings from meta-analyses examining the associations between various sleep measures and age across both the full adult life-span (19-102 yrs) and the older adult life-span (60-102 yrs)

	Adults 19–102 y	Older adults 60–102 y
Total sleep time	⇓	⇔
Sleep latency	⇔	⇔
WASO	⇑	⇔
Sleep efficiency	⇓	⇓
Percent stage 1	⇑	⇔
Percent stage 2	⇑	⇔
Percent SWS	⇓	⇔
Percent REM	⇓	⇔
REM latency	⇔	⇔

Abbreviations: REM, rapid eye movement; SWS, slow wave sleep; WASO, wake after sleep onset; ⇔, unchanged; ⇓, decreased; ⇑, increased.
(*From* Ohayon MM, Carskadon M, Guilliminault C, et al. Meta-analysis of quantitative sleep parameters from childhood to old age in healthy individuals: developing normative sleep values across the human lifespan. Sleep 2004:27:1255–73; with permission.)

All of these significant age changes in objectively assessed sleep architecture, however, were found only when the full adult life span was examined. When the sleep of only older (60+ years) adults was examined, meta-analyses demonstrated that only sleep efficiency declined significantly from ages 60 to 70 to ages ≥70 years, and even then at a modest rate of approximately 3% per decade. None of the other eight sleep measures showed any significant age-related change within the older adult portion of the study sample. It is of interest to note that these findings were comparable for both older men and older women.

These findings seem counterintuitive, and fly against the wind of commonly held concepts of sleep-changes with aging. It is important to remember, however, that Ohayon and colleagues [15] used very rigorous selection criteria in choosing the study subjects for their meta-analyses. The approximately 2400 subjects were not representative of the older population, but rather were in excellent health and more likely represent individuals who are "optimally" or "successfully" aging. Ohayon and coworkers [15] findings report normative sleep architecture data representing only those older adults who are in very good health and not average data for the overall older adult population, an extremely important distinction.

To illustrate this crucial point better, it is informative to contrast the findings of Ohayon and colleagues [15] with those of a recent large (2685 subjects) cross-sectional study of objective sleep measures of adults (37–92 years), the Sleep Heart Health Study cohort [16]. In this large and well-conducted study, Redline and colleagues [16] concluded that "...sleep architecture varies with sex, (and) age..." and that "Men, but not women, show evidence of poorer sleep with aging...." These conclusions seem at odds with those of Ohayon and colleagues [15]. Several important differences in the two studies need to be considered, however, beyond the obvious one of Ohayon and coworkers [15] being a meta-analysis and Redline and coworkers [16] being the report of a prospective cohort study. First, and perhaps most importantly, the Sleep Heart Health Study cohort was "...recruited from 9 existing epidemiological studies in which data on cardiovascular risk factors had been collected..." forming a cohort that "...met the inclusion criteria (age ≥40 years), no history of sleep apnea, no tracheotomy, and no current home oxygen therapy..." This relatively mild screening is in marked contrast to the extensive screening criteria used to develop Ohayon and coworkers study sample [15]. Second, Redline and colleagues [16], when examining possible age effects, did not break down their sample to see if there were any age effects in the older half of their sample, but rather examined such effects across the full age range available.

Essentially, the two studies are complementary with Ohayon and coworkers [15] reporting on the impact of age in individuals who are aging "successfully," whereas Redline and coworkers [16], with their much more liberal selection criteria, reporting on the impact of age in a group of individuals who are likely much more representative of the older population as a whole, are reporting on "average" aging. It is of particular interest that Redline concludes that men, but not women, tend to show poorer sleep with aging. Likely, this is the result of excess subclinical morbidity in men, because when such morbidity is screened out, as in the case of Ohayon and coworkers [15], there are minimal sex differences in the sleep of men and women across the adult life span.

What all of these finding suggest is that sleep clearly changes significantly across the human life span. When the comorbidities that typically accompany the aging process are controlled for and "optimal" aging examined, however, then the bulk of age-related sleep changes occurs in early and middle adulthood (years 19–60) and that after age 60, assuming one is in good health, further age-related sleep changes are modest. Conversely, if comorbidities are present, it is clear that normal age-related sleep changes may well be exacerbated.

Circadian rhythms in normal aging

Not only does the quality of sleep change across the human life span, but the timing of that sleep also changes with aging. Circadian rhythms are those that occur within a period of 24 hours (from the Greek "about [circa] a day [dies]"), such as the adult human sleep-wake cycle. The impact of aging on human circadian rhythms has recently been comprehensively reviewed by Monk [17]. Interestingly, as with sleep, there is a considerably disparity with what is the conventional wisdom concerning circadian rhythms and aging, and what is the evidence supporting or not supporting those conventionally held beliefs. Monk [17] summaries the conventional wisdom regarding what happens to human circadian processes with aging as (1) circadian amplitude is reduced; (2) there is a circadian phase advance (ie, the circadian rhythm moves earlier relative to the environment); (3) there is a shortening of the circadian free-running period (tau); and (4) the ability to tolerate rapid phase-shifts (eg, shift work, or rapid transmeridian travel [jet lag]) declines [17].

The available evidence, however, convincingly supports only two of these assumptions: older people tend to have earlier circadian phases, with a corresponding tendency to go to and arise from bed earlier than younger adults (eg; 7); and, older people have more trouble than younger adults adjusting to the rapid phase shifts of shift work and jet lag, at least in terms of sleep quality, subjective complaint, and performance measures (e.g.; 8–9). Interestingly, the data in support of diminished circadian amplitudes and shortened circadian taus in healthy older adults are equivocal [17].

Napping and excessive daytime sleepiness in normal aging

Two other commonly held assumptions about sleep and aging are that older adults typically nap more than younger adults and report more EDS. Although numerous community-based epidemiologic studies have reported prevalence rates for sleep disturbances, daytime sleep-related complaints, such as EDS, and possibly undiagnosed sleep disorders among older adults to be as high as 20% to 30% [1,18,19], few of these have reported the prevalence of regular napping and its association with sleep complaints and other mental and physical health problems, especially in relation EDS [18]. Perhaps surprisingly, although epidemiologic studies typically show a significant increase in the prevalence of regular napping with advancing age, EDS does not demonstrate a similar increase in prevalence among older adults [18,20].

Consistent with the findings described previously for nighttime sleep measures, very recent findings indicate that the presence of comorbidities (medical illness, depression, and so forth) is highly associated with the likelihood of an older adult reporting regular napping or EDS [21,22]. Healthy older adults, even those complaining of significant nighttime sleep disturbance, are much less likely to report regular napping or EDS than their more health burdened cohorts.

Regarding napping behavior, there is also considerable debate as to whether regular napping among older adults, particularly those in good health, may be beneficial to daytime wakefulness or perhaps detrimental to their nighttime sleep propensity [23–25]. The two studies that examined the impact of daytime napping on the nighttime sleep quality of healthy older adults found that napping had only a mild to moderate impact on nighttime sleep quality [24,25]; one of them further demonstrated that such napping resulted in improved cognitive performance postnap [24]. These results need to be interpreted with caution, however, because it must be emphasized that the subjects involved were healthy older adults without significant sleep complaints and neither older adults unhappy with their sleep quality nor geriatric insomniacs. It is unclear if similar results can be obtained, for example, with a sample of older insomniacs.

Causes of disturbed sleep in older adults

Much has been made of the often repeated fact that epidemiologic studies report as much as 50% of older adults complain of significant, chronic sleep disturbance. It is important to keep in mind, however, that 50% of older adults do not. Ohayon and coworkers [15] demonstrated that the bulk of age-related sleep changes occur in early to middle adulthood and that the sleep of very healthy older adults changes only very slowly across the later human life span. It has correspondingly been demonstrated that older adults who do not complain of any sleep problems nevertheless have objective sleep quality that is markedly compromised (eg, less total sleep time, sleep efficiency, slow wave sleep, and more wake after sleep onset) compared with that of healthy, non–sleep-complaining, younger adults. Nevertheless, there are many factors over and above age-related sleep (both sleep homeostatic and circadian) changes that can and do contribute to the significant sleep disturbance reported by nearly half of all older adults. These can include (1) medical and psychiatric comorbidities and their treatments, such as cardiovascular disease, arthritis, gastroesophageal reflux, or depression, and many of the drugs used to treat them; (2) primary sleep disorders, many of which, such as sleep apnea, restless legs syndrome, and rapid eye movement behavior disorder, tend to occur with

Table 2:   Causes of poor sleep in older adults

Cause or problem	Examples
Physiologic	Age-related sleep change
	Age-related circadian rhythm change (phase advance)
Medical illnesses	Arthritis or other conditions causing chronic or intermittent pain
	Chronic cardiac or pulmonary disease
	Gastroesophageal reflux disorder
Psychiatric illnesses	Depression
Medications	Diuretics (leading to nocturnal awakenings)
	Inappropriate use of OTC medications
Primary sleep disorders	Sleep disordered breathing (sleep apnea)
	Restless legs syndrome
	REM behavior disorder
Behavioral or social	Retirement or lifestyle change reducing need for regular bed and rise times
	Death of a family member or friend
	Inappropriate use of social drugs
	Transmeridian air travel
	Napping
Environmental	Bedroom environment (eg, ambient noise, temperature, light, bedding)
	Moving to a new home or downsizing to a smaller space or a retirement community or related facility
	Institutionalization

Abbreviations: OTC, over-the-counter; REM, rapid eye movement.

increasing frequency in older adults; (3) the many behavioral, environmental, and social factors, often collectively referred to as "sleep hygiene," that can maximize or compromise an individual's sleep quality; or (4) some combination of these factors [12,13,26]. A more comprehensive listing of these factors is found in Table 2, and many of these issues are explored elsewhere in this issue.

Summary

There is no reason to assume, a priori, that the sleep of an older adult is necessarily disturbed or of poor quality; many high-functioning older adults are satisfied with their sleep, even though it is of objectively poorer quality compared with younger adults. It seems that, when the various factors that can disrupt sleep (health burden, primary sleep disorders, poor sleep hygiene practices, and so forth) are screened out, "optimally" or "successfully" aging adults can expect to undergo little change in their sleep, relative to those in the early to middle adult life span, and are not likely to experience EDS and the concomitant need to nap regularly during the day. Nevertheless, even successfully aging older adults can expect on average to be earlier to bed and to rise and to be less tolerant of circadian phase shifts, such as those induced by jet lag, than younger similarly healthy adults.

References

[1] Foley DJ, Monjan AA, Brown SL, et al. Sleep complaints among older persons: an epidemiological study of three communities. Sleep 1995; 18:425–32.

[2] Foley DJ, Monjan A, Simonsick EM, et al. Incidence and remission of insomnia among elderly adults: an epidemiologic study of 6,800 persons over three years. Sleep 1999;22(Suppl 2): S366–72.

[3] Vitiello MV, Foley D, Stratton KL, et al. Prevalence of sleep complaints and insomnia in the Vitamins And Lifestyle (VITAL) Study cohort of 77,000 older men and women [abstract]. Sleep 2004;27:120.

[4] Dijk DJ, Duffy JF, Riel E, et al. Ageing and the circadian and homeostatic regulation of human sleep during forced desynchrony of rest, melatonin and temperature rhythms. J Physiol 1999; 516(Pt 2):611–27.

[5] Dijk DJ, Duffy JF, Czeisler CA. Age-related increase in awakenings: impaired consolidation of nonREM sleep at all circadian phases. Sleep 2001;24:565–77.

[6] Zepelin H, McDonald CS, Zammit GK. Effects of age on auditory awakening thresholds. J Gerontol 1984;39:294–300.

[7] Duffy JF, Zeitzer JM, Rimmer DW, et al. Peak of circadian melatonin rhythm occurs later within the sleep of older subjects. Am J Physiol Endocrinol Metab 2002;282:E297–303.

[8] Harma MI, Hakola T, Akerstedt T, et al. Age and adjustment to night work. Occup Environ Med 1994;51:568–73.

[9] Bonnefond A, Harma M, Hakola T, et al. Interaction of age with shift-related sleep-wakefulness, sleepiness, performance, and social life. Exp Aging Res 2006;32:185–208.

[10] Buysse DJ, Reynolds CF III, Monk TH, et al. Quantification of subjective sleep quality in healthy elderly men and women using the Pittsburgh Sleep Quality Index (PSQI). Sleep 1991; 14:331–8.

[11] Vitiello MV, Larsen LH, Moe KE. Age-related sleep change: gender and estrogen effects on the subjective-objective sleep quality relationships of healthy, non-complaining older men and women. J Psychosom Res 2004;56: 503–10.

[12] Vitiello MV. Normal versus pathological sleep changes in aging humans. In: Kuna ST, Suratt PM, Remmers JE, editors. Sleep and respiration in aging adults. New York: Elsevier; 1991. p. 71–6.

[13] Vitiello MV. Effective treatment of sleep disturbances in older adults. Clin Cornerstone 2000; 2:16–27.

[14] Roffwarg HP, Muzio JN, Dement WC. Ontogenetic development of the human sleep-dream cycle. Science 1966;152:604–19.

[15] Ohayon MM, Carskadon MA, Guilleminault C, et al. Meta-analysis of quantitative sleep parameters from childhood to old age in healthy individuals: developing normative sleep values across the human lifespan. Sleep 2004; 27:1255–73.

[16] Redline S, Kirchner HL, Quan SF, et al. The effects of age, sex, ethnicity, and sleep-disordered breathing on sleep architecture. Arch Intern Med 2004;164:406–18.

[17] Monk TH. Aging human circadian rhythms: conventional wisdom may not always be right. J Biol Rhythms 2005;20:366–74.

[18] Young TB. Epidemiology of daytime sleepiness: definitions, symptomatology, and prevalence. J Clin Psychiatry 2004;65(Suppl 16):12–6.

[19] Ohayon MM. Epidemiology of insomnia: what we know and what we still need to learn. Sleep Med Rev 2002;6:97–111.

[20] Metz ME, Bunnell DE. Napping and sleep disturbances in the elderly. Fam Pract Res J 1990; 10:47–56.

[21] Vitiello MV, Larsen LH, Bliwise DL, et al. Relationship of regular napping to health and self-reported sleep quality in older adults: results from the 2003 NSF Sleep in America poll [abstract]. Sleep 2004;27:A126.

[22] Foley DJ, Vitiello MV, Bliwise DL, et al. Frequent napping is associated with excessive daytime sleepiness, depression, pain and nocturia in older adults: findings from the national sleep

foundation "2003 sleep in America" poll. Am J Geriatr Psychiatry, in press.

[23] Tamaki M, Shirota A, Tanaka H, et al. Effects of a daytime nap in the aged. Psychiatry Clin Neurosci 1999;53:273–5.

[24] Campbell SS, Murphy PJ, Stauble TN. Effects of a nap on nighttime sleep and waking function in older subjects. J Am Geriatr Soc 2005;53: 48–53.

[25] Monk TH, Buysse DJ, Carrier J, et al. Effects of afternoon "siesta" naps on sleep, alertness, performance, and circadian rhythms in the elderly. Sleep 2001;24:680–7.

[26] Vitiello MV, Moe KE, Prinz PN. Sleep complaints co-segregate with illness older adults: clinical research informed by and informing epidemiological studies of sleep. J Psychosom Res 2002; 53:555–9.

SLEEP
MEDICINE
CLINICS

Sleep Med Clin 1 (2006) 177–186

Napping in Older Adults

Jennifer L. Martin, PhD[a,b],*, Sonia Ancoli-Israel, PhD[c]

- Prevalence of napping in older adults
- Prevalence of daytime sleepiness in older adults
- Causes of daytime sleepiness and napping
  - *Disruption of nighttime sleep*
  - *Circadian rhythm changes*
  - *Medical and psychiatric factors*
- Correlates and consequences of napping and daytime sleepiness

- *Napping and nighttime sleep quality*
- *Napping and health outcomes*
- *Daytime sleepiness and health outcomes*
- Beneficial effects of napping among older adults
- Summary
- References

Older adults commonly report napping, yet the extent to which it may affect sleep at night, functioning during the day, or overall well-being is unclear. Some studies have suggested an association between napping and adverse health outcomes [1–8], whereas some have shown that napping may have beneficial effects [9–13]. This article reviews available literature on the prevalence, correlates, and consequences of napping and daytime sleepiness among older adults. Four different aspects of daytime sleep are considered: (1) napping; (2) total daytime sleeping (including napping and unintentional dozing); (3) subjective daytime sleepiness; and (4) objective daytime sleepiness or sleep propensity. In general, different methods of assessment are required to measure each of these daytime sleep-related constructs. Table 1 lists the advantages and disadvantages of each methodology commonly used to measure these constructs.

Prevalence of napping in older adults

Older adults around the world report sleeping more than younger adults during the daytime hours [14–17]. Prevalence rates for habitual napping range from 22% to 61% depending on the location of the study, characteristics of the study population, and the definition of napping used.

It remains unclear whether there are gender differences in napping. Two studies have found higher rates of napping among older men compared with older women. An Icelandic study (N = 800, aged 65–84 years) [18] found that 50% of men napped regularly compared with 31% of women

Supported by the UCLA Claude Pepper Older Americans Independence Center (AG-10415, Career Development Award, Martin); NIA AG08415 (Ancoli-Israel); the VAGLAHS Geriatric Research, Education and Clinical Center; and the research service of the VASDHS.

[a] UCLA Department of Medicine, San Fernando Valley Program (111), 16111 Plummer St., North Hills, CA 91007 USA

[b] Geriatric Research, Education and Clinical Center–Sepulveda, VA Greater Los Angeles Healthcare System (11E), 16111 Plummer Street, North Hills, CA 19343, USA

[c] Department of Psychiatry, University of California San Diego, 9500 Gilman Drive #0603, La Jolla, CA 92093, USA

* Corresponding author.
E-mail address: jennifer.martin@va.gov (J.L. Martin).

Table 1: Daytime sleep-related constructs and their measurement

Construct	Measurement techniques and tools	Advantages	Disadvantages
Napping	Self-report questionnaires	Easy to administer Low-cost	Subject to interpretation by individual
Total daytime sleeping[a]	Self report questionnaires Wrist actigraphy Polysomnography	Easy to administer Low cost Enables recording in natural environment Moderate cost Moderate patient or participant burden Precisely reflects sleep	May underestimate total daytime sleep May underestimate total daytime sleep Moderate cost Moderate patient or participant burden May overestimate total daytime sleep Most costly
Subjective daytime sleepiness	Self-report measures	Easy to administer Low cost	May be unrelated to objective daytime sleep
Objective daytime sleepiness or sleep propensity	Multiple Sleep Latency Test Maintenance of Wakefulness Test	Accurately reflects sleep propensity	Requires sleep laboratory and Polysomnography Does not measure sleep in the natural environment Most costly

[a] Including napping, dozing off unintentionally, and so forth.

($P < .001$). A Swedish study (N = 876, aged 65–79 years) [19] also observed a significantly higher napping prevalence among older men than older women (29% versus 15%, respectively; $P < .001$). Studies in other countries, however, have not found significant gender differences and most studies have reported combined prevalence rates [15–17].

Several napping studies have been conducted in the United States. In a study using daily sleep diaries, Buysse and coworkers [16] compared napping patterns between younger (mean age = 30 years) and older (mean age = 78 years) healthy adults. They found that over a 2-week period, younger adults reported taking an average of 1.1 naps, whereas older adults reported taking 3.4 naps. In a study of daytime sleepiness and napping, Hayes and coworkers [6] found that 25.2% of older adults over age 65 reported feeling so sleepy during the day or evening that they had to nap.

Metz and Bunnell [15] found that "older old" subjects (mean age = 80 years) took an average of five naps per week, whereas "younger old" subjects (mean age = 65 years) took an average of four naps per week ($P < .05$). "Older old" subjects also napped for a significantly longer mean duration (67.5 minutes) compared with "younger old" subjects (51.3 minutes; $P <. 05$). More recently, the 2003 National Sleep Foundation survey found that 10% of respondents aged 55 to 64 years reported taking naps regularly (defined as four to seven times per week), compared with 24% of respondents aged 75 to 84 years [14]. These studies suggest that a substantial minority of older adults in the United States nap on a regular basis.

Using wrist actigraphy to assess daytime napping, Yoon and coworkers [20] found that even very healthy older adults were slightly more likely to nap during the day than younger (college-aged) adults (77% versus 62% of participants, respectively; $P = .064$), but did not sleep more in total during the daytime hours compared with younger adults ($P > .10$).

Bursztyn and colleagues conducted a study of napping and mortality among adults over age 70 years living in Israel [3,7,21]. They reported the prevalence of regular "siesta" among 70 year olds to be approximately 60%, with an additional 23% reporting a daytime rest period without sleep. The higher prevalence of routine napping in Israel compared with the United States is likely caused by differences in cultural norms and lifestyle.

Although the literature on the prevalence of napping suggests that it is more common and perhaps occurs at different times of day from early to late adulthood, studies have not systematically distinguished between intentional (ie, planned) and unintentional naps (ie, dozing off when sleep was not planned). Although both intentional and unintentional naps may have negative consequences, the causes may differ considerably. Intentional planned naps may be caused by either sleepiness or by lifestyle changes, such as retirement, that allow for sleep during the daytime hours. Unintentional sleep during the day is most likely related to pathologic daytime sleepiness.

Most older adults are not aware of unintentional naps, such as falling asleep during sedentary, solitary activities (eg, watching television). It is possible that epidemiologic data in which older adults were asked about the frequency of napping may underestimate the total amount of sleep obtained during the daytime hours. This is particularly relevant because studies with wrist actigraphy (a methodology for distinguishing wake from sleep) show older adults may doze for brief periods during the day, which they may not report when asked about napping [20]. A pattern of frequent, brief sleep episodes intruding on wakefulness throughout the day may represent serious underlying pathology (eg, sleep-disordered breathing) [22].

Prevalence of daytime sleepiness in older adults

Although daytime sleepiness and napping are not synonymous, the two constructs are clearly related. Daytime sleepiness is most often assessed with subjective report questionnaires. Commonly, investigators use the Epworth Sleepiness Scale [23], which assesses an individual's reported likelihood of falling asleep in eight different situations. This measure, however, may be problematic for use among older adults, some of whom may not engage in one or more of the eight activities queried in the Epworth Sleepiness Scale (eg, driving). In addition, this measure was developed for use in sleep clinic populations and has not been validated with older adults in the community. Other subjective measures assess sleepiness in slightly different ways (eg, by asking about how the individual feels at the moment, or on a typical day) [24]. Subjective daytime sleepiness is an important clinical issue, because individuals who feel sleepy are presumably more likely to actually sleep during the day. Although sleep propensity is one important aspect of the subjective experience of sleepiness, other factors that are also likely to play a roll, such as mood, expectations about sleepiness, and motivation, must also be considered.

Two studies have examined the prevalence of reports of daytime sleepiness among older adults, and have found that between one in five and one in seven older adults experience significant daytime sleepiness. Ohayon and Vecchierini [25] interviewed over 1000 older adults in France and found that 13.6% of the sample reported excessive daytime sleepiness. As part of the Cardiovascular Health Study, Whitney and coworkers [26] examined daytime sleepiness among 4578 adults in the United States over age 65 and found that 20% reported significant daytime sleepiness on the Epworth Sleepiness Scale.

Daytime sleepiness can also be considered the objective propensity to fall asleep. In this case, daytime sleepiness is assessed objectively with laboratory studies, such as the Multiple Sleep Latency Test [27]. During a Multiple Sleep Latency Test the individual is instructed to go to sleep at 2-hour intervals during the day, with the amount of time needed to fall asleep being measured. In a second objective measure of daytime sleepiness, the Maintenance of Wakefulness Test [28], the individual is instructed to remain awake while in a dark, quiet environment. Although the results of these tests do differ for some individuals [29], both are considered reliable, objective measures of daytime sleep propensity. These tests are conducted in sleep laboratories, and are difficult to perform in the home environment. These objective methods have not been used to examine the prevalence of daytime sleepiness among older adults, which is likely because of the cost; the time required to complete the assessment (1 full day); and the need for participants to be in a sleep laboratory or other controlled environment during the testing.

It is important to consider that some older adults may experience sleepiness during the daytime hours without actually sleeping during the day. This sleepiness may have negative consequences even if the person does not actually nap on a regular basis.

Causes of daytime sleepiness and napping

There are several possible underlying causes of napping and multiple factors may interact to contribute to the overall likelihood that an older person sleeps during the day. Box 1 depicts the multitude of factors that may contribute to both daytime sleepiness and napping among older adults. Underlying daytime sleepiness likely leads to daytime napping, with factors causing daytime sleepiness including disruption of nighttime sleep, age-related changes in underlying circadian rhythms, and medical and psychiatric comorbidities. Although the relationship of these topics to nighttime sleep is discussed at length elsewhere in this issue, a brief summary is provided here to highlight the relationship between nighttime sleep, circadian rhythms, and napping.

Box 1:   Factors that contribute to daytime sleepiness and daytime napping among older adults
Sociocultural factors   Customary "siesta" period   Beliefs about aging and sleep   Changes in daily activities (eg, retirement)
Sleep and circadian factors   Nighttime sleep disruption   Shift in timing (phase advance) and amplitude of circadian rhythms   Increase in daytime sleep propensity
Medical and psychiatric factors   Depression or anxiety   Dementia   Pain

Disruption of nighttime sleep

With advancing age, nighttime sleep is often disrupted by underlying sleep disorders or by medical and psychiatric difficulties that increase in prevalence as people grow older (eg, depression, dementia). Numerous studies have found an association between napping and nighttime sleep disruption including symptoms of insomnia [18,30,31]; sleep fragmentation [32,33]; poor sleep quality [34]; use of long-acting hypnotics or other sedating medications [15,32]; and circadian rhythm disturbance (eg, advanced sleep phase) [32,35,36]. Individuals who nap regularly are more likely to report chronic difficulty maintaining sleep than individuals who do not nap (40% versus 28%, respectively; $P < .05$) [18]. Frisoni and coworkers [31] found a significant, positive, and independent association between napping and not feeling rested in the morning; however, there are also studies that did not find a significant association between degree of nighttime sleep disruption and daytime sleepiness [16,17,19,37–40]. Some of these studies were small in size and may have had insufficient statistical power to detect relationships.

Insufficient nighttime sleep is, nonetheless, likely to lead to increased daytime sleepiness across age groups. Disruption of nighttime sleep may lead some older people to become sleep deprived, impairing their ability to sustain wakefulness throughout the day. It is difficult to determine the direction of the causal relationship between napping and nighttime sleep disruption and the direction of the relationship may vary across individuals. Some individuals may begin sleeping more during the day to "make up for lost sleep" at night, whereas others may begin napping, then as a result, develop difficulties with nighttime sleep.

Circadian rhythm changes

A second important factor is changes in underlying circadian rhythms with advancing age. Older adults typically show a lower amplitude and an advance (ie, shift earlier) of endogenous circadian rhythms. This advance in circadian rhythms may lead older adults to feel sleepier earlier in the evening and awaken earlier in the morning. This can impact daytime sleeping in two ways. First, it may lead to insufficient nighttime sleep if the older adult attempts to stay up late, but is biologically awakened early in the morning. Obtaining insufficient nighttime sleep because of an advance of circadian rhythms and compensating with napping creates a vicious cycle. The daytime napping may enable the older adult to stay up later into the evening, perpetuating the problem of shorter nighttime sleep and early morning awakenings. Second, advanced circadian rhythms can lead to evening dozing and unintentional sleeping. In the Yoon and coworkers [20,36] wrist actigraphy study of a small group of healthy older (age 60–75 years) and younger (age 18–32 years) adults mentioned previously, there was no difference in the duration of daytime sleeping overall, but the older adults were more likely to sleep within 2 hours of bedtime, whereas the younger adults were more likely to nap earlier in the day. They also found differences between age groups in underlying circadian rhythms of melatonin, cortisol, and body temperature.

Medical and psychiatric factors

Some medical conditions and psychiatric disorders impact daytime alertness. Although there is less work on the impact of medical and psychiatric conditions on daytime sleepiness than on nighttime sleep, research suggests these issues are interrelated. In the 2003 National Sleep Foundation survey of 1506 adults age 65–84 years mentioned previously, depression, heart disease, bodily pain, and memory problems were associated with more symptoms of insomnia. In addition, pain, depression, diabetes, stroke, and lung diseases were associated with daytime sleepiness [41]. One important unanswered question is whether medical and psychiatric disorders directly impact daytime sleepiness or whether daytime sleepiness is increased because of a reduced ability to obtain sufficient sleep at night.

Correlates and consequences of napping and daytime sleepiness

Napping and nighttime sleep quality

Theoretically, napping may perpetuate a vicious cycle of sleep fragmentation, decreased sleep efficiency, fatigue, and subsequent napping [30,32].

Some studies show that extended daytime napping can negatively impact nighttime sleep (Table 2). Monk and coworkers [42] found that a 1.5-hour daytime nap shortened nighttime sleep, decreased sleep efficiency, and led to earlier morning rise times among nine healthy older individuals studied in a sleep laboratory. The Yoon and coworkers [20,36] wrist actigraphy study mentioned previously found that healthy older adults who napped in the evening hours awoke and got out of bed earlier in the morning, spent less time in bed, and had a shorter sleep period. They also fell asleep more quickly in the evening. One possibility is that, because these older adults napped close to bedtime, they had obtained sufficient total sleep by their morning rise time. Another possibility is that these older adults had more phase-advanced circadian rhythms, which led to an overall earlier sleep period.

Studies examining the general population of older adults have reported an association between napping and nocturnal sleep difficulties, although the duration of daytime naps seems to be a key factor. Metz and Bunnell [15] reported a potential association (not statistically significant) between increased sleep-onset latency and nap duration in group of older adults and suggested that duration of naps had more influence than frequency of naps on difficulty initiating sleep. Longer naps have also been implicated as contributing to frequent nocturnal awakenings among older adults [42,43].

Findings across studies, however, have not been consistent. Bliwise and coworkers [40] examined factors related to sleep quality in healthy older women (mean age, 68 years) identifying themselves as good (N = 22) or poor (N = 16) sleepers. Poor sleepers were characterized by shorter objectively

Table 2: Napping and nighttime sleep disturbance among community-dwelling older adults

Study	Study sample N (women); age	Study design (location)	Assessment method	Main findings
Hays et al 1996 [6]	N = 3962 (2581 W) Age range: 65–101 y	Prospective cohort study (USA)[a]	Interview	Frequent daytime nappers reported more problems with nighttime sleep versus infrequent or nonnappers
Campos and Siles, 2004 [4]	MI survivors N = 505 (131 W) M (SD) age = 57 (11) y No MI controls N = 522 (136 W) M (SD) age = 57 (11) y	Case control; seeking medical care at community facility (Costa Rica)	In-person interview	Siesta associated with poorer nighttime sleep quality across groups
Monk et al 2001 [42]	N = 9 (5W) Age = 74–87 y	Within-subject experiment (nap versus no-nap); (USA)	Polysomnography	1.5 = h daytime nap led to decreased nighttime sleep efficiency and earlier morning rise times
Yoon et al 2003 [20,36]	Older (60–70 y) N = 60 (38 W) M (SD) age = 66 (5) Younger (18-32 y) N = 73 (47 W) M (SD) age = 24 (4) y	Cross-sectional comparison (USA)	Wrist actigraphy with sleep diary	Trend for more napping among older versus young group Older group more likely to nap within 2 h of bedtime Older adults who napped within 2 h of bedtime awoke and got out of bed earlier, spent less time in bed, and had shorter sleep periods versus older adults who did not nap

Abbreviations: M, mean; MI, myocardial infarction; SD, standard deviation.
[a] *Data from* EPESE study.

measured nighttime total sleep time and more subjective nonrestorative sleep; however, no differences were found between good and poor sleepers in the number of daily naps. Mallon and Hetta [19] found no difference in total sleep time or sleep problems between individuals who napped and those who did not nap (N = 876 Swedish adults aged 65–79 years), and Metz and Bunnell [15] found no significant relationship between napping and number of nocturnal awakenings, sleep-onset latency, total sleep time, or quality of sleep, although a trend was noted toward more sleep-onset difficulty and longer duration of napping. Hsu [44] also found no correlation between naps and quality of sleep among 80 community-dwelling Chinese elders, and Campbell and Dawson [11] found that an afternoon nap had no effect on subsequent nighttime sleep.

Napping and health outcomes

Several studies have found that daytime sleepiness and napping are related to increased risk for mortality (Table 3). In a large study of nearly 6000 older adults (mean age = 73 years), Newman and coworkers [5] found that reported napping was associated with increased risk for both mortality and cardiovascular disease after controlling for other known risk factors (adjusted odds ratio = 2.34; 95% confidence interval, 1.66–3.29). Campos and Siles [4] studied a cohort of 505 survivors of myocardial infarction and compared their siesta-taking behavior with a cohort of 522 matched controls without a history of myocardial infarction. They found that individuals with a history of myocardial infarction were more likely to take daily siestas and to take longer siestas on average than those without a history of myocardial infarction. Individuals with the shortest siesta period were least likely to have a subsequent myocardial infarction after controlling for known myocardial infarction risk factors including lipids; smoking; body mass index; light physical activity; night sleep; and history of diabetes, hypertension, and angina. The prevalence of daily siestas among myocardial infarction survivors was 44%, compared with 35% in controls ($P = .01$). This study, however, did not control for depression or cognitive impairment, both of which may be confounding variables.

Burazeri and coworkers [8] studied a cohort of older adults (over age 50 years) in Israel using self-reported amount of sleep per 24 hours (including nighttime sleep and daytime sleep). They found that reported sleep duration of more than 8 hours per 24 hours was related to increased mortality risk among men. This finding suggests that longer reported sleeping, whether at night or during the day, is associated with higher mortality risk. In the study by Hays and coworkers [6], the authors found that

older adults who reported frequent daytime napping were more likely to report problems with nighttime sleep, and had a higher mortality risk than those who napped less frequently. In the study by Bursztyn and colleagues [3,7,21] mortality rates were doubled among older adults in Israel who slept during the day compared with those who rested but did not sleep and with those who did not rest or sleep during the day. They also found that individuals who slept during the day had higher rates of myocardial infarction and were more likely to have cancer or vascular causes of death compared with those who did not sleep during the day. Brassington and coworkers [2], however, found that although there was a significant bivariate correlation between reported daytime sleepiness that led to napping and risk of falling, after controlling for other known fall risk factors, there was no additional increase in risk associated with reported napping.

Direct causal links between napping and negative health outcomes cannot be drawn based on available data. It is likely that older people with underlying health conditions are both more likely to sleep during the day and to have shorter survival. It is also possible, however, that daytime sleeping may lead to reduced daytime activities, less exposure to light during the day, fewer social interactions, and other changes that may increase mortality risk. Studies are needed to understand the potential mechanisms underlying the relationship between napping and increased mortality risk.

Daytime sleepiness and health outcomes

Daytime sleepiness, independent of napping, can have life-threatening consequences. This is reflected in the findings from a 1991 National Sleep Foundation survey in which 5% of respondents with difficulty sleeping at night reported having an automobile accident because of daytime sleepiness, compared with 2% of those with no problems sleeping [45]. Fifty percent reported frequently waking up feeling drowsy or tired. These findings also highlight the impact of nighttime sleep disturbance on increased daytime sleepiness.

Gooneratne and coworkers [46] studied a group of older adults (>65 years) in an assisted living facility. Those who reported daytime sleepiness were more likely to report functional impairments related to their sleepiness than individuals who did not report daytime sleepiness. This study assessed the subjective experience of sleepiness, but did not assess whether or not the individual slept during the daytime hours, and it is unclear whether the effect of sleepiness on functional impairment was related to actual sleeping during the daytime hours or to other factors that led to the subjective feeling of sleepiness; nonetheless, these findings

Table 3: Napping and health outcomes among community-dwelling older adults

Study	Study sample N (women); age	Study design (location)	Assessment method	Main findings
Hays et al 1996 [6]	N = 3962 (2581 W) Age range: 65–101 y	Prospective cohort study (USA)[a]	Interview	Frequent daytime nappers had higher mortality risk versus infrequent or nonnappers
Bursztyn et al 1999 [3,7] Burstyn and Stessman 2005 [21]	N = 455 (249 W) Age = all 70 y	Prospective cohort study (Israel)	In-person interview	60.7% took siestas (men > women; MI survivors > no MI) Lower 6-y survival rates for siesta takers versus for nonsiesta takers; increased risk persisted in adjusted analyses Mortality risk elevated only among those who slept versus those who "rested without sleep" and nonsiesta takers
Newman et al 2000 [5]	N = 5888 M age = 73 y	Prospective cohort study (USA)[b]	In-person interview	Daytime sleeping associated with increased mortality and Cardiovascular disease risk among men and women, after controlling for known risk factors Daytime sleeping associated with increased MI risk among women, after controlling for known risk factors
Campos and Siles 2000 [4]	MI survivors N = 505 (131 W) M (SD) age = 57 (11) y No MI controls N = 522 (136 W) M (SD) age = 57 (11) y	Case control (all seeking medical care at community facility [Costa Rica])	In-person interview	MI survivors more likely to take regular siesta versus no-MI controls MI survivors took longer siestas versus no-MI controls More frequent siesta associated with MI status in adjusted analyses
Brassington et al 2000 [2]	N = 1526 (971 W) Age 64–199 y	Descriptive study (USA)	Telephone interview	Daytime sleepiness and napping associated with increased fall risk Only napping (not sleepiness) associated with increased risk in adjusted analyses
Burazeri et al 2003 [8]	N = 1842 (1001 W) Age > 50 y	Prospective cohort study (11 y); (Israel)	In-person interview	More than 8 h sleep in 24 h associated with increased mortality among men only Relationship strong among those who reportedly took siesta

Abbreviation: MI, myocardial infarction.
[a] *Data from* EPESE study.
[b] Cardiovascular Health Study.

do suggest that reported sleepiness could be an important indicator for risk of functional impairment.

Daytime sleepiness may also be related to cognitive deficits. Ohayon and Vecchierini [25] found that older adults who reported excessive daytime sleepiness were more likely to report cognitive impairment across several dimensions, even after controlling for other known risk factors for cognitive impairment. A study by Asada and coworkers [1] examined reported napping and later development of Alzheimer's disease and found that whereas napping under 1 hour had some protective effects, napping over 1 hour per day was associated with higher risk of Alzheimer's disease among individuals with the APOEε 4 genotype (which is associated with elevated Alzheimer's disease risk).

Beneficial effects of napping among older adults

Although this issue has received relatively little attention in the research literature, there is some evidence that napping can be beneficial if it takes place at the appropriate time of day and is of appropriate duration. Fig. 1 depicts a hypothetical relationship between daytime sleeping and outcomes. The figure reflects a hypothetical inverted "U" function, in which brief naps may be more beneficial than no naps (eg, by increasing evening alertness), but lengthy daytime sleep may have adverse consequences (eg, shortened or fragmented nighttime sleep).

Most research on the beneficial effects of napping has been conducted with younger adults, shift workers, and long-distance drivers. Findings do suggest beneficial effects of napping on performance and alertness in these populations [47–49]. In young adults, short naps have been shown to reduce subjective sleepiness; increase daytime alertness; improve neurobehavioral performance (particularly in sleep-deprived subjects) [50]; and improve mood [51].

In 2003, Takahashi [9] reviewed the literature on prescribed napping in sleep medicine and concluded that laboratory findings suggest napping can be beneficial if properly timed and short in duration. One study showed that older adults may benefit in terms of increased alertness and reduced fatigue from a short (about 30 minute) nap in the afternoon (1:00 PM). The authors did not find that this short daytime nap negatively impacted nighttime sleep [10]. The study by Asada and coworkers [1] found that a reported history of short naps (less than 1 hour) was associated with lower risk of Alzheimer's disease among individuals with the APOEε 4 genotype.

In a laboratory study of naps among 32 healthy older adults, Campbell and Dawson [11] found that an afternoon nap (mean duration = 81 minutes) had no negative effect on subsequent nighttime sleep but increased total sleep time per 24 hours and enhanced cognitive and psychomotor performance immediately after the nap and throughout the next day.

It is somewhat unclear whether napping has beneficial effects in terms of health outcomes. Data from two case-control studies of Greek men across age groups suggested a protective effect of afternoon rests or naps against coronary heart disease [12,13]. Findings from these studies have not been confirmed or duplicated in other countries and contradict the numerous recent reports of increased cardiovascular mortality associated with daytime sleepiness or napping [3–7,21].

Summary

Napping and subjective feelings of daytime sleepiness are more common among older than among younger adults. This increase in napping is likely caused by changes in nighttime sleep, circadian rhythms, and lifestyle factors. Although a brief sleep period during the day may have some benefit in terms of increased evening alertness, longer periods of daytime sleep may negatively impact nighttime sleep quality and may be associated with negative health outcomes, cognitive impairment, and increased mortality risk among older persons. Additional research is needed on the timing and characteristics of napping among older people and to explore further the mechanisms underlying the relationship between napping and negative health outcomes.

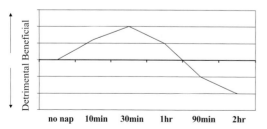

Fig. 1. The hypothetical relationship between duration of napping and overall impact on older adults. Although short naps may provide some benefit in terms of increased alertness, longer naps are more likely to result in sleep inertia and to interfere with the duration and quality of nighttime sleep.

References

[1] Asada T, Motonaga T, Yamagata Z, et al. Associations between retrospectively recalled napping behavior and later development of Alzheimer's disease: association with APOE genotypes. Sleep 2000;23:629–34.

[2] Brassington GS, King AC, Bliwise DL. Sleep problems as a risk factor for falls in a sample of community-dwelling adults aged 64–99 years. J Am Geriatr Soc 2000;48:1234–40.

[3] Bursztyn M, Ginsberg G, Stessman J. The siesta and mortality in the elderly: effect of rest without sleep and daytime sleep duration. Sleep 2002; 25:187–91.

[4] Campos H, Siles X. Siesta and the risk of coronary heart disease: results from a population-based, case-control study in Costa Rica. Int J Epidemiol 2000;29:429–37.

[5] Newman AB, Spiekerman CF, Enright P, et al. Daytime sleepiness predicts mortality and cardiovascular disease in older adults. The Cardiovascular Health Study Research Group. J Am Geriatr Soc 2000;48:115–23.

[6] Hays JC, Blazer DG, Foley DJ. Risk of napping: excessive daytime sleepiness and mortality in an older community population. J Am Geriatr Soc 1996;44:693–8.

[7] Bursztyn M, Ginsberg G, Hammerman-Rozenberg R, et al. The siesta in the elderly: risk factor for mortality? Arch Intern Med 1999; 159:1582–6.

[8] Burazeri G, Gofin J, Kark JD. Over 8 hours of sleep–marker of increased mortality in Mediterranean population: follow-up population study. Croat Med J 2003;44:193–8.

[9] Takahashi M. The role of prescribed napping in sleep medicine. Sleep Med Rev 2003;7:227–35.

[10] Tamaki M, Shirota A, Hayashi M, et al. Restorative effects of a short afternoon nap (<30 min) in the elderly on subjective mood, performance and EEG activity. Sleep Res Online 2000; 3:131–9.

[11] Campbell SS, Dawson D. Aging young sleep: a test of the phase advance hypothesis of sleep disturbance in the elderly. J Sleep Res 1992; 1:205–10.

[12] Trichopoulos D, Tzonou A, Christopoulos C, et al. Does a siesta protect from coronary heart disease? Lancet 1987;2:269–70.

[13] Kalandini A, Tzonou A, Toupadaki N, et al. A case-control-study of coronary heart disease in Athens, Greece. Int J Epidemiol 1992;21: 1074–80.

[14] National Sleep Foundation. 2003 Sleep in America poll. Available at: www.sleepfoundation.org/polls/2003SleepPollExecutiveSumm.pdf. Accessed September 12, 2005.

[15] Metz ME, Bunnell DE. Napping and sleep disturbance in the elderly. Fam Pract Res J 1990; 10:47–56.

[16] Buysse DJ, Browman KE, Monk TH, et al. Napping and 24-hour sleep/wake patterns in healthy elderly and young adults. J Am Geriatr Soc 1992; 40:779–86.

[17] Dinges DF. Napping patterns and effects in human adults. In: Dinges DF, Broughton RJ, editors. Sleep and alertness: chronobiological, behavioral and medical aspects of napping. New York: Raven Press; 1989. p. 171–204.

[18] Gislason T, Reynisdottir H, Kristbjarnarson H, et al. Sleep habits and sleep disturbances among the elderly: an epidemiological survey. J Intern Med 1993;234:31.

[19] Mallon L, Hetta J. A survey of sleep habits and sleeping difficulties in an elderly Swedish population. Ups J Med Sci 1997;102:185–97.

[20] Yoon IY, Kripke DF, Youngstedt SD, et al. Actigraphy suggests age-related differences in napping and nocturnal sleep. J Sleep Res 2003;12:87–93.

[21] Bursztyn M, Stessman J. The siesta and mortality: twelve years of prospective observations in 70-year-olds. Sleep 2006;28:345–7.

[22] Schmitt FA, Phillips BA, Cook YR, et al. Self report of sleep symptoms in older adults: correlates of daytime sleepiness and health. Sleep 1996;19:59–64.

[23] Johns MW. A new method for measuring daytime sleepiness: The Epworth sleepiness scale. Sleep 1991;14:540–5.

[24] Mitler MM, Carskadon MA, Hirshkowitz M. Evaluating sleepiness. In: Kryger MH, Roth T, Dement WC, editors. Principles and practice of sleep medicine. Philadelphia: Elsevier Saunders; 2005. p. 1417–23.

[25] Ohayon MM, Vecchierini MF. Daytime sleepiness and cognitive impairment in the elderly population. Arch Intern Med 2002;162:201–8.

[26] Whitney CW, Enright PL, Newman GC, et al. Correlates of daytime sleepiness in 4578 elderly persons: the Cardiovascular Health Study. Sleep 1998;21:27–36.

[27] Carskadon MA, Dement WC, Mitler MM, et al. Guidelines for the multiple sleep latency test (MSLT): a standard measure of sleepiness. Sleep 1986;9:519–24.

[28] Mitler MM, Gujavarty KS, Browman CP. Maintenance of wakefulness test: a polysomnographic technique for evaluating treatment efficacy in patients with excessive somnolence. Electroencephalogr Clin Neurophysiol 1982;53:658–61.

[29] Sangal RB, Thomas L, Mitler MM. Disorders of excessive sleepiness: treatment improves ability to stay awake but does not reduce sleepiness. Chest 1992;102:699–703.

[30] Carskadon MA, Brown ED, Dement WC. Sleep fragmentation in the elderly: relationship to daytime sleep tendency. Neurobiol Aging 1982; 3:321–7.

[31] Frisoni GB, De Leo D, Rozzini R, et al. Napping in the elderly and its association with night sleep and psychological status. Int Psychogeriatr 1996; 8:477–87.

[32] Ancoli-Israel S, Kripke DF. Prevalent sleep problems in the aged. Biofeedback Self Regul 1991; 16:349–59.

[33] Ohayon MM, Caulet M, Philip P, et al. How sleep and mental disorders are related to complaints of daytime sleepiness. Arch Intern Med 1997;157:2645–52.

[34] Pilcher JJ, Schoeling SE, Prosansky CM. Self-report sleep habits as predictors of subjective sleepiness. Behav Med 2000;25:161.

[35] Ancoli-Israel S. Insomnia in the elderly: a review for the primary care practitioner. Sleep 2000; 23(Suppl 1):S23–30.

[36] Yoon IY, Kripke DF, Elliott J, et al. Age-related changes of circadian rhythms and sleep-wake cycles. J Am Geriatr Soc 2003;51:1085–91.

[37] Asplund R. Sleep disorders in the elderly. Drugs Aging 1999;14:91–103.

[38] Wauquier A, Van Sweden B, Lagaay AM, et al. Ambulatory monitoring of sleep-wakefulness patterns in healthy elderly males and females (>88 years): the "Senieur" protocol. J Am Geriatr Soc 1992;40:109–14.

[39] Morin CM, Gramling SE. Sleep patterns and aging: comparison of older adults with and without insomnia complaints. Psychol Aging 1989; 4:290–4.

[40] Bliwise NG. Factors related to sleep quality in healthy elderly women. Psychol Aging 1992; 7:83–8.

[41] Foley D, Ancoli-Israel S, Britz P, et al. Sleep disturbance and chronic disease in older adults: results of the 2003 National Sleep Foundation Sleep in America survey. J Psychosom Res 2004; 56:497–502.

[42] Monk TH, Buysse DJ, Carrier J, et al. Effects of afternoon "siesta" naps on sleep, alertness, performance, and circadian rhythms in the elderly. Sleep 2001;24:680–7.

[43] Floyd JA. Sleep and aging. Nurs Clin North Am 2002;37:719–31.

[44] Hsu HC. Relationship between quality of sleep and its related factors among elderly Chinese immigrants in the Seattle area. J Nurs Res 2001; 9:179–90.

[45] Roth T, Ancoli-Israel S. Daytime consequences and correlates of insomnia in the United States: results of the 1991 National Sleep Foundation Survey. II. Sleep 1999;22(Suppl 2):S354–8.

[46] Gooneratne NS, Weaver TE, Cater JR, et al. Functional outcomes of excessive daytime sleepiness in older adults. J Am Geriatr Soc 2003; 51:642–9.

[47] Purnell MT, Feyer AM, Herbison GP. The impact of a nap opportunity during the night shift on the performance and alertness of 12-h shift workers. J Sleep Res 2002;11:219–27.

[48] Macchi MM, Boulos Z, Ranney T, et al. Effects of an afternoon nap on nighttime alertness and performance in long-haul drivers. Accid Anal Prev 2002;34:825–34.

[49] Takahashi M, Arito H. Maintenance of alertness and performance by a brief nap after lunch under prior sleep deficit. Sleep 2000;23:813–9.

[50] Taub JM. Effects of scheduled afternoon naps and bedrest on daytime alertness. J Neurosci 1982;16:107–27.

[51] Daiss SR, Bertelson AD, Benjamin LT. Napping versus resting: effects on performance and mood. Psychophysiology 1986;23:82–8.

SLEEP
MEDICINE
CLINICS

Sleep Med Clin 1 (2006) 187–196

Circadian Rhythm Alterations with Aging

Erik Naylor, PhD, Phyllis C. Zee, MD, PhD*

Changes in both sleep timing and quality have been documented to occur with advancing age [1–4]. A recent survey conducted by the National Sleep Foundation reported that 36% of respondents aged 65 years and older experienced sleep disturbances [5]. These complaints include habitually earlier bedtimes and wake times, inability to maintain sleep at night, undesired early morning awakenings, and frequent daytime sleepiness [6–9]. When nocturnal sleep does occur in older patients, it contains less slow wave activity and prolonged periods of wakefulness, particularly during the second half of the night, possibly indicating a decreased homeostatic sleep load [10,11].

Alterations of the circadian system are also known to occur with advancing age [12–16]. In humans, the aging circadian system has been observed to exhibit changes in both amplitude and phase [17,18]. Additionally, the elderly have reduced exposure to external entraining agents, such as light, socialization, and physical activity [19]. These age-related changes in circadian clock functions or reduced exposure to synchronizing agents, such as

light and social and physical activity, may contribute to the development of sleep disturbances, such as insomnia, irregular sleep-wake patterns, and advanced sleep phase syndrome [20]. This article discusses the current knowledge and theory underlying circadian changes with age and their possible contribution to decreased sleep quality in this population.

Neurobiology of circadian rhythms

Circadian rhythms are generated by a circadian pacemaker located in the suprachiasmatic nuclei (SCN) of the hypothalamus [21,22]. These daily rhythms are intrinsic to the organism and observed in virtually every physiologic and behavioral parameter including sleep-wakefulness, daily temperature fluctuations, and endocrine cycling. The SCN also controls the timing of the melatonin rhythm through a multisynaptic pathway terminating at the pineal gland [23].

Circadian rhythms are synchronized, or entrained, to the environmental light-dark and

Department of Neurology, Northwestern University Medical School, 11th Floor Abbott Hall, 710 North Lake Shore Drive, Chicago, IL 60611, USA
* Corresponding author.
E-mail address: p-zee@northwestern.edu (P.C. Zee).

1556-407X/06/$ – see front matter © 2006 Elsevier Inc. All rights reserved.
sleep.theclinics.com

doi:10.1016/j.jsmc.2006.04.006

social-activity cycles by daily adjustments in the timing and phase of the internal rhythm [24]. These adjustments occur through the presentation of stimuli that signal the time of day or state of activity, known as "zeitgebers," derived from the German word for "time-giver." Although light is the most effective zeitgeber for the clock, exercise is also an important synchronizing agent in humans [25,26]. In the absence of synchronizing stimuli, rhythms continue to repeat with a period of approximately 24 hours [24].

Evidence for a circadian process regulating sleep initiation and duration was first obtained in the temporal isolation studies conducted by Aschoff [27]. Based on the results of these and subsequent studies, it has been suggested that a primary role of the human circadian pacemaker is to facilitate the consolidation of sleep and wakefulness [28–32]. The duration of sleep episodes and architecture, including the distribution of rapid eye movement sleep and sleep spindles, are all correlated with the phase of circadian rhythms [33].

The sensation of sleepiness, increased propensity to fall asleep, and increased sleep time and depth once sleep ensues are hallmarks of the compensatory response to sleep loss [30,34]. This drive toward sleep and the tendency to sleep longer and more deeply after sleep deprivation [30,34] is referred to as "sleep homeostasis." The homeostatic process for the expression of sleep need is based on the amount of prior wakefulness and prior hours of sleep [35,36]. The process of sleeping is currently the only known way to reduce the homeostatic drive to sleep after extended waking. In rats and humans, the depth of sleep (as indexed by electroencephalogram delta power during non–rapid eye movement sleep) and amount of sleep during recovery are proportional to the duration of prior wakefulness [37–39]. At present, the neural mechanisms responsible for compensatory sleep after extended waking are poorly understood, although recent studies suggest that the cholinergic basal forebrain and adenosine may play an important role in this physiologic drive [40].

Age-related changes in the circadian system

The circadian timing system is conceptualized as three distinct components: (1) a circadian oscillator with a rhythm approximating 24 hours; (2) input pathways for light and other stimuli that synchronize the pacemaker to the environmental light-dark cycle, and (3) output rhythms that are regulated by the pacemaker. All of these have been shown to be affected by aging.

Circadian clock

Within the circadian oscillator itself, animal studies have shown a reduced amplitude in the expression of the immediate early gene c-fos and a deficit in cyclic-AMP response element-binding protein phosphorylation in the SCN following light exposure [41,42]. Photic-induced expression of *Per1* and *Per2*, genes important for clock control, are likewise reduced [43]. Other studies of specific clock-related genes have found alterations in the expression profile of *Clock* and *Bmal1* [44], along with reduced Per1 [44] and *Per2* gene expression [45] within the SCN of aged animals. Old animals demonstrate a reduced temperature rhythm and fragmented activity patterns [46], which are similar to changes observed in young animals with SCN ablation surgery. A study by Van Reeth and colleagues [47] showed a reversal in this effect by demonstrating that old animals could regain much of their ability to adjust to a light pulse after receiving an implant of fetal SCN tissue.

Physical degeneration of the SCN including decreased cell numbers [48,49] and decreased vasopressin neuronal activity [50,51] has been directly observed in human studies. Age-related neurodegeneration caused by dementia or Alzheimer's disease may also contribute to circadian breakdown. Alzheimer's disease patients have been noted to have higher mean body temperature and a delayed sleep phase when compared with age-matched controls [52–54]. There is also some evidence that vasopressin gene expression within the SCN is decreased in this population, [55] suggesting that the neurodegeneration associated with aging or exacerbated by Alzheimer's disease may be directly affecting the circadian clock mechanisms and contributing to sleep disturbances noted in aging. It is likely that the lower amplitude and difficulty in adjusting to phase shifts observed in aging individuals may be caused by reduced cell numbers, insufficient clock-controlled cell function, or a combination of the two.

Responsiveness of the circadian clock to photic and nonphotic stimuli

It has been suggested that aging may decrease the responsiveness of the circadian clock to light and contribute to changes in circadian amplitude and entrainment. Special melanopsin-containing photoreceptors in retinal ganglion cells are thought to provide the primary photic input to the circadian clock [56]. Light information transmitted from these photoreceptors is then integrated by the neurons of the SCN. Regulatory signals are sent to other areas of the brain including sleep-wake centers in the ventrolateral preoptic nucleus and lateral hypothalamic area by connections through the dorsomedial hypothalamus (for review see [57]). In later age, light transmission may be decreased by cataracts or yellowing of the lens, which has been demonstrated to reduce blue light transmittance by as much as 80% in primates [58]. Lens yellowing may be particularly significant because melanopsin-containing retinal ganglion cells are sensitive to short wavelength (blue) light [59].

Within the clock system, specific neurotransmitter systems that are involved with circadian regulation, such as serotonin and melatonin, also change in old age. For example, Penev and coworkers [60] found that administration of a serotonin agonist was only partially effective in blocking the phase-shifting effects of light in older hamsters when compared with younger animals. Human studies have shown a decline in melatonin levels with age [16,61] and other studies have demonstrated that suppression of nighttime melatonin release by light is significantly reduced in elderly subjects [62]. These changes in neurotransmitter systems affected by the circadian clock may be contributing to sleep difficulties in this population.

Circadian amplitude

Age-related reductions in the circadian amplitude of body temperature rhythms were first observed in animal studies. McDonald and coworkers [46] found that the temperature amplitude of old rats with a stable body weight body was significantly less than that of young rats. Likewise, Satinoff [63] reported that, "In almost all old rats there is a clear decrease in the amplitude of the circadian temperature rhythm." It should be noted, however, that a great deal of variability was present in the older cohort. Human studies have demonstrated decreased amplitudes of body temperature rhythms in the elderly under both entrained [64,65] and free-running [17,18,66] circumstances. These reductions in core body temperature amplitude seem to be less evident in women [67,68].

Age-related changes in various circadian endocrine rhythms have also been observed. One study reported that mean cortisol levels in an elderly sample showed reduced circadian amplitude [16]. The dampened circadian amplitude is thought primarily to be caused by an elevation in the nocturnal nadir of cortisol levels [69]. Decreased amplitude of circulating growth hormone, thyroid-stimulating hormone [69], prolactin, and melatonin [16] have also been reported to be reduced in the elderly. These age-related changes, however, are not universally seen in older adults. Several other studies failed to demonstrate a difference in the amplitude of core body temperature [70–72] or melatonin rhythms in very healthy older adults. Zeitzer and coworkers [73] found no difference in the endogenous amplitude of the plasma melatonin rhythm between a group of young men and a cohort of healthy, drug-free men and women over 65. These results suggest that factors other than chronologic age, such as comorbid disorders, level of light exposure, or physical activity, are likely also to play a role in the observed circadian rhythm alterations.

Circadian phase

A consistent finding in the study of aging populations is a phase advance of many circadian-related measures. The nadir of the endogenous body temperature rhythm in old subjects has been found to be significantly advanced during both normal routine [70,74] and constant conditions [18,75]. Like temperature, advances in hormone rhythms are also common. Van Coevorden and coworkers [16] noted that the rhythms of cortisol, thyroid-stimulating hormone, and melatonin all occurred 1 to 1.5 hours earlier in the elderly as compared with younger subjects. A representative melatonin curve showing the differences between a young and old subject is shown in Fig. 1. Another study by Van Cauter and coworkers [11,69] found similar advances in the rhythms of cortisol and growth hormone. The advance of the growth hormone rhythm is mainly evident in men where the primary growth hormone pulse is seen during the first third of the nightly sleep episode [76] and is likely a result of an earlier sleep-onset rather than a circadian-related advance in the growth hormone rhythm itself.

One possible hypothesis for the phase advance of many rhythms seen in aging suggests that the endogenous period or tau (τ) shortens over the lifespan. This idea postulates that a shortened tau leads to an alteration of the phase relationship where the external light-dark cycle falls more on the advancing portion of the phase-response curve to light resulting in a chronic phase advance of internal rhythms. Support of this idea comes primarily from animal studies. Mice have been reported to lengthen their circadian period with age [77–79], whereas hamsters [80,81] and rats [82] may shorten their tau. Recent animal findings, however, have reported no change in tau of Syrian hamsters when they are maintained in constant conditions throughout their lifespan [83,84].

In humans, the period of the core body temperature rhythm of older adults has been found to be reduced when studied under a free-running sleep-wake protocol [17]. More recent studies, however, have called this idea into question. Czeisler and coworkers [29] carefully observed the free-running period of young and elderly subjects under a free-running protocol and found no difference in their rhythms. In another experiment, 10 elderly subjects

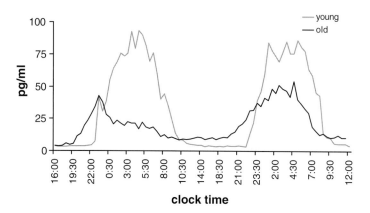

Fig. 1. Plasma melatonin rhythm collected at 30-minute intervals over a 44-hour period from a young (27 year old) subject (*shown in gray*) and old (63 year old) subject (*shown in black*). Melatonin amplitude is reduced and the phase of melatonin onset is advanced in the elderly subject.

studied under free-running conditions also showed no difference in tau from that commonly reported for young subjects [85]. One study in totally blind individuals has reported rhythms lengthening with age [86]. It remains unclear whether age-related changes in circadian period are species specific or what effect such changes might have on the development of sleep disturbances in older adults.

Entrainment of circadian rhythms

Aging of the circadian system may also alter the ability to phase shift in response to zeitgebers, such as light or exercise. A study by Zee and coworkers [80] demonstrated that 16-month-old hamsters took longer to re-entrain to an 8-hour phase delay of the light dark cycle than young hamsters. Interestingly, the old hamsters re-entrained more quickly to an 8-hour phase advance than the young hamsters, further supporting the idea of a shortened circadian period. When Van Reeth and colleagues [87,88] administered two stimuli known to cause phase shifts by increasing activity (benzodiazepines and dark pulses) to aged hamsters, they noted the expected increase in locomotor activity; however, no concurrent phase-shifting effect was seen. They also reported being unable to entrain old hamsters through benzodiazepine injections alone. Another study examining glucose use within the SCN found that aged rats use less glucose in response to light-dark transitions under normally entrained conditions [89,90].

In humans, the inability to respond to changing zeitgebers is most evident in shift workers and those suffering from jet lag. Measurements of temperature and subjective sleepiness in late middle-aged shift workers found that young subjects were better able to delay their temperature phase and reported decreased sleepiness during the wake period than the older subjects [91]. Furthermore, in a study of crewmembers flying long haul flight operations, subjects aged 50 to 60 averaged 3.5 times more

sleep loss per day than subjects aged 20 to 30 [92]. It should come as no surprise to find that older shift workers report more sleep difficulties than younger shift workers [93].

Results of laboratory experiments on phase shifting in older subjects show similar difficulties. When Monk and coworkers [94] induced a 6-hour phase advance or delay on 15 elderly subjects living in time isolation they found that, "circadian rectal temperature rhythms confirmed that phase adjustment was slow in both directions." Furthermore, significantly more sleep and circadian rhythm disruption was present after the phase advance than after the phase delay. They concluded that sleep disruption (and daytime sleepiness) seemed to be longer lived in the elderly, showing little of the recovery over time observed in younger subjects [95]. Another study looking at phase shifts in response to ocular light exposure reported that the magnitude of phase advances was significantly attenuated in the older group [96]. One contrasting study found that when administered a bright light pulse, elderly were not significantly different from young subjects in their phase-delay response [97]. Phase-advance response, however, was not tested. Finally, Baehr and coworkers [98] concluded that the phase shifts in response to exercise, as measured by dim light melatonin onset, is preserved in older adults. Although contradictory to the animal studies, human data indicate that the elderly do have some difficulty readjusting to a shift of the light-dark cycle; however, exercise may still elicit a strong phase-shifting effect.

Decreased exposure to circadian synchronizing agents

Aging is associated with decreased exposure to external cues, which are known to entrain and strengthen the circadian clock. Exposure to bright light, which most receive on a daily basis, has been found to be significantly reduced in the aged [99,100]. Additionally, elderly have been reported to have more sedentary lifestyles [101] resulting in lower mean activity levels [52]. Furthermore, this group are much more likely to be socially disengaged and participate in fewer social interactions [102]. Both light and sociopsychologic clues, such as daily contact with other individuals and structured schedules of activity, are thought to play roles as zeitgebers for the circadian system [31,103]. Decreased activity and light exposure in an elderly subject as compared with a younger control can be seen in Fig. 2. It may be that this age-related reduction in external zeitgeber exposure, possibly combined with an age-related decline in clock function, is contributing to the sleep difficulties seen in the elderly.

Those elderly in nursing home facilities or afflicted with dementia may be especially at risk. Sleep patterns in nursing home residents have been shown to be more disrupted than normal elderly [104–106], although sleep in those with moderate

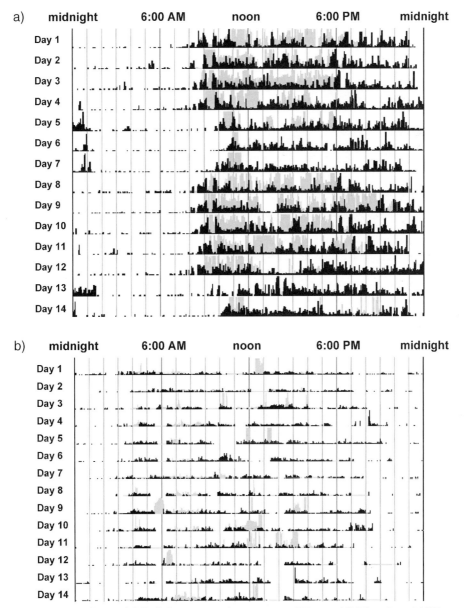

Fig. 2. Wrist activity recording and daily light exposure from a young (27 year old) (*A*) and an old (75 year old) (*B*) subject. Black bars represent activity counts and gray bars represent light exposure. Both the young and old subjects are plotted on identical scales. The activity rhythm and daily light exposure in the elderly subject is significantly reduced, whereas daily activity onset shows a notable advance.

to severe dementia has been shown to be worse still [53]. Compared with independently living elderly, those in nursing homes receive a paucity of adequate bright light exposure, suffer from a lack of structured lifestyle, and typically spend more time in bed [15,53,104]. Taken together, these factors contribute to poor circadian regulation in this population. At least one study has shown that severely demented nursing home patients have a blunted activity rhythm and were more phase delayed than normal elderly [53]. When combined with other comorbid complaints, such as medical conditions, psychiatric disorders, and excessive medication use, the lack of adequate zeitgeber exposure may play a large role in contributing to poor sleep quality in this population.

Manipulation of circadian rhythms and therapeutic implications

The findings of age-related changes in circadian rhythms have led to circadian-based interventions to treat sleep disturbances in the elderly. Some studies have shown that bright light exposure can improve circadian activity rhythms, nighttime sleep, and daytime alertness in elderly suffering from sleep maintenance insomnia [107] and early morning awakening [108]. Work by Ancoli-Israel and coworkers [109,110] has demonstrated that increasing exposure to morning bright light in mild to severely demented elderly living in nursing homes can delay the acrophase of the activity rhythm, improve the robustness of the circadian rhythm, and enhance sleep consolidation at night. Although studies are limited, current outcomes suggest that bright light exposure, especially in the evening, is beneficial in alleviating sleep maintenance insomnia in a healthy elderly population and those suffering from behavioral disturbance or dementia [111].

Exercise or lightly structured physical activity may also provide some benefit for the elderly. Studies of independently living elderly have shown improved nighttime sleep and daytime neuropsychologic performance after only 2 weeks of daily sessions consisting of mild exercise and social activity [112,113]. King and coworkers [114] also reported improved subjective sleep quality following 16 weeks of moderate intensity exercise. It may be that a combination of these factors yields greater results than any one alone. In a study by Alessi and coworkers [115], elderly subjects reduced their time in bed during the day, followed a structured bedtime routine at night, got 30 minutes or more of sunlight exposure a day, and increased their physical activity. After 5 days of intervention, subjects reported decreased daytime sleeping and increased participation in social and physical activities and social conversation. Although more studies are needed to assess fully the positive effects of activity programs in the elderly, these early results are encouraging.

There are some reports that melatonin administration before bedtime can improve sleep quality in older adults [116,117]. Likewise, the melatonin agonist agomelatine has been found to phase-shift circadian rhythms of temperature, cortisol, and thyroid-stimulating hormone in older adults [118]. One large-scale trial of 157 individuals, however, found no statistically significant differences in actiwatch-derived sleep measures between a control group and those taking melatonin [119]. Overall, the efficacy of melatonin treatment for circadian and sleep disorders is still undetermined (for review see Brzezinski and coworkers [120]); however, it has been suggested to be effective in patients with known melatonin deficiencies [121].

Summary

Sleep disturbances, specifically early morning awakenings, insomnia, and increased daytime napping, show higher prevalence with advanced age. Age-related circadian changes are seen at all levels, from molecular and cellular within the SCN to physiologic, hormonal, and behavioral output of the circadian clock. Modifications in circadian rhythms alone do not fully explain common age-related difficulties, such as advanced sleep phase or the decrease in the amplitude of the sleep-wake activity cycle. It is likely that changes in both circadian and sleep homeostatic processes, or the interaction between the two, are responsible for the impaired sleep of older adults.

Although age-related changes have been reported in healthy "usual" older adults, evidence suggests that, in addition to age, health status, medications, social structure, and physical environment are perhaps even more important contributors to the high prevalence of circadian-related sleep disturbances. As Ohayon and coworkers [19] noted

> …the aging process per se is not responsible for the increase of insomnia often reported in older people. Instead, inactivity, dissatisfaction with social life, and the presence of organic diseases and mental disorders were the best predictors of insomnia, age being insignificant. Healthy older people (i.e., without organic or mental pathologies) have a prevalence of insomnia symptoms similar to that observed in younger people.

Increasing evidence suggests that alterations in the circadian system, which are evident later in life, may begin to appear during the middle years and that this is the time to begin to take measures to prevent or delay their onset.

Advances in understanding of the circadian system and its interactions with sleep have resulted in some promising treatment options. Interventions that target the circadian system, such as selective application of bright light, structuring daily activities, increased exercise, and in some studies administration of melatonin, have been shown to improve circadian rhythm–based sleep disorders.

References

[1] Bliwise DL. Sleep in normal aging and dementia. Sleep 1993;16:40–81.

[2] Brock MA. Chronobiology and aging. J Am Geriatr Soc 1991;39:74–91.

[3] Van Gool WA, Mirmiran M. Effects of aging and housing in an enriched environment on sleep-wake patterns in rats. Sleep 1986;9:335–47.

[4] Vitiello MV. Sleep disorders and aging: understanding the causes. J Gerontol A Biol Sci Med Sci 1997;52:M189–91.

[5] Foley D, Ancoli-Israel S, Britz P, et al. Sleep disturbances and chronic disease in older adults: results of the 2003 National Sleep Foundation Sleep in America Survey. J Psychosom Res 2004; 56:497–502.

[6] Dement WC, Miles LE, Carskadon MA. White paper on sleep and aging. J Am Geriatr Soc 1982;30:25–50.

[7] Mellinger GD, Balter MB, Uhlenhuth EH. Insomnia and its treatment: prevalence and correlates. Arch Gen Psychiatry 1985;42:225–32.

[8] Middelkoop HA, Smilde-van den Doel DA, Neven AK, et al. Subjective sleep characteristics of 1,485 males and females aged 50–93: effects of sex and age, and factors related to self-evaluated quality of sleep. J Gerontol A Biol Sci Med Sci 1996;51:M108–15.

[9] Prinz PN. Sleep and sleep disorders in older adults. J Clin Neurophysiol 1995;12:139–46.

[10] Ohayon MM, Carskadon MA, Guilleminault C, et al. Meta-analysis of quantitative sleep parameters from childhood to old age in healthy individuals: developing normative sleep values across the human lifespan. Sleep 2004;27: 1255–73.

[11] Van Cauter E, Leproult R, Plat L. Age-related changes in slow wave sleep and REM sleep and relationship with growth hormone and cortisol levels in healthy men. JAMA 2000; 284:861–8.

[12] Gislason T, Reynisdottir H, Kristbjarnarson H, et al. Sleep habits and sleep disturbances among the elderly: an epidemiological survey. J Intern Med 1993;234:31–9.

[13] Monane M. Insomnia in the elderly. J Clin Psychiatry 1992;53:23–8.

[14] Foley DJ, Monjan AA, Brown SL, et al. Sleep complaints among elderly persons: an epidemiologic study of three communities. Sleep 1995;18:425–32.

[15] Ancoli-Israel S, Kripke DF. Prevalent sleep problems in the aged. Biofeedback Self Regul 1991; 16:349–59.

[16] van Coevorden A, Mockel J, Laurent E, et al. Neuroendocrine rhythms and sleep in aging men. Am J Physiol 1991;260(4 Pt 1):E651–61.

[17] Weitzman ED, Moline ML, Czeisler CA, et al. Chronobiology of aging: temperature, sleep-wake rhythms and entrainment. Neurobiol Aging 1982;3:299–309.

[18] Czeisler CA, Dumont M, Duffy JF, et al. Association of sleep-wake habits in older people with changes in output of circadian pacemaker. Lancet 1992;340:933–6.

[19] Ohayon MM, Zulley J, Guilleminault C, et al. How age and daytime activities are related to insomnia in the general population: consequences for older people. J Am Geriatr Soc 2001;49:360–6.

[20] Reid KJ, Chang AM, Zee PC. Circadian rhythm sleep disorders. Med Clin North Am 2004; 88:631–51.

[21] Edgar DM. Functional role of the suprachiasmatic nucleus in the regulation of sleep and wakefulness. In: Guilleminault C, Montagna P, Lugaresai E, et al, editors. Fatal familial insomnia: inherited prion diseases, sleep and the thalamus. New York: Raven Press; 1994. p. 203–13.

[22] Edgar DM. Circadian control of sleep/wakefulness: implications in shiftwork and therapeutic strategies. In: Shiraki S, Sagawa S, Yousef MK, editors. Physiological basis of occupational health: stressful environments. Amsterdam: Academic Publishing; 1996. p. 253–65.

[23] Cassone VM, Warren WS, Brooks DS, et al. Melatonin, the pineal gland, and circadian rhythms. J Biol Rhythms 1993;8:S73–81.

[24] Moore-Ede MC, Sulzman FM, Fuller CA. The clocks that time us. Cambridge: Harvard University Press; 1982.

[25] Buxton OM, Frank SA, L'Hermite-Balériaux M, et al. Roles of intensity and duration of nocturnal exercise in causing phase delays of human circadian rhythms. Am J Physiol 1997;273: E536–42.

[26] Van Reeth O, Sturis J, Byrne MM, et al. Nocturnal exercise phase delays circadian rhythms of melatonin and thyrotropin secretion in normal men. Am J Physiol 1994;266(6 Pt 1):E964–74.

[27] Aschoff J. Circadian rhythms in man. Science 1965;148:1427–32.

[28] Akerstedt T, Gillberg M. The circadian variation of experimentally displaced sleep. Sleep 1981; 4:159–69.

[29] Czeisler CA, Duffy JF, Shanahan TL, et al. Stability, precision, and near-24-hour period of the human circadian pacemaker. Science 1999; 284:2177–81.

[30] Dijk DJ, Czeisler CA. Paradoxical timing of the circadian rhythm of sleep propensity serves to

consolidate sleep and wakefulness in humans. Neurosci Lett 1994;166:63–8.

[31] Wever RA. Influence of physical workload on freerunning circadian rhythms of man. Pflugers Arch 1979;381:119–26.

[32] Zulley J, Wever R, Aschoff J. The dependence of onset and duration of sleep on the circadian rhythm of rectal temperature. Pflugers Arch 1981;391:314–8.

[33] Czeisler CA, Weitzman E, Moore-Ede MC, et al. Human sleep: its duration and organization depend on its circadian phase. Science 1980; 210:1264–7.

[34] Borbely AA. Sleep: circadian rhythm vs. recovery process. In: Koukkou M, Loehmann D, Angst J, editors. Functional states of the brain: their determinants. Amsterdam: Elsevier/North Holland; 1980. p. 151–61.

[35] Daan S, Beersma DG, Borbely AA. Timing of human sleep: recovery process gated by a circadian pacemaker. Am J Physiol 1984;246(2 Pt 2): R161–83.

[36] Kronauer RE, Czeisler CA, Pilato SF, et al. Mathematical model of the human circadian system with two interacting oscillators. Am J Physiol 1982;242:R3–17.

[37] Benoit O, Foret J, Bouard G, et al. Habitual sleep length and patterns of recovery sleep after 24 hour and 36 hour sleep deprivation. Electroencephalogr Clin Neurophysiol 1980; 50:477–85.

[38] Dijk DJ, Beersma DG. Effects of SWS deprivation on subsequent EEG power density and spontaneous sleep duration. Electroencephalogr Clin Neurophysiol 1989;72:312–20.

[39] Dijk DJ, Brunner DP, Beersma DG, et al. Electroencephalogram power density and slow wave sleep as a function of prior waking and circadian phase. Sleep 1990;13:430–40.

[40] Porkka-Heiskanen T, Strecker RE, Thakkar M, et al. Adenosine: a mediator of the sleep-inducing effects of prolonged wakefulness. Science 1997;276:1265–8.

[41] Sutin EL, Dement WC, Heller HC, et al. Light-induced gene expression in the suprachiasmatic nucleus of young and aging rats. Neurobiol Aging 1993;14:441–6.

[42] Zhang Y, Kornhauser JM, Zee PC, et al. Effects of aging on light-induced phase-shifting of circadian behavioral rhythms, fos expression and CREB phosphorylation in the hamster suprachiasmatic nucleus. Neuroscience 1996;70: 951–61.

[43] Asai M, Yoshinobu Y, Kaneko S, et al. Circadian profile of Per gene mRNA expression in the suprachiasmatic nucleus, paraventricular nucleus, and pineal body of aged rats. J Neurosci Res 2001;66:1133–9.

[44] Kolker DE, Fukuyama H, Huang DS, et al. Aging alters circadian and light-induced expression of clock genes in golden hamsters. J Biol Rhythms 2003;18:159–69.

[45] Weinert H, Weinert D, Schurov I, et al. Impaired expression of the mPer2 circadian clock gene in the suprachiasmatic nuclei of aging mice. Chronobiol Int 2001;18:559–65.

[46] McDonald RB, Hoban-Higgins TM, Ruhe RC, et al. Alterations in endogenous circadian rhythm of core temperature in senescent Fischer 344 rats. Am J Physiol 1999;276(3 Pt 2): R824–30.

[47] Van Reeth O, Zhang Y, Zee PC, et al. Grafting fetal suprachiasmatic nuclei in the hypothalamus of old hamsters restores responsiveness of the circadian clock to a phase shifting stimulus. Brain Res 1994;643(1–2):338–42.

[48] Swaab DF, Fliers E, Partiman TS. The suprachiasmatic nucleus of the human brain in relation to sex, age and senile dementia. Brain Res 1985;342:37–44.

[49] Swaab DF, Van Someren EJ, Zhou JN, et al. Biological rhythms in the human life cycle and their relationship to functional changes in the suprachiasmatic nucleus. Prog Brain Res 1996; 111:349–68.

[50] Hofman MA. The human circadian clock and aging. Chronobiol Int 2000;17:245–59.

[51] Hofman MA, Swaab DF. Alterations in circadian rhythmicity of the vasopressin-producing neurons of the human suprachiasmatic nucleus (SCN) with aging. Brain Res 1994;651:134–42.

[52] Harper DG, Volicer L, Stopa EG, et al. Disturbance of endogenous circadian rhythm in aging and Alzheimer disease. Am J Geriatr Psychiatry 2005;13:359–68.

[53] Ancoli-Israel S, Klauber MR, Jones DW, et al. Variations in circadian rhythms of activity, sleep, and light exposure related to dementia in nursing-home patients. Sleep 1997;20: 18–23.

[54] Satlin A, Volicer L, Stopa EG, et al. Circadian locomotor activity and core-body temperature rhythms in Alzheimer's disease. Neurobiol Aging 1995;16:765–71.

[55] Liu RY, Zhou JN, Hoogendijk WJ, et al. Decreased vasopressin gene expression in the biological clock of Alzheimer disease patients with and without depression. J Neuropathol Exp Neurol 2000;59:314–22.

[56] Rollag MD, Berson DM, Provencio I. Melanopsin, ganglion-cell photoreceptors, and mammalian photoentrainment. J Biol Rhythms 2003; 18:227–34.

[57] Saper CB, Scammell TE, Lu J. Hypothalamic regulation of sleep and circadian rhythms. Nature 2005;437:1257–63.

[58] Dillon J, Zheng L, Merriam JC, et al. Transmission of light to the aging human retina: possible implications for age related macular degeneration. Exp Eye Res 2004;79:753–9.

[59] Hattar S, Liao HW, Takao M, et al. Melanopsin-containing retinal ganglion cells: architecture, projections, and intrinsic photosensitivity. Science 2002;295:1065–70.

[60] Penev PD, Turek FW, Wallen EP, et al. Aging alters the serotonergic modulation of light-induced phase advances in golden hamsters. Am J Physiol 1997;272(2 Pt 2):R509–13.

[61] Sharma M, Palacios-Bois J, Schwartz G, et al. Circadian rhythms of melatonin and cortisol in aging. Biol Psychiatry 1989;25:305–19.

[62] Herljevic M, Middleton B, Thapan K, et al. Light-induced melatonin suppression: age-related reduction in response to short wavelength light. Exp Gerontol 2005;40:237–42.

[63] Satinoff E. Patterns of circadian body temperature rhythms in aged rats. Clin Exp Pharmacol Physiol 1998;25:135–40.

[64] Touitou Y, Reinberg A, Bogdan A, et al. Age-related changes in both circadian and seasonal rhythms of rectal temperature with special reference to senile dementia of Alzheimer type. Gerontology 1986;32:110–8.

[65] Richardson GS, Carskadon MA, Orav EJ, et al. Circadian variation of sleep tendency in elderly and young adult subjects. Sleep 1982;5:S82–94.

[66] Vitiello MV, Smallwood RG, Avery DH, et al. Circadian temperature rhythms in young adult and aged men. Neurobiol Aging 1986;7:97–100.

[67] Campbell SS, Gillin JC, Kripke DF, et al. Gender differences in the circadian temperature rhythms of healthy elderly subjects: relationships to sleep quality. Sleep 1989;12:529–36.

[68] Moe KE, Prinz PN, Vitiello MV, et al. Healthy elderly women and men have different entrained circadian temperature rhythms. J Am Geriatr Soc 1991;39:383–7.

[69] Van Cauter E, Leproult R, Kupfer DJ. Effects of gender and age on the levels and circadian rhythmicity of plasma cortisol. J Clin Endocrinol Metab 1996;81:2468–73.

[70] Monk TH, Buysse DJ, Reynolds CF, et al. Circadian temperature rhythms of older people. Exp Gerontol 1995;30:455–74.

[71] Monk TH, Buysse DJ, Reynolds CF, et al. Rhythmic vs homeostatic influences on mood, activation, and performance in young and old men. J Gerontol 1992;47:221–7.

[72] Buysse DJ, Monk TH, Reynolds CF, et al. Patterns of sleep episodes in young and elderly adults during a 36-hour constant routine. Sleep 1993;16:632–7.

[73] Zeitzer JM, Daniels JE, Duffy JF, et al. Do plasma melatonin concentrations decline with age? Am J Med 1999;107:432–6.

[74] Duffy JF, Dijk DJ, Hall EF, et al. Relationship of endogenous circadian melatonin and temperature rhythms to self-reported preference for morning or evening activity in young and older people. J Investig Med 1999;47:141–50.

[75] Dijk DJ, Duffy JF, Riel E, et al. Ageing and the circadian and homeostatic regulation of human sleep during forced desynchrony of rest, melatonin and temperature rhythms. J Physiol 1999;516:611–27.

[76] Van Cauter E, Copinschi G. Interrelationships between growth hormone and sleep. Growth Horm IGF Res 2000;10(Suppl B):S57–62.

[77] Benloucif S, Masana MI, Dubocovich ML. Light-induced phase shifts of circadian activity rhythms and immediate early gene expression in the suprachiasmatic nucleus are attenuated in old C3H/HeN mice. Brain Res 1997; 747:34–42.

[78] Valentinuzzi VS, Scarbrough K, Takahashi JS, et al. Effects of aging on the circadian rhythm of wheel-running activity in C57BL/6 mice. Am J Physiol 1997;273(6 Pt 2):R1957–64.

[79] Possidente B, McEldowney S, Pabon A. Aging lengthens circadian period for wheel-running activity in C57BL mice. Physiol Behav 1995; 57:575–9.

[80] Zee PC, Rosenberg RS, Turek FW. Effects of aging on entrainment and rate of resynchronization of circadian locomotor activity. Am J Physiol 1992;263(5 Pt 2):R1099–103.

[81] Morin LP. Age-related changes in hamster circadian period, entrainment and rhythm splitting. J Biol Rhythms 1988;3:237–48.

[82] Van Gool WA, Witting W, Mirmiran M. Age-related changes in circadian sleep-wakefulness rhythms in male rats isolated from time cues. Brain Res 1987;413:384–7.

[83] Davis FC, Viswanathan N. Stability of circadian timing with age in Syrian hamsters. Am J Physiol 1998;275:R960–8.

[84] Duffy JF, Viswanathan N, Davis FC. Free-running circadian period does not shorten with age in female Syrian hamsters. Neurosci Lett 1999;271:77–80.

[85] Monk TH, Moline ML. Removal of temporal constraints in the middle-aged and elderly: effects on sleep and sleepiness. Sleep 1988; 11:513–20.

[86] Kendall AR, Lewy AJ, Sack RL. Effects of aging on the intrinsic circadian period of totally blind humans. J Biol Rhythms 2001;16: 87–95.

[87] Van Reeth O, Zhang Y, Reddy A, et al. Aging alters the entraining effects of an activity-inducing stimulus on the circadian clock. Brain Res 1993;607:286–92.

[88] Van Reeth O, Zhang Y, Zee PC, et al. Aging alters feedback effects of the activity-rest cycle on the circadian clock. Am J Physiol 1992;263(4 Pt 2): R981–6.

[89] Wise PM, Cohen IR, Weiland NG, et al. Aging alters the circadian rhythm of glucose utilization in the suprachiasmatic nucleus. Proc Natl Acad Sci U S A 1988;85:5305–9.

[90] Wise PM, Walovitch RC, Cohen IR, et al. Diurnal rhythmicity and hypothalamic deficits in glucose utilization in aged ovariectomized rats. J Neurosci 1987;7:3469–73.

[91] Harma MI, Hakola T, Akerstedt T, et al. Age and adjustment to night work. Occup Environ Med 1994;51:568–73.

[92] Gander PH, Nguyen D, Rosekind MR, et al. Age, circadian rhythms, and sleep loss in flight crews. Aviat Space Environ Med 1993;64(3 Pt 1): 189–95.

[93] Foret J, Bensimon G, Benoit O, et al. Quality of sleep as a function of age and shift work. In: Reinberg A, editor. Night and shift work: biological and social aspects. Oxford: Pergamon Press; 1981. p. 149–54.

[94] Monk TH, Buysse DJ, Carrier J, et al. Inducing jet-lag in older people: directional asymmetry. J Sleep Res 2000;9:101–16.

[95] Monk TH, Buysse DJ, Reynolds CF, et al. Inducing jet lag in older people: adjusting to a 6-hour phase advance in routine. Exp Gerontol 1993; 28:119–33.

[96] Klerman EB, Duffy JF, Dijk DJ, et al. Circadian phase resetting in older people by ocular bright light exposure. J Investig Med 2001;49:30–40.

[97] Benloucif S, Green K, L'Hermite-Baleriaux M, et al. Responsiveness of the aging circadian clock to light. Neurobiol Aging 2005, in press.

[98] Baehr EK, Eastman CI, Revelle W, et al. Circadian phase-shifting effects of nocturnal exercise in older compared with young adults. Am J Physiol Regul Integr Comp Physiol 2003; 284:R1542–50.

[99] Campbell SS, Kripke DF, Gillin JC, et al. Exposure to light in healthy elderly subjects and Alzheimer's patients. Physiol Behav 1988;42:141–4.

[100] Shochat T, Martin J, Marler M, et al. Illumination levels in nursing home patients: effects on sleep and activity rhythms. J Sleep Res 2000;9:373–9.

[101] Bortz WM. Disuse and aging. JAMA 1982; 248:1203–8.

[102] Bassuk SS, Glass TA, Berkman LF. Social disengagement and incident cognitive decline in community-dwelling elderly persons. Ann Intern Med 1999;131:165–73.

[103] Aschoff J, Fatranska M, Giedke H, et al. Human circadian rhythms in continuous darkness: entrainment by social cues. Science 1971; 171:213–5.

[104] Ancoli-Israel S, Parker L, Sinaee R, et al. Sleep fragmentation in patients from a nursing home. J Gerontol 1989;44:M18–21.

[105] Jacobs D, Ancoli-Israel S, Parker L, et al. Twenty-four-hour sleep-wake patterns in a nursing home population. Psychol Aging 1989; 4:352–6.

[106] Martin JL, Webber AP, Alam T, et al. Daytime sleeping, sleep disturbance, and circadian rhythms in the nursing home. Am J Geriatr Psychiatry 2006;14:121–9.

[107] Campbell SS, Dawson D, Anderson MW. Alleviation of sleep maintenance insomnia with timed exposure to bright light. J Am Geriatr Soc 1993;41:829–36.

[108] Lack L, Wright H, Kemp K, et al. The treatment of early-morning awakening insomnia with 2 evenings of bright light. Sleep 2005;28: 616–23.

[109] Ancoli-Israel S, Martin JL, Kripke DF, et al. Effect of light treatment on sleep and circadian rhythms in demented nursing home patients. J Am Geriatr Soc 2002;50:282–9.

[110] Ancoli-Israel S, Gehrman P, Martin JL, et al. Increased light exposure consolidates sleep and strengthens circadian rhythms in severe Alzheimer's disease patients. Behav Sleep Med 2003;1:22–36.

[111] Van Someren EJ, Kessler A, Mirmiran M, et al. Indirect bright light improves circadian rest-activity rhythm disturbances in demented patients. Biol Psychiatry 1997;41:955–63.

[112] Naylor E, Penev PD, Orbeta L, et al. Daily social and physical activity increases slow-wave sleep and daytime neuropsychological performance in the elderly. Sleep 2000;23:87–95.

[113] Benloucif S, Orbeta L, Ortiz R, et al. Morning or evening activity improves neuropsychological performance and subjective sleep quality in older adults. Sleep 2004;27:1542–51.

[114] King AC, Oman RF, Brassington GS, et al. Moderate-intensity exercise and self-rated quality of sleep in older adults: a randomized controlled trial. JAMA 1997;277:32–7.

[115] Alessi CA, Martin JL, Webber AP, et al. Randomized, controlled trial of a nonpharmacological intervention to improve abnormal sleep/wake patterns in nursing home residents. J Am Geriatr Soc 2005;53:803–10.

[116] Garfinkel D, Laudon M, Nof D, et al. Improvement of sleep quality in elderly people by controlled-release melatonin. Lancet 1995;346: 541–4.

[117] Leger D, Laudon M, Zisapel N. Nocturnal 6-sulfatoxymelatonin excretion in insomnia and its relation to the response to melatonin replacement therapy. Am J Med 2004;116:91–5.

[118] Leproult R, Van Onderbergen A, L'Hermite-Baleriaux M, et al. Phase-shifts of 24-h rhythms of hormonal release and body temperature following early evening administration of the melatonin agonist agomelatine in healthy older men. Clin Endocrinol (Oxf) 2005;63: 298–304.

[119] Singer C, Tractenberg RE, Kaye J, et al. A multicenter, placebo-controlled trial of melatonin for sleep disturbance in Alzheimer's disease. Sleep 2003;26:893–901.

[120] Brzezinski A, Vangel MG, Wurtman RJ, et al. Effects of exogenous melatonin on sleep: a meta-analysis. Sleep Med Rev 2005;9:41–50.

[121] Pandi-Perumal SR, Zisapel N, Srinivasan V, et al. Melatonin and sleep in aging population. Exp Gerontol 2005;40:911–25.

**ELSEVIER
SAUNDERS**

SLEEP
MEDICINE
CLINICS

Sleep Med Clin 1 (2006) 197–205

Sleep in Midlife Women

Kathryn A. Lee, PhD, RN

- What is menopause?
- Literature search strategy
- Subjective sleep complaints
  Cross-sectional studies
  Longitudinal studies
- Objective sleep disturbance

Cross-sectional studies
Longitudinal intervention studies
- Clinical assessment guide
- Summary
- Acknowledgements
- References

Women between 40 and 60 years of age are considered midlife, and are a rapidly growing group in the United States, representing about 27% of the population [1]. Some midlife women are starting families, whereas others are becoming grandmothers, but most are employed, and find themselves at a stage in life when caregiving for spouses or aging parents is an additional role demand. Most of what is known about women's sleep during this period in their lives is based on retrospective self-reports or large cross-sectional epidemiologic surveys related to menopause. As part of the ongoing Study of Women's Health Across the Nation (SWAN), Kravitz and coworkers [2] reported their community survey results on prevalence of sleep difficulty in United States women between 40 and 55 years of age. In this multiethnic sample of over 12,600 women, 38% reported difficulty sleeping in the past 2 weeks, with the lowest rate of difficulty among Japanese Americans (28%) and premenopausal women (31%), and the highest rates among whites (40%), those after surgical menopause (48%), and those experiencing natural menopausal transition (45%) [2].

In broad surveys of symptom experience, midlife women are as likely to complain about hot flashes and trouble sleeping as they are to complain about their weight gain [3–6]. Most of the research on women in these earlier studies was conducted with educated white women, however, and many of these participants were recruited from menopause clinics, which creates bias in the ability to generalize these research findings to the typical midlife woman in the United States. The sleep disturbance occurring from menopausal vasomotor symptoms, including nocturnal hot flashes and night sweats, has been inadequately studied in controlled laboratory settings, and it remains unclear whether a history of sleep complaints exists before menopause, or whether the sleep disturbance is unique to menopause or unique to aging [6,7].

This article describes the types of sleep disturbance reported by women as they experience menopausal transition. The menopausal transition is viewed as a normal developmental stage for midlife women during which ovarian hormone secretion either diminishes over time or abruptly stops. Sleep patterns related to this biologic transition, however, can be influenced by many psychologic and sociocultural factors unrelated to cessation of menstruation and ovarian hormone production. Although disturbed sleep associated with menopausal hot

This work was supported in part by Grant No. R01 NR04259 from the National Institute of Nursing Research Department of Family Health Care Nursing, School of Nursing, University of California, San Francisco, Box 0606, Room N411Y, 2 Kirkham Avenue, San Francisco, CA 94143–0606, USA
E-mail address: kathryn.lee@nursing.ucsf.edu

flashes or night sweats should be a transient experience, it is of unknown severity and duration, and has potential for adverse health outcomes and poor quality of life. The current knowledge about the sleep of midlife women is presented within a biopsychosocial framework and gaps in knowledge and areas for future research are delineated.

What is menopause?

Menopause occurs at 51.4 years of age for the average woman, but hormonal fluctuations and irregular menstrual cycles can begin as early as 7 to 10 years before the actual cessation of menstrual cycles. With such highly variable menstrual cycles during this transition, menopause is only definitive after 12 consecutive months of amenorrhea. In 2001, the National Institute on Aging, the North American Menopause Society, and others sponsored a workshop to establish a staging system to categorize midlife women, and experts at this Stages of Reproductive Aging Workshop disseminated their executive summary and recommendations for nomenclature [8]. During the early phase of menopause transition, there may be periodic ovarian function, but lack of estrogen and progesterone secretion from the ovary results in a negative feedback response to the hypothalamus, whereby follicle-stimulating hormone secretion is increased. During the later phase of menopausal transition, follicle-stimulating hormone is consistently elevated, and amenorrhea has been at least 60 days, reflecting at least two missed menstrual cycles. Early postmenopause is defined as the first 5 years after the last menstrual period, and late postmenopause starts with the sixth year after the final menstrual period and continues into old age [8].

The vasomotor symptoms associated with menopause, such as hot flashes and night sweats, vary to such a great extent that they are not specified as one of the Stages of Reproductive Aging Workshop staging criteria for ascertaining phases of menopause

[8]. These particular symptoms, however, occur on average of five times per day in most women in Western society, whereas they are rare in some Asian cultures and nonexistent in others [9,10]. Regardless of how common it is among women, hot flashes can be very disruptive of nighttime sleep. The pattern for hot flashes across the 24-hour day for a group of 12 postmenopausal women monitored for 24 hours is shown in Fig. 1, where there is a peak at 10:00 PM and very few from 6:00 AM to 1:00 PM [11]. An excellent review of the physiology of hot flashes was recently published [12].

The perimenopausal transition and postmenopausal experience for an individual woman arises from a complex interaction of biologic, cultural, psychologic, and environmental factors. The timing and duration of this midlife transition cannot be easily predicted. As a result, very few longitudinal studies with minimal attrition rates can be conducted and most of what is known about sleep in midlife women is based on cross-sectional studies with self-report recall measures of sleep problems.

Literature search strategy

Studies for this literature review were obtained by using PubMed and the following key words: menopause, sleep, hot flashes, night sweats, perimenopause, and symptoms. There have been fewer than 450 studies and 12 reviews published on this topic since 1964, and most (250 studies) have been published since 2000, with 56 citations in 2005, but no meta-analysis has been done. For this article, research studies and review articles in English were reviewed. Most were descriptive reports, and a few were clinical trials in which hormone-replacement therapy or other pharmacologic therapies were tested as an intervention to relieve menopausal symptoms, including sleep disturbance. Because the incidence of specific sleep disorders like narcolepsy, restless legs, or sleep apnea, does not significantly increase during midlife after accounting for

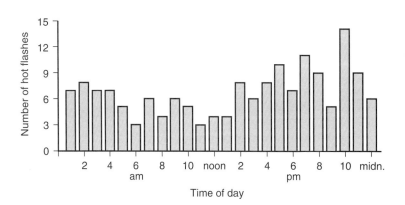

Fig. 1. Pattern of hot flash frequency monitored across 24 hours in 12 women. (*Modified from* Woodward S, Freedman RR. The thermoregulatory effects of menopausal hot flashes on sleep. Sleep 1994;17:499; with permission.)

body weight [13–16], the focus of this article is on subjective sleep complaints by self-report and sleep disturbances assessed by more objective polysomnography or actigraphy measures.

Subjective sleep complaints

Cross-sectional studies

In a large survey of Swedish women, it was nocturnal micturition, not menopause or age, which was related to disturbed sleep [17]. Nocturnal micturition was the most common (53%) reason for disrupted sleep in women 40 to 49 years of age, and it was the frequent nightly awakenings for urination that impaired sleep and resulted in poor daytime performance; decreased sense of well-being; more physician visits; and more frequent use of medications, including estrogen and medications for sleep. Table 1 [17–20] depicts the increasing prevalence of reported sleep problems in population studies of Australian [19] and Swedish women by age cohorts and the increasing use of sleep medications in midlife [17,18,20]. It seems to stabilize at about 50 to 60 years of age. Fewer than half of women who reported sleep problems actually used a sleep medication or sought medical treatment for their insomnia [20].

In the large SWAN survey of women in the United States, women between 40 and 55 years of age were asked by telephone whether or not they had difficulty sleeping in the past 2 weeks. The prevalence was 38%, very similar to that reported for Australian women [19] and Swedish women [20]. It was white ethnicity, higher education, poor health behaviors, such as smoking and inactivity, psychologic symptoms (feeling nervous, irritable, or depressed), and higher perceived stress levels that were associated with difficulty sleeping [2]. Over time, mood state has been shown to be highly stable during menopausal transition, and it is the premenopausal levels of stress and attitudes about aging reported by women that best predicted their postmenopausal mood state, not menopause or changes in hormones [21]. In this sample of

Australian midlife women, trouble sleeping was predicted by mood state and well-being [19].

These studies support the conclusion that sleep becomes problematic for women as they transition from premenopausal to postmenopausal life, yet the specific type of sleep problem was not ascertained. As part of the Wisconsin Sleep Cohort Study, Young and colleagues [13] asked about specific types of sleep problems and found that it was difficulty falling asleep (initiation insomnia) that distinguished premenopausal women from postmenopausal women, after controlling for age and body mass index. Those who reported hot flashes also experienced more self-reported sleep problems and more dissatisfaction with their sleep. In this cross-sectional study, however, it was postmenopausal women taking hormone-replacement therapy who had more sleep complaints than postmenopausal women not taking hormone therapy. This supports previous reports in other cross-sectional studies [5].

Longitudinal studies

From annual assessments of many symptoms over a 7-year period in Australian women, it was clear that severity of "trouble sleeping in the past 2 weeks" was the outstanding symptom that increased over time as women transitioned from premenopausal to early postmenopausal [19]. In a longitudinal study of 522 midlife women in the Pittsburgh area who were 42 to 50 years of age when they began the study, Owens and Matthews [22] used an investigator-developed sleep questionnaire to also assess how they were sleeping 3 years later. They found that 42% of the 213 available cases had "trouble sleeping" that was specific to waking up during the night. Although 25% had trouble sleeping at both time points, 38% had no problems at either time point. Interestingly, they found no relationship between sleep complaints and body weight, nutritional intake, or family and social variables. The participants were recruited from a health care clinic, and validity and reliability estimates of their sleep and nutrition measures were not included.

Hollander and coworkers [23] studied a cohort of 218 black and 218 white women in the Philadelphia area who were between 35 and 47 years of age and regularly menstruating at time of enrollment into the study. After four assessments over a 2-year period, they found that sleep complaints were stable at about 17% over the course of their study. They assessed sleep with the St. Mary's Hospital Sleep Questionnaire, which asks about the last night's sleep and is less subject to recall bias. Unlike Owens and Mathews [22], Hollander and colleagues' [23] findings support the SWAN [2]

Table 1: Prevalence of sleep problems in midlife women

Age group	% Sleep problem	% Use sleep medication
38 years of age	20	2–3
50 years of age	37–38	8–15
60 years of age	37	15–25

Based on prevalence data from Sweden and Australia [17–20].

findings that poor sleep in midlife women is associated with many biologic and psychosocial factors, including report of hot flashes; use of sleep medication; higher body mass index; high caffeine intake; and high stress, anxiety, and depression. In this cohort of women on the east coast of the United States, however, the sleep complaints were more common in African American women than whites, in unemployed women, and in women with less education [23]. Kripke and coworkers [24] suggest that poor sleep among ethnic minority postmenopausal women may be associated with minimal light exposure and depression rather than circadian rhythms of melatonin hormone secretion. The most recent published findings from the SWAN study indicate that sleep problems increase just before menses and just after menses compared with the rest of the menstrual cycle in both premenopausal and early perimenopausal women, with more perimenopausal women consistently reporting trouble with sleep compared with premenopausal women after controlling for age [25].

Using a well-established and validated self-report measure, Kloss and coworkers [26] did not find any differences in sleep quality on the Pittsburgh Sleep Quality Index by income, education, use of hormones, or ethnicity, even though more African American women reported hot flashes and night sweats than whites. In this group of perimenopausal women in the Philadelphia area, 67% had a Pittsburgh Sleep Quality Index score greater than 5 (0–21 scale), the cut-point for determining poor sleep quality. The Pittsburgh Sleep Quality Index asks participants to consider the past month when responding to each item, and may be subject to recall bias. The most common problem was sleep maintenance insomnia (53%), however, followed by early morning awakening (32%) and not feeling rested on wakening (25%). Poor sleep quality was associated with depressed mood, higher trait anxiety, and dysfunctional beliefs and attitudes about sleep.

Objective sleep disturbance

Cross-sectional studies

Shaver and coworkers [7] found more disrupted sleep in midlife women who experienced hot flashes compared to women without hot flashes. There was only 13% wake time during the night for the symptomatic women, however, compared with 10% wake time for the asymptomatic women. These low rates of wake time were supported in subsequent laboratory sleep studies using polysomnography [11,13,27].

Sleep efficiency, which includes the time initially to fall asleep and time asleep during the night,

likewise does not differ for menopausal women compared with premenopausal women or asymptomatic menopausal women of the same age in laboratory comparisons. In the Wisconsin Sleep Cohort Study, average sleep onset was 10 to 14 minutes, sleep efficiency was 84% to 87%, total sleep time was 375 to 390 minutes, and deep sleep stages were 13% to 17% for all groups of midlife women after controlling for age and body mass index [13]. Results were similar in a small group of premenopausal women (N = 13) compared with postmenopausal women (N = 12) [14]. In this sample, however, the latency to the first interval of deep sleep was shorter on both nights (17 and 20 minutes) in postmenopausal women compared with premenopausal women (27 and 54 minutes), but there was high variability in both groups.

After healthy women were recruited from the community by newspaper advertisements and rigorously screened for sleep disorders, major depression, drug use, and obesity, Freedman and Roehrs [27] found no relationship between hot flashes and sleep. They recorded both polysomnography for standard sleep measures and sternal skin conductance for measuring hot flashes in the laboratory for 3 nights. An average of 5.2 ± 2.9 hot flashes occurred per night in the symptomatic women (range 1–18 with a median of 5). There were no recorded hot flashes in the women who were asymptomatic by self-report, but six women who indicated no vasomotor symptoms actually had hot flashes in the laboratory and were excluded from further analyses. Hot flashes occurred less in deep sleep stages 3 and 4 (8%) and rapid eye movement (REM) (0.83%) than in stage 2 non-REM light sleep (40%) or when awake (34%). When awakenings were examined within 2 minutes of a hot flash, 55% of the awakenings occurred before the hot flash and 40% occurred after the hot flash. Only 5% of the hot flashes occurred simultaneously with an awakening of 60 seconds or longer, and only 6% of the hot flashes occurred simultaneously with a brief arousal defined as 3 to 14 seconds in duration [27].

In these studies, midlife women with menopausal symptoms have subjective and objective sleep disturbance, yet many of the research findings about self-reported sleep complaints and objective sleep disturbance were associated with psychosocial factors rather than menopausal status [13,17–24,26–29]. Those who controlled for age and body weight, or included only a healthy, nondepressed sample, typically found no difference in sleep by menopausal status and relatively high sleep efficiency in laboratory studies. These studies all speak to the need for longitudinal assessments of women's sleep patterns to determine whether sleep problems are pre-existing for women entering midlife and menopausal transition.

Longitudinal intervention studies

Hormone-replacement therapy

Thompson and Oswald [30] were the first to conduct a study to test the effects of estrogen therapy on sleep, psychologic mood, and hot flashes. Women between 45 and 55 years of age who had amenorrhea for at least 3 months were asked to participate if they also experienced insomnia, negative affect symptoms, and hot flashes. Of the 42 who started the protocol, 34 completed the 2-month study period. Both the placebo group and the group receiving estrogen had a similar improvement in the measures of anxiety and depression, and both groups experienced similar decreases in their report of hot flashes. Those taking estrogen, however, had fewer arousals during sleep and less wake time (15 minutes compared with 2 minutes less for the placebo group). They also had an increase in REM sleep in the later part of the night, but no changes in non-REM light or deep sleep stages [30].

Other small sample studies of postmenopausal women support Thompson and Oswald's [30] findings. Sleep researchers at Harvard examined the effects of estrogen on sleep in eight women who had experienced natural menopause and eight women who had experienced surgical menopause [6,31]. In a double-blind crossover design, each woman spent a total of 10 nights in the sleep laboratory undergoing polysomnography, including 2 nights of adaptation before receiving placebo or low-dose estrogen (0.625 mg/day). Only 10 of the 16 women complained of hot flashes, and although hot flashes decreased with estrogen treatment, there was no change in any of their psychologic mood parameters. With estrogen therapy, sleep-onset latency was shorter (12 minutes, compared with 19 minutes on placebo), and more time was spent in REM sleep (22% of total sleep time, compared with 16.5% on placebo). This small sample of women was recruited from a menopause clinic and ranged in age from 31 to 65 years; the duration of menopause was also quite variable (2–22 years), but these results supported findings about exogenous estrogen administration and its effect on REM sleep and mood state [31]. Objective measures of hot flashes, however, were not part of the study design.

A similar estrogen dose in a pilot study with seven women also showed a significant reduction in sleep-onset latency (down from 29–18 minutes), improvement in sleep efficiency (up from 80%–86%), and an increase in REM sleep [32] after 1 month of estrogen therapy. In this small pilot study, it is not clear how participants were recruited, but hot flashes were also monitored during the 3 nights in the sleep laboratory under each placebo and estrogen condition, and hot flash frequency was also significantly decreased during sleep [32].

Erlik and coworkers [33] were the first to record hot flashes in a laboratory study of sleep using finger temperature and skin resistance. After the standard protocol of 2 nights of adaptation to the laboratory, sleep and flashes were recorded from 2200 hours to 0700 hours in nine postmenopausal women who complained of severe hot flashes. They ranged in age from 30 to 55 years and were 1 to 5 years after surgical or natural menopause. Most (45 of 47) of the recorded hot flashes were within a 5-minute period of wake time. Of note, however, was the finding that most awakenings occurred 20 to 30 seconds prior to the measurable hot flash. Rather than awakening from the discomfort resulting from a hot flash, this finding suggested a central, hypothalamic function for both vasomotor symptoms and arousal from sleep [33].

In a British study of 33 postmenopausal women randomized to placebo or estrogen, 0.625 mg/day, neither the subjective sleep quality measure nor objective polysomnographic sleep measures differed between the two groups. Although neither REM sleep nor number of awakenings differed by group, both groups consistently improved over the 12 weeks of the study and both groups experienced a reduction in vasomotor symptoms by self-report and laboratory measures. There was a larger reduction in hot flashes associated with arousals from sleep for the estrogen-treated group ($P = .07$), but it did not reach statistical significance in the small sample of 17 women allocated to the estrogen group. The estrogen-treated group also had significant improvement in well-being and anxiety measures [34].

The type and dose of hormone therapy is one factor that may account for differences in study findings related to sleep efficiency and wake time during the night or self-reported improvement in symptoms. After 6 months of hormone therapy in a randomized clinical trial, subjective measures of hot flashes and sleep improved more so than the objective sleep measures assessed in the sleep laboratory for 2 consecutive nights, but there was no difference in anxiety or mood after 6 months of hormone treatment [35]. Those 11 women randomized to estrogen, 0.625 mg, with medroxyprogesterone acetate, 5 mg, had no improvement in any objective sleep measure and their sleep efficiency remained at 87% $\pm$ 6.5%, whereas the 10 women randomized to receive the same dose of estrogen but with a shorter half-life progestogen compound, 200 mg, had a significant improvement in sleep efficiency (from 81% $\pm$ 11.5% to 89% $\pm$ 5.5%).

Unfortunately, the two groups were not similar on sleep efficiency at their baseline measures, so it remains questionable whether the latter group really improved, or whether there were a few participants in this small sample who were outliers at the baseline measurement. Notable in this study was the finding of very few apnea episodes or periodic limb movements in this sample during the 3 nights of sleep recordings at baseline or 6 months after hormone therapy. Women in this study were carefully screened for the presence of sleep disorders before enrollment, but the researchers commented that no potential participant met their exclusion criteria for sleep apnea syndrome or restless legs syndrome [35].

Non-hormonal alternative therapies

Because of the possible side effects related to hormone-replacement therapy and the desire to offer alternatives for sleep disturbances related to menopause, Dorsey and coworkers [36] conducted a multisite randomized clinical trial in which symptomatic midlife women were randomized to receive placebo or a hypnotic medication, zolpidem, 10 mg each night for 4 weeks. Compared with placebo, those taking the hypnotic reported improvements in total sleep time (60 minutes more than placebo group) and less wake time (40 minutes less than placebo group) and fewer awakenings during the night. There was no group difference in latency to sleep onset, but these sleep measures were all by self-reported diary entries over the month in their home environments rather than objective laboratory measures.

Very limited research has been conducted on nonpharmacologic interventions to improve sleep in menopausal women, but a thorough review of alternative medicine approaches to treating menopausal symptoms has been done and concluded that black cohosh and foods with phytoestrogens (in soy products and other types of legumes) show promise in reducing hot flashes when used for longer than 6 weeks [37,38]. Current research is underway to examine the potential use of herbal remedies in a large randomized clinical trial of midlife women in the Pacific Northwest area of the United States [39]. None of these trials involving alternative herbal therapies, however, specifically address outcomes focused on women's sleep.

Previous reviews have confirmed that chronic sleep problems are better managed with behavioral therapies compared with pharmacologic intervention, and these behavioral therapies are better tolerated and more satisfying over long-term assessments [40–42]. Studies included in these reviews, however, typically include only chronic insomnia in older adults with no pre-existing medical conditions. Whether cognitive behavioral therapies apply to midlife women and sleep problems associated with menopause remains to be studied. These behavioral therapies range from classic sleep hygiene strategies to 8 weekly sessions of cognitive behavioral therapy. Components of these strategies include sleeping in a safe and comfortable bed, getting adequate light exposure and exercise, stress reduction, smoking and alcohol cessation, and keeping a consistent bed time and wake time. The ability to implement many of these strategies may be limited for women of low socioeconomic status, women exposed to physical or sexual abuse, or women with multiple roles to juggle.

To test the effects of moderate exercise on subjective sleep, a sample of obese sedentary postmenopausal women living in the Seattle, Washington, area was randomized to aerobic exercise (N = 87) or stretching (N = 86) and completed questionnaires every 3 months for 1 year [42]. Subjective sleep quality was assessed with six items from the Women's Health Initiative Insomnia Rating Scale that asked women to consider the past month and respond about frequency of particular sleep behaviors in a typical week, including use of sleep medication or alcohol to help with sleep. There was very little effect of exercise on self-reported sleep as assessed in this study. Falling asleep at night improved somewhat for the morning exercisers, but not for the evening exercisers, who were more likely to be employed. There was also a suggestion that less medication or alcohol was used for sleep, but the self-report measures may not be sensitive to change over time [42]. Weight gain was more stable for the women taking hormone-replacement therapy, but there is a wide range of weight gain during menopausal transition unrelated to obvious health behaviors, such as smoking, alcohol consumption, or exercise. The Australian longitudinal study data indicate that the average midlife woman gains about 2.1 ± 5.1 kg weight over the key 5 years of menopausal transition regardless of level of activity [43].

Clinical assessment guide

Based on the literature reviewed in this article, Table 2 provides a summary of some initial guidelines for clinical assessment and interventions for midlife women with a chief complaint of problems sleeping.

All measures of sleep, including one-item self-reports for the past day or week, the Pittsburgh Sleep Quality Index, and objective monitoring with either actigraphy [29] or polysomnography, support some level of difficulty with falling asleep or staying asleep during the night. Racial or cultural

Table 2: **Clinical assessment of sleep problems in midlife women**

What is her sleep complaint?	
Difficulty falling asleep—*why*?	
Restless legs	Assess for anemia or family history
Mind racing	Assess for stress or depression
	Assess for posttraumatic stress or history of violence or abuse
Difficulty staying asleep—*why*?	
Herself	Assess bladder function
Bed partner	Assess partner snoring or leg kicking
Child	Assess for cosleeping and bed sharing or ages of children
Insufficient amount of sleep to feel rested or stay awake during the day	Assess total sleep time for >7 h
	Assess falling asleep in hazardous situations, like driving and refer to accredited sleep disorders center
	Assess for temporal-mandibular joint problems
	Ask bed partner or obtain videotape to assess her snoring, kicking, teeth grinding
Differential Diagnoses	
Assess menopausal status and date of last menstrual period	Confirm menopausal status with follicle stimulating hormone level regardless of age
Assess for frequency and severity of hot flashes and other vasomotor symptoms associated with menopause	
Assess for obesity, diabetes	Obtain nutrition or diet consult
Evaluate health behaviors	
Smoking pattern	Provide information about healthy sleep habits
Alcohol consumption	
Caffeine consumption	
Exercise	Prescribe formal exercise program
Napping	
Amount of daylight exposure	
Rule out depression	Ask about sources of stress
	Ask about supportive relationships
	Differentiate depressive symptoms from fatigue or sleepiness

differences in the experience of menopausal symptoms are likely to be similar to racial or cultural differences in sleep, but studies that compare sleep by women's race or ethnicity are just beginning [2,44,45]. Sleep is much more disrupted as a function of body weight and psychiatric symptoms, such as anxiety or depression [46–50], than a function of menopausal status. Some women with objectively recorded hot flashes during sleep deny experiencing hot flashes [27], whereas others are annoyed by hot flashes during the day and extremely bothered by hot flashes during the night while trying to sleep, particularly if they place high value on sleeping at least 8 hours every night and worry about how less sleep will affect their ability to maintain a high level of function during the day [26]. The SWAN data [2] also indicate that higher education and white ethnicity are related to poor sleep rather than body weight, marital status, or

employment. These initial results may differ from other studies by ways in which body weight and sedentary lifestyle are controlled, by differences in how menopausal status or sleep difficulty [51] are operationalized, or by sample selection or response rates [2,52].

Summary

Sleep problems in midlife women should not necessarily be attributed to menopausal changes. The extent to which menopausal symptoms change over time and influence sleep during the perimenopausal and postmenopausal phases of midlife women's lives remains to be determined in larger longitudinal types of studies. Further research is needed to ascertain the extent to which obesity, depressive symptoms, sedentary lifestyle, or poor sleep behaviors may precede or overlap with the menopausal transition.

Acknowledgments

The author thanks Margaret Taffe for her administrative assistance with this manuscript.

References

[1] United States Census Bureau. United States Census 2000. Table 3. Female population by age, race and Hispanic or Latino origin for the United States:2000. Available at: http://www.census.gov/population/www/cen2000/phc-t9.html. Accessed December 20, 2005.

[2] Kravitz HM, Ganz PA, Bromberger J, et al. Sleep difficulty in women at midlife: a community survey of sleep and the menopausal transition. Menopause 2003;10:19–28.

[3] Matthews K, Wing R, Kuller L, et al. Influences of natural menopause on psychological characteristics and symptoms of middle-aged healthy women. J Consult Clin Psychol 1990;58:345–51.

[4] Hunter M. The south-east England longitudinal study of the climacteric and post menopause. Maturitas 1992;14:117–26.

[5] Lee K, Taylor D. Is there a generic midlife woman? The health and symptom experience of employed midlife women. Menopause 1996; 3:154–64.

[6] Schiff I, Regestein Q, Tulchnisky D, et al. Effects of estrogens on sleep and psychological state of hypogonadal women. JAMA 1979;242:2405–7.

[7] Shaver J, Giblin E, Lentz M, et al. Sleep patterns and stability in perimenopausal women. Sleep 1988;11:556–61.

[8] Soules MR, Sherman S, Parrott E, et al. Executive summary: stages of reproductive aging workshop (STRAW). Fertil Steril 2001;76:874–8.

[9] Beyene Y, Martin MC. Menopausal experiences and bone density of Mayan women in Yucatan, Mexico. Am J Hum Biol 2001;13:505–11.

[10] Beyene Y. Menopause: a biocultural event. In: Dan AJ, Lewis LL, editors. Menstrual health in women's lives. Chicago: University of Illinois Press; 1992. p. 169–77.

[11] Woodward S, Freedman RR. The thermoregulatory effects of menopausal hot flashes on sleep. Sleep 1994;17:497–501.

[12] Freedman RR. Hot flashes: behavioral treatments, mechanisms, and relation to sleep. Am J Med 2005;118:124S–30S.

[13] Young T, Rabago D, Zgierska A, et al. Objective and subjective sleep quality in premenopausal, perimenopausal, and postmenopausal women in the Wisconsin sleep cohort study. Sleep 2003;26:667–72.

[14] Sharkey KM, Bearpark HM, Acebo C, et al. Effects of menopausal status on sleep in midlife women. Behav Sleep Med 2003;1:69–80.

[15] Bixler EO, Vgontzas AN, Lin H, et al. Prevalence of sleep-disordered breathing in women: effects of gender. Am J Respir Crit Care Med 2001; 163:608–13.

[16] Resta O, Caratozzolo G, Pannacciulli N, et al. Gender, age and menopause effects on the prevalence and the characteristics of obstructive sleep apnea in obesity. Eur J Clin Invest 2003; 33:1084–9.

[17] Asplund R, Aberg HE. Body mass index and sleep in women aged 40 to 64 years. Maturitas 1995;22:1–8.

[18] Asplund R, Aberg H. Nocturnal micturition, sleep and well-being in women of ages 40-64 years. Maturitas 1996;24:73–81.

[19] Dennerstein L, Dudley EC, Hopper JL, et al. A prospective population-based study of menopausal symptoms. Obstet Gynecol 2000;96: 351–8.

[20] Bjorkelund C, Bengtsson C, Lissner L, et al. Women's sleep: longitudinal changes and secular trends in a 24-year perspective. Results of the population study of women in Gothenburg, Sweden. Sleep 2002;25:894–6.

[21] Dennerstein L, Lehert P, Dudley E, et al. Factors contributing to positive mood during the menopausal transition. J Nerv Ment Dis 2001;189: 84–9.

[22] Owens JF, Matthews KA. Sleep disturbance in healthy middle-aged women. Maturitas 1998; 30:41–50.

[23] Hollander LE, Freeman EW, Sammel MD, et al. Sleep quality, estradiol levels, and behavioral factors in late reproductive age women. Obstet Gynecol 2001;98:391–7.

[24] Kripke DF, Jean-Louis G, Elliott JA, et al. Ethnicity, sleep, mood, and illumination in postmenopausal women. BMC Psychiatry 2004;4:8.

[25] Kravitz HM, Janssen I, Santoro N, et al. Relationship of day-to-day reproductive hormone levels to sleep in midlife women. Arch Intern Med 2005;165:2370–6.

[26] Kloss JD, Tweedy K, Gilrain K. Psychological factors associated with sleep disturbance among perimenopausal women. Behav Sleep Med 2004;2:177–90.

[27] Freedman RR, Roehrs TA. Lack of sleep disturbance from menopausal hot flashes. Fertil Steril 2004;82:138–44.

[28] Shaver JLF, Giblin E, Paulsen V. Sleep quality subtypes in midlife women. Sleep 1991;14: 18–23.

[29] Baker A, Simpson S, Dawson D. Sleep disruption and mood changes associated with menopause. J Psychosom Res 1997;43:359–69.

[30] Thompson J, Oswald I. Effect of oestrogen on the sleep, mood, and anxiety of menopausal women. BMJ 1977;2:1317–9.

[31] Regestein QR, Schiff I, Tulchinsky D, et al. Relationships among estrogen-induced psychophysiological changes in hypogonadal women. Psychosom Med 1981;43:147–55.

[32] Scharf MB, McDannold MD, Stover R, et al. Effects of estrogen replacement therapy on rates of cyclic alternating patterns and hot-flush events during sleep in postmenopausal women: a pilot study. Clin Ther 1997;19:304–11.

[33] Erlik Y, Tataryn IV, Meldrum DR, et al. Association of waking episodes with menopausal hot flushes. JAMA 1981;245:1741–4.

[34] Purdie DW, Empson JA, Crichton C, et al. Hormone replacement therapy, sleep quality, and psychological wellbeing. Br J Obstet Gynaecol 1995;102:735–9.

[35] Montplaisir J, Lorraine J, Denesle R, et al. Sleep in menopause. differential effects of two forms of hormone replacement therapy. Menopause 2001;8:10–6.

[36] Dorsey CM, Lee KA, Scharf MB. Effect of zolpidem on sleep in women with perimenopausal and postmenopausal insomnia: a 4-week, randomized, multicenter, double-blind, placebo-controlled study. Clin Ther 2004;26:1578–86.

[37] Kronenberg F, Fugh-Berman A. Complementary and alternative medicine for menopausal symptoms: a review of randomized, controlled trials. Ann Intern Med 2002;137:805–13.

[38] Kessel B, Kronenberg F. The role of complementary and alternative medicine in management of menopausal symptoms. Endocrinol Metab Clin North Am 2004;33:717–39.

[39] Newton KM, Reed SD, Grothaus L, et al. The herbal alternatives for menopause (HALT) study: background and study design. Maturitas 2005; 52:134–46.

[40] Murtaugh DR, Greenwood KM. Identifying effective psychological treatments for insomnia: a meta-analysis. J Consult Clin Psychol 1995; 63:79–89.

[41] Morin CM, Culbert JP, Schwartz SM. Non-pharmacological intervention for insomnia: a meta-analysis of treatment efficacy. Am J Psychiatry 1994;151:1172–80.

[42] Harvey AG, Tang NKY. Cognitive behavior therapy for primary insomnia: can we rest yet? Sleep Med Rev 2003;7:237–62.

[43] Tworoger SS, Yasui U, Vitiello MV, et al. Effects of a yearlong moderate-intensity exercise and stretching intervention on sleep quality in postmenopausal women. Sleep 2003;26:830–6.

[44] Guthrie JR, Dennerstein L, Dudley EC. Weight gain and the menopause: a 5-year prospective study. Climacteric 1999;2:205–11.

[45] Shin C, Lee S, Lee T, et al. Prevalence of insomnia and its relationship to menopausal status in middle-aged Korean women. Psychiatry Clin Neurosci 2005;59:395–402.

[46] Lock M. Cross-cultural vasomotor symptom reporting: conceptual and methodological issues. Menopause 2005;12:239–41.

[47] Parry BL, Meliska CJ, Martinez F, et al. Menopause: neuroendocrine changes and hormone replacement therapy. J Am Med Womens Assoc 2004;59:135–45.

[48] Polo-Kantola P, Erkkola R, Irjala K, et al. Climacteric symptoms and sleep quality. Obstet Gynecol 1999;94:219–24.

[49] Ohayon MM. Prevalence and correlates of non-restorative sleep complaints. Arch Intern Med 2005;165:35–41.

[50] Cohen LS, Soares CN, Joffe H. Diagnosis and management of mood disorders during the menopausal transition. Am J Med 2005;118: 93S–7S.

[51] Ford K, Sowers M, Crutchfield M, et al. A longitudinal study of the predictors of prevalence and severity of symptoms commonly associated with menopause. Menopause 2005;12: 308–17.

[52] Gold EB, Sternfeld B, Kelsey JL, et al. Relation of demographic and lifestyle factors to symptoms in a multi-racial/ethnic population of women 40–55 years of age. Am J Epidemiol 2000; 152:463–73.

SLEEP
MEDICINE
CLINICS

Sleep Med Clin 1 (2006) 207–220

Sleep and Cognition in Older Adults

Amanda Schurle Bruce, MS, Mark S. Aloia, PhD*

- Sleep and aging
- Normal aging and cognition
- Sleep and cognition
- Perceived poor sleep quality and excessive daytime sleepiness
- Sleep deprivation
- Napping and cognition
- Diagnosed sleep disorders
- Insomnia and cognition
- Obstructive sleep apnea
- Potential mechanisms
- Summary
- References

There has long been interest in the relationship between sleep and cognitive functioning. The literature demonstrating a negative effect of sleep abnormalities on cognitive functioning has developed rapidly over the past decade. This association has functional relevance, reminding one of the importance of sufficient, consolidated sleep. The relation between sleep and cognition is even more salient as it applies to older adults. Cognitive decline is a part of the normal aging process. This decline, however, may be exaggerated by extraneous factors, such as abnormal sleep. A large body of literature has shown that sleep, like cognition, is also affected by age. The goal of this line of research is often to identify modifiable sleep-related factors that can maximize functioning throughout the otherwise normal process of aging. This article addresses questions designed to summarize the existing literature and to theorize about the mechanisms behind the findings and their implications for future research. Addressed are questions of specificity, including which aspects of cognition are most affected by different types of sleep changes in the elderly. Also addressed is functionality, asking how sleep might interfere with functional abilities. For sleep-related topics with no published research specific to older adults, general findings

from other samples may be discussed. This article focuses primarily on sleep and cognition in normal older adults. Dementing illnesses are known negatively to impact both sleep and cognition; however, these topics are not reviewed here, but are covered elsewhere in this issue.

Sleep and aging

The process of normal aging affects both the quality and quantity of sleep in older adults. Studies suggest that half of the elderly experience sleep disturbances [1–5]. Sleep disturbances can take the form of medical disorders; sleep-wake pattern abnormalities (ie, circadian rhythm disorders); limited quantity of sleep (ie, insomnia); or limited quality of sleep (ie, perceived poor sleep and sleep fragmentation). On average, older adults get one or fewer less hours sleep per night than younger adults [6–9]. A common belief is that older individuals simply need less sleep. This myth is predicated on the observation that less consolidated sleep is common in older adults. In reality, the need for sleep does not decrease as an individual ages; rather, it is the ability to sleep that diminishes with age [10]. Frequent sleep complaints from older adults include difficulty initiating or maintaining sleep, nocturnal

Department of Psychiatry and Human Behavior, Brown Medical School, Duncan Building, Butler Hospital, 700 Butler Drive, Providence, RI 02906, USA
* Corresponding author.
E-mail address: aloia@brown.edu (M.S. Aloia).

1556-407X/06/$ – see front matter © 2006 Elsevier Inc. All rights reserved.
doi:10.1016/j.jsmc.2006.04.008
sleep.theclinics.com

waking, daytime napping, and waking feeling un-rested [11]. In addition, it is now known that poor sleep in older adults can lead to a variety of conse-quences, including excessive daytime sleepiness, difficulties sustaining attention, memory problems, slowed response time, and impaired performance in general during waking hours [10–12].

Older adults often report sleep problems to their physicians [13]. Sleep problems can cause chronic fatigue, daytime functional impairments, and in-creased risk of accidents and falls [6]. Sleep prob-lems also have the potential negatively to impact the individual's and spouse's or caregiver's quality of life [14,15]. Reported sleep problems can be the result of a variety of factors, such as chronic bed rest, regular napping, circadian rhythm de-synchronization, medication use, psychiatric disor-ders, or comorbid medical disorders [11,16,17]. Although these sleep-related problems often coexist with cognitive and functional problems, the nature of this relationship remains unclear. It is possible that sleep disturbances are the primary cause for some cognitive problems that accompany aging. Al-ternatively, sleep disturbances may simply exist as an epiphenomenon of other, comorbid medical or psychiatric conditions that affect cognitive and functional abilities.

Normal aging and cognition

Just as some sleep difficulties are relatively common in the older adult, it is true that some degree of de-cline in cognitive ability is a part of the normal ag-ing process for most individuals. Cognitive decline is not global, however, and it is not inevitable for every aging person. It is estimated that the preva-lence of clinically significant cognitive deficits ranges from 4% to 10% in community-dwelling older adults [18–21]. Cognitive problems can have a profound impact on one's ability to function on a daily basis. Difficulties with concentration, mem-ory, and decision making can contribute to func-tional instability and dependency. There are some factors considered to be protective for the preserva-tion of cognitive functioning, such as higher levels of education, good physical health, higher activity levels, and the absence of certain genetic markers of vulnerability to cognitive decline [22]. It is also important to note that the stability of cognitive functioning with advancing age depends on which cognitive ability is being assessed. Numerous stud-ies have shown that cognitive change is not unitary and that some abilities decline more rapidly than others, making an understanding of the various common cognitive functions important [22–25].

Cognition can be examined as a unitary function or it can be divided into several specific domains (eg, memory, attention, executive functioning, and so forth). The use of each type of examination de-pends on the question being asked and the degree to which each approach adequately addresses a given hypothesis. Studies of global impairment may be better suited for addressing the overall ef-fects of a particular independent variable on global ability. A common way to measure global cognition in the elderly is the Mini-Mental Status Exam [26]. Studies have shown that scores on the Mini-Mental Status Exam decrease slightly with age [27–29]. The decline is more pronounced for individuals over the age of 85 [30,31]. Research studies have shown that when considering cognition to be a unitary con-struct, aging indeed impairs overall global cognitive functioning. Studies that limit themselves to global functioning, however, cannot have a true apprecia-tion for the various components of cognition that contribute to this global score. Domain-specific questions, however, can help uncover specific defi-cits that are otherwise masked by studies of global cognitive functioning. Domains can be divided in several ways but common domain names include executive functioning, memory, attention, vigi-lance, visuospatial ability, constructional ability, psychomotor functioning, and language. One must remember, however, that each of these domains may also have subdomains that further break apart their complex nature (eg, executive functioning), and that domains are not mutually exclusive in their functions.

Research has demonstrated that some cognitive abilities are more affected by normal aging than others. For example, although global cognitive functioning can sometimes predict functional abil-ity, recent studies have suggested that the more spe-cific domain of executive function may be better suited for this purpose [32,33]. Executive function-ing is an integral aspect of cognition, described as "those capacities that enable a person to engage suc-cessfully in independent, purposive, self-serving be-havior" [34]. It is reasonable that such a broad, complex construct that encompasses abstract rea-soning, initiation, strategizing, and planning in-deed predicts functional status. There are other cognitive functions that are also affected by aging. Cognitive domains, such as working memory, speed of information processing, reaction time, and controlled attention, tend to decline with age [35,36]. Memory and information processing speed typically show a linear decline beginning in mid-adulthood [22,24,25,37,38]. Normal aging also slows an individual's reaction time. Some cognitive abilities, however, are thought to be more crystal-lized throughout adulthood. Crystallized abilities, including accumulated factual knowledge and vo-cabulary, tend to be the least affected by age [22].

Many studies of cognitive functioning take a battery approach, using several measures of each domain to get a broad appreciation for the areas that are most associated with manipulations of the independent variable. Theory-driven domain-specific studies, however, use cognitive domains that are informed by the theoretical questions addressed within the study. For example, a study of sleep deprivation that proposes a model of frontal susceptibility is likely to test executive functions and those memory or other functions that incorporate executive ability than measures of visuospatial or motor functioning per se. Such studies are not designed to be comprehensive but rather focused on supporting or refuting a particular theory or model. In this way, models can be adjusted and new studies conducted in a systematic manner to identify the likely complex nature of sleep's relation to cognition.

Sleep and cognition

Studies of the effects of sleep aberrations on cognition have increased dramatically over the past decade. With several potential methods for measuring sleep and cognition, there seems to be an infinite number of permutations to study. This article, however, provides structure to the published studies, especially where older adults are concerned. Specifically, the authors examined the literature related to sleep and cognition in older adults in the following sleep-related categories: perceived poor sleep quality and excessive daytime sleepiness; sleep deprivation; napping; and various diagnosable sleep disorders including narcolepsy, circadian rhythm sleep disorders (CRSD), insomnia, and obstructive sleep apnea (OSA).

Perceived poor sleep quality and excessive daytime sleepiness

Perceived sleep quality is a complex concept. Although objective measurements of sleep quantity and quality are the gold standard, many studies have been published using only subjective measures of sleep or daytime sleepiness. These studies deserve mention, but the reader should also keep in mind that the mechanisms underlying poor sleep or daytime sleepiness may involve diagnosable sleep disorders not assessed within any given study. Importantly, the perceived quality of one's sleep, or the perception of daytime sleepiness, has the potential to impact a person's cognitive performance. A significant relationship has been found between perceived sleep quality and cognitive functioning in older adults [13,39,40]. Sustained attention, reaction time, and memory are particularly affected by poor sleep quality [11]. Psychomotor

performance is also commonly impaired during the day following a night of reported disturbed sleep [41].

Excessive daytime sleepiness, which can be caused by a wide range of conditions, has been found to impair daily functioning in older adults [42]. Excessive sleepiness can be measured in multiple ways. Ideally, studies should include both subjective reports and objective measures to characterize best the construct of sleepiness. Subjective sleepiness measures, such as the Stanford Sleepiness Scale [43] or the Epworth Sleepiness Scale [44], represent the most economic and time-efficient means of collecting information about introspective sleepiness. Subjective reports of sleepiness do not always correlate, however, with objective measures of sleepiness or with performance testing [45,46]. The Multiple Sleep Latency Test and the Maintenance of Wakefulness Test [47] are widely used objective measures of physiologic sleepiness. Excessive daytime sleepiness in older adults has been shown to be associated with poor cognitive performance [40]. Global cognition, assessed using the Mini-Mental Status Exam, was found to be significantly impaired in over 4500 older adults reporting daytime sleepiness with the Epworth Sleepiness Scale [48]. More recently, Ohayon and Vecchierini [18] corroborated this finding in a study using over 1000 participants. These investigators also administered a self-report measure of cognitive difficulties, and found that daytime sleepiness was a significant, independent predictor of impaired cognition above and beyond age, sex, physical activity, occupation, or organic diseases [18]. The self-report measure, the Cognitive Difficulties Scale, assessed six dimensions of cognition: (1) attention-concentration, (2) praxis, (3) delayed recall, (4) difficulty in orientation for person, (5) difficulty in temporal orientation, and (6) difficulty in prospective memory. Individuals reporting significant daytime sleepiness were significantly more impaired on all six of the subscales [18]. Differences were also found across specific age groupings. Sleepy individuals ages 75 and older were impaired on all six subscales, whereas those ages 60 to 64 and 70 to 74 were not impaired on praxis or prospective memory. Interestingly, sleepy individuals ages 65 to 69 were only impaired on temporal orientation. This study suggests an interaction between age and sleepiness on perceived cognitive functioning. Some investigators have even suggested that daytime sleepiness may be an early precursor to cognitive decline and the onset of dementia [49].

Interestingly, studies have shown that in experimentally fragmented sleep, the elderly may be less sensitive to sleep fragmentation compared with younger adults [50–53]. Specifically, one study reported that older adults' performance on tests of arithmetic was less affected by experimentally fragmented sleep (14 times per hour) compared with young controls [50]. This finding suggests that sleep fragmentation may not have as profound an affect on cognitive functioning in old age. It remains possible, however, that older individuals perform poorly enough on this test under conditions of adequate sleep to limit the degree to which they can show decrements under fragmentation. Additional studies are required to determine the validity of this finding and the age at which this potential effect begins.

Sleep deprivation

The quantity of sleep at night can also dramatically affect cognition. Sleep deprivation studies, either complete or partial, in healthy normal controls consistently show behavioral, psychologic, and physiologic consequences that can seriously impair functioning [41,54–57]. In a recent review of this literature, Durmer and Dinges [54] highlight the significant research conducted on the behavioral effects of sleep deprivation. The authors clarify the relationship between sleep deprivation and cognitive dysfunction, marked partly by metabolic changes in the prefrontal cortex. These studies, however, are often the culmination of up to 36 hours of experimentally sustained wakefulness. To account for this issue, Durmer and Dinges [54] also review the significant increase in data to suggest that chronic partial sleep deprivation, mimicking what might be seen in normal individuals within society, can dramatically affect functioning over time. In one seminal study, Dinges and colleagues [58] showed that 7 consecutive nights of 33% reduction in normal sleep time resulted in significant increases in subjective sleepiness and decreases in vigilance.

Rapid eye movement–specific deprivation has been demonstrated to have specific negative effects on memory. Recent investigations using animal models have begun to offer an underlying neural mechanism involving long-term potentiation in the hippocampus to explain how rapid eye movement–specific sleep deprivation interferes with memory consolidation [59]. Hornung and colleagues [60] have recently reported on effective methods that can be used to manipulate rapid eye movement sleep in older adults. Although they did not include cognition in their study, future studies using these methods will likely include cognitive tasks as outcome measures.

Stimulant medication may potentially mute some of the cognitive impairment associated with sleep deprivation. Several studies have consistently shown that treatment with stimulants, such as modafinil, caffeine, and dextroamphetamine, can improve cognitive performance in adults tested under conditions of acute sleep deprivation [61–63]. It is unknown, however, whether the same findings also apply to older adult samples.

Consistent with general results that sleep deprivation causes functional impairment, studies focusing specifically on older adult samples have reported that sleep deprivation can cause cognitive impairment [64]. Older adults who have difficulties sleeping often report daytime sleepiness and a decline in waking performance [12]. Investigators also determined that perceived cognitive impairment was positively associated with a nighttime sleep duration of 6 hours or less and daytime sleep duration of 1 hour or more [1]. Psychophysiologic studies have reported that younger adults are more likely to demonstrate an expected frontal predominance in electroencephalogram delta activity after sleep deprivation when compared with older adults. In one study, older adults demonstrated a significant increase in delta power, but it was located more in parietal regions than in the expected frontal regions. The investigators of this study suggest that this finding may represent a frontal susceptibility to the aging process [65]. Together, these findings invalidate the common belief that older individuals need less sleep.

There is, however, some disagreement as to the specific cognitive effects of sleep deprivation across the adult life span. Investigators initially reported that individuals' response to sleep deprivation was consistent across age groups [66]. Other studies, however, have reported that older adults' cognitive functioning may perhaps be more resilient when compared with younger adults under conditions of experimentally induced sleep deprivation. Interestingly, studies have shown that the elderly are also less sensitive than younger adults to sleep deprivation [50–53]. Most of these studies were conducted over a decade ago. Recent studies, however, have corroborated these earlier findings. One study by Philip and colleagues [67] demonstrated that the reaction times of older adults were less affected by sleep loss when compared with younger controls. Stenuit and Kerkhofs [68] have also found consistent results in their study of women undergoing sleep deprivation. In fact, the negative effects of 3 nights of sleep restricted to 4 hours per night were more prominent in young women than in older women on measures including the Maintenance of Wakefulness Test, Stanford Sleepiness Scale, and the Psychomotor Vigilance Test. It seems that older adults' perceptual abilities may also be more resilient to restrictions in sleep. Similar results have been found on simulated driving tasks. In one study, older adults' were not as negatively affected by sleep deprivation when compared with younger adults on the useful visual field of view test [69]. This finding has implications for motor vehicle accidents, in that older adults may have a higher tolerance to driving-related fatigue than younger adults [67,70]. Although older adults with a reduced amount of sleep report disturbances in waking performance, their impairment may be relatively less of a decrease from normal sleeping conditions when compared with younger adults. It should be noted that findings of resiliency to sleep loss in older adults may be an effect of the overall lower scores of older adults under conditions of normal sleep. Younger adults have more room for error than older adults. At this point there is not enough research to speculate as to the mechanisms underlying these associations.

Napping and cognition

Intuitively, if a lack of sleep leads to a decrease in performance on cognitive tests, increasing sleep, whether at night or during the day, would have the potential to improve performance. Indeed, some studies using younger adults have consistently shown that daytime napping leads to enhanced cognitive and psychomotor performance [71–74]. Fewer studies with less consistent results have attempted to discover if the same holds true for older adults. One study reported that there was no improvement on several performance tasks after 2 weeks of daily naps for a group of older adults [75]. Some evidence even suggests that napping may be detrimental to performance on cognitive tests. In Bliwise and Swan's [76] recent study with elderly individuals, a greater frequency of self-reported napping was associated with worse performance on a test of executive functioning. Although they acknowledge that self-reported napping may not be as accurate as other types of sleep measures, the findings are intriguing. Other investigators have found that naps do improve cognitive performance in older adults. One study reported that a 30-minute afternoon nap improved reaction time and accuracy of visual detection [77]. More recently, investigators corroborated these findings, demonstrating that immediately after a nap, older adults' performance improved on both reaction time and executive function tasks [12]. Additionally, their performance improved on a logical reasoning task on the following day [12].

Because the evidence is mixed, further studies are needed to evaluate whether napping in older adults is helpful or harmful. The large body of evidence from studies using younger adults suggests that napping can be beneficial for cognitive functioning, but this relationship has reason to be questioned in older adults. If napping were found to be helpful, it could be considered as a tool to aid in the cognitive performance of older adults. A long-term bias exists against napping, however, with the thought that naps can disrupt effective nighttime sleep [78,79]. Monk and colleagues [75] have demonstrated that a daily nap regimen between 13:30 and 15:00 did reduce sleep efficiency and cause earlier wake times in older adults. Data from the Multiple Sleep Latency Test also revealed that there was larger sleep latency for individuals adhering to the nap regimen [75]. Further evidence supporting this claim is scattered, with many studies reporting no significant negative impact of napping [73,75,77,80,81]. In fact, Campbell and colleagues [12] recommended that healthy older adults may benefit from napping as a supplement to shortened nighttime sleep. If so, napping should be scheduled so as to minimize the potential for disrupting nighttime sleep patterns. Future studies should be designed to address this interesting question experimentally, with consideration given to potential differential effects caused by age.

Diagnosed sleep disorders

Diagnosed sleep disorders are very common among older adults [82,83]. Frequent complaints of individuals with sleep disorders include daytime fatigue, sleepiness, and cognitive difficulties. The most common sleep disorders are insomnia and OSA, but additional disorders like narcolepsy and CRSD also exist in older adults. Because some of these disorders are less common, they have not been studied as extensively, particularly relating to cognition. Consequently, the studies reported next discuss the relationship between the disorder and cognition in general and are sometimes not specific to older adults.

Narcolepsy is a relatively rare, yet disabling sleep disorder that causes patients to experience excessive sleepiness throughout their waking hours accompanied by involuntary sleep attacks. It usually begins before age 25 and persists throughout one's life, with men and women equally affected [84]. There is evidence to suggest that narcolepsy can present slightly differently depending on a person's age. One study showed that as a narcolepsy patient ages, there are relatively fewer sleep-onset rapid eye movement periods and longer sleep latency duration [85]. Cognitive difficulties have been found to be associated with narcolepsy. In adult patients diagnosed with narcolepsy, excessive sleepiness has been associated with impairments in cognitive function [86–89]. Complex cognitive tasks seemed to be the most affected by the disorder [87]. Tests of vigilance also display consistent impairment in narcoleptic patients [90]. There is mixed evidence regarding whether memory is impaired from neuropsychologic and electrophysiologic data, but studies have consistently reported that individuals with narcolepsy complain of forgetfulness and perceive their memory to be worse than it actually is when tested objectively [91,92]. Stimulants, such as amphetamines, methylphenidate, and modafinil, are commonly used to manage narcolepsy [84]. One study demonstrated that modafinil significantly improved executive functioning in a group of patients with narcolepsy [86]. This is consistent with the finding that modafinil improves cognitive performance in individuals tested under conditions of acute sleep deprivation [61,62]. These studies were not specific to older adult populations; future studies should examine the effects of stimulants on narcolepsy and sleep deprivation on cognitive performance in elderly samples. Therapeutic napping can also serve to enhance daytime alertness in addition to reducing one's dependence on high doses of stimulants [84]. It would be interesting to discover whether napping in narcolepsy patients produces similar cognitive improvements as seen in healthy young individuals.

CRSD are also rarely identified, although they may not be uncommon in older adults [93,94]. Many individuals suffering from a CRSD are misdiagnosed as having insomnia and treated ineffectively [95]. The authors could find no published studies that have examined the specific effects of diagnosed CRSD on cognition in the elderly. They found no published studies examining cognition in CRSD in any age group. The most relevant finding is that there is a high prevalence of learning disorders (19.3%) in people who have CRSD [96]. More research is necessary to gain a better understanding of these rare disorders.

There has been some research on nondisordered circadian rhythms and cognition not specific to aging. A relationship has been found between daily circadian patterns and cognitive functioning. Individuals tested during peak circadian periods show better performance on tests of strategic processing [97]. Evidence from studies specific to older adults has been inconsistent. One study demonstrated that the negative effect of nighttime work on cognitive function is greater for older adults when compared with young adults [98]. Other investigators, however, report that age-related cognitive abilities are not affected by the time of day [99,100]. Fewer studies have been conducted recently, highlighting the need for additional research to clarify the complex relationship between circadian rhythms, age, and cognition.

Insomnia and cognition

Insomnia is a very common sleep disorder, affecting up to 20% of patients who consult general physicians [101,102]. As many as 12% to 25% of individuals over the age of 65 complain of regular difficulties with insomnia [103,104]. Insomnia is often associated with psychologic distress and is accompanied by a variety of conditions, such as depression, a medical condition, another sleep disorder, substance use, or medication use. It can, however, exist as a primary condition, in isolation of other potential causes. The clinical features of insomnia tend to vary based on age. Insomnia in younger adults typically manifests itself as a difficulty to initiate sleep, whereas in older adults, insomnia tends to cause a difficulty in maintaining sleep [105,106]. Pharmacotherapy is the most frequently used treatment for elderly insomnia sufferers [107].

Not surprisingly, individuals who complain of insomnia tend to report worse sleep during the night than "good sleepers." They also tend to perceive more functional impairment during the day than "good sleepers" [108]. One specific complaint involves "cognitive inefficiency" accompanied by sleepiness during the day [109]. Individuals who report experiencing poor sleep also rate their subjective performance as more negative than "good sleepers." Insomnia patients tend to have weaker expectations of their performance, evaluate their performance more negatively, and report having performed less well than individuals of similar age and actual capability level [110]. In general, the duration of sleep is positively correlated with their subjective evaluation of performance [110]. The subjective self-report of patients with insomnia has been found to be consistent with objective measures of cognitive functioning.

Neuropsychologic tests have shown that there are also objective impairments in older adult insomnia sufferers relative to "good sleepers" [111]. Specifically, studies have demonstrated that individuals with insomnia experience difficulties with attention, concentration, and retrieval of information from semantic memory [112–114]. In addition, for insomnia patients 55 years and older, subjectively rated poor sleep quality is associated with reduced performance in tasks measuring vigilance, psychomotor speed, recall, problem resolution, and speed and accuracy in complex decision making [115]. Evidence linking insomnia to reaction time is mixed [110,112].

Long-term effects of insomnia on older adults have also been reported. A longitudinal study examined the long-term effects of poor sleep quality for over 6000 cognitively intact men and women age 65 and older [116]. Results indicated that a report of chronic insomnia was found to be a significant and independent risk factor for cognitive decline [116]. Specifically, for men, a self-report of chronic insomnia was found to be a significant and independent risk factor for global cognitive decline [116]. For women, a self-report of chronic insomnia was related to global cognitive decline only in women who also had depressive symptoms [116]. Unfortunately, this study did not administer any domain-specific measures to elucidate further these findings. This study suggests that although perceived poor sleep quality can have a powerful impact on cognition in older adults, depressive symptoms also likely play a role in self-reported sleep quality. Not all studies have shown, however, that insomnia negatively impacts cognition. Some investigators report no differences for psychomotor functioning, episodic memory, divided attention, verbal learning, and figure-word recognition [110,112,113,117]. It should be noted, however, that one of these studies used a small sample size of 10 participants per group, a high percentage of who were experiencing psychologic distress [113].

A common method for treating insomnia in the elderly is through sedative medications like benzodiazepines; the newer hypnotic medications like zolpidem, eszopiclone, zaleplon; and the melatonin agonist, ramelteon [118]. Between 5% and 33% of older adults in North America and the United Kingdom are prescribed such a medication [119,120]. In addition to influencing sleep, evidence suggests that sedative medications can also impact cognition. Glass and colleagues' [118] meta-analysis of risks and benefits of sedative hypnotics in the elderly determined that although there were statistically significantly improvements in sleep, the magnitude of the effect was small. There were clinically significant risks of falls and cognitive impairment, however, associated with sedative hypnotic use [118]. It has been recommended that for older adults the benefits of such medications be weighed carefully against the risks [118,121]. Several studies, including two meta-analyses, have demonstrated the effectiveness of behavioral interventions for insomnia in older adults [122,123]. To minimize side effects and cognitive impairment in older adults, it is worthwhile to consider alternative nonpharmacologic treatments for insomnia.

Finally, it should be noted that there is an increased likelihood of elderly individuals suffering from insomnia to be concurrently experiencing some form of psychologic distress. The distress can take the form of anxiety or depression. The relationship between anxiety and depression and cognitive dysfunction is also established [124–128]. It is possible that the relationship between insomnia and impaired neuropsychologic test performance could be mediated by the presence of psychologic distress.

Obstructive sleep apnea

OSA affects at least 2% to 4% of middle-aged women and men, respectively [129]. Although these numbers are compelling, they may be underestimates because they are based on a study from over a decade ago when the rates of obesity, a disorder associated with OSA, were lower. The prevalence of OSA is known to increase dramatically with age, with as many as 42% of individuals over the age of 65 demonstrating evidence of the disorder [130]. OSA is characterized by repeated complete (apnea) or partial (hypopnea) cessation and reinitiation of breathing during sleep. These breathing disturbances occur during the body's attempt to achieve normal restorative sleep and often result in disturbances of the normal sleep architecture. The end result is fragmented sleep, potential loss of blood oxygenation, and notable disruption of the restorative sleep process.

Daytime sequelae of OSA can include excessive sleepiness; depression; irritability; functional impairments, such as slowed reaction time; and impairments in various cognitive domains, such as attention, concentration, and memory [131–134]. The functional impairments related to sleep apnea can be severe, because patients are more likely to be involved in motor vehicle accidents than normal controls [135,136]. In fact, the risk of having a motor vehicle accident increases with the severity of OSA [137]. OSA can also contribute to physical health consequences, such as hypertension, increased risk of heart disease, and stroke [138–141]. Because of these psychologic problems, cognitive impairments, functional impairments, and serious medical risks, individuals with undiagnosed or untreated OSA are at an increased risk of mortality [142,143].

Cognitive sequelae are commonly associated with OSA [131,144]. Impaired cognition, however, is not global. The domains of cognitive functioning are affected differentially. Vigilance, including sustained attention, controlled attention, efficiency of information processing, and reaction time, is the most commonly assessed cognitive construct in OSA and has been found to be the most consistently affected cognitive domain in apnea patients [131]. Executive functioning, which includes processes involved in planning, initiation, and execution of goal-oriented behavior and mental flexibility, is another affected domain. Some argue that it is the most prominent area of cognitive impairment in untreated sleep-disordered breathing [145]. It should be noted that the broad construct of executive functioning makes it somewhat difficult accurately to describe the deficits and to construct a model explaining causes of the impairment. Examples of executive functioning range from working memory, set-shifting, perseveration, planning, abstract reasoning, and verbal fluency. Even more, executive functions are in part supported by adequate attention. Attentional problems could represent the root cause of executive dysfunction. Verstraeten and Cluydts [146] have proposed this very model of cognitive dysfunction in OSA. Despite it being a broad construct, OSA patients clearly perform consistently more poorly on tests of executive functioning than matched controls [131]. Similar to executive function, but perhaps to a lesser degree, learning and memory constitute a broad, complex domain that includes verbal memory, visual memory, short-term memory, and long-term memory. Memory performance deficits can be attributed to several areas: initial learning, free recall, or forgetfulness, each of which has different implications [131]. OSA patients perform more poorly on tests of memory and learning than matched controls [131,147,148]. Psychomotor performance is a domain that has been assessed less frequently than the aforementioned types of cognition. Many studies, however, show OSA patients to be impaired relative to controls [131]. Specifically, OSA patients perform relatively poorer on tests of fine motor coordination [149–152]. Not all studies have reported impairment on tests of motor speed [152,153]. Overall, there has been relatively little discussion of this domain as a primary source of impairment [131].

Few studies have been conducted examining cognitive dysfunction associated with OSA in older adults. A large-scale study in France reported that participant reports of snoring or breathing cessation during sleep were associated with greater impairment on tests of attention and information processing, even after controlling for several extraneous variables. These findings were significantly associated with cognition only when daytime sleepiness was also reported. Another recent, longitudinal study used more stringent criteria for diagnosing OSA. The Ancoli-Israel laboratory examined the sleep and global cognitive functioning of 46 community-dwelling older adults over the course of 4 years, finding that increases in apnea severity and daytime sleepiness were associated with respective decreases in global cognitive functioning over time [154]. Moreover, the findings seemed to be driven by daytime sleepiness when regression models were used. An intriguing study by Antonelli-Incalzi and colleagues [155] compared older apneics with patients with either Alzheimer's disease or multi-infarct dementia on a battery of neuropsychologic tests. This study suggested that the cognitive profile of apnea is most like that seen in multi-infarct dementia. They relate this finding to the probable involvement of subcortical brain regions in apnea, a relationship that has also been posited by other investigators [131]. Indeed, the mechanism for cognitive dysfunction in OSA among older adults is not clear. It may be associated primarily with daytime sleepiness, or nocturnal hypoxemia may be a more direct cause of impairments to certain cognitive functions. It is certainly reasonable to assume that the outcome of such studies may be specific to the cognitive tests and sleep measures used.

The most effective treatment for OSA is positive airway pressure. When properly used, positive airway pressure has been shown dramatically to reduce morbidity and mortality [156–158]. There is also a substantial positive effect that continuous positive airway pressure treatment of sleep apnea has on cognition. Investigators have reported a significant positive correlation between treatment adherence and improvement in performance on a variety of neuropsychologic tests, even in older adults [159,160]. Despite its effectiveness, long-term adherence to positive airway pressure treatment is less than optimal, with approximately 25% of patients discontinuing use within a year [161].

Potential mechanisms

The relationship between sleep and cognition in older adults can be seen as either causal or coincidental. The causal model suggests that sleep is disrupted and subsequently results in impairments in cognitive functioning. Perhaps the most obvious example of this type of relationship exists in apnea. In this case, it remains possible that upper airway muscle tone decreases with age, contributing the potential for obstructive events to develop. It is further possible that the development of hypoxemia and sleep fragmentation in apnea can lead to cognitive and functional compromise. Although this is plausible, data are not presently sufficient to secure this as the single model for the relationship between sleep and cognition in older adults. For example, several individuals do not present with cognitive impairment or even sleepiness associated with apnea [129,162].

An alternative model suggests that the relationship is coincidental. Under this model, age-related changes to the structure or function of the brain can lead to both sleep disturbances and cognitive dysfunction. This model is supported in part by the several studies that demonstrate a change in the function of the suprachiasmatic nucleus with aging [163,164]. The suprachiasmatic nucleus is known to play a central role in the maintenance of circadian rhythms and in the release of melatonin. Both of these have implications for the relationship between sleep and cognition in the aging process. Disrupted circadian rhythms can result in disturbed and nonrestorative sleep. Decrements in melatonin can also impair cognition more directly. Melatonin is a powerful antioxidant. It is the only endogenous antioxidant known to decrease substantially past middle age [163]. This has obvious implications for neuronal survival and the protection of cells from toxic free radicals. The loss of melatonin in older adults may have a direct effect on cognition and sleep. Moreover, the suprachiasmatic nucleus itself has been shown to demonstrate functional changes during the aging process, which can affect cognition during aging [163]. The suprachiasmatic nucleus receives input from the basal forebrain cholinergic complex, which in turn is part of the ascending reticular activating system, a known contributor to sleep [165]. The basal forebrain cholinergic complex is a common area for cell loss in aging and is notably involved in cognitive disorders of aging like Alzheimer's disease. Cholinergic innervation has been most consistently associated with this bundle, but new studies have also implicated GABAergic involvement. Loss of these neurons can have implications for both cognition and sleep by associations with the suprachiasmatic nucleus.

Yet another potential mechanism for the relationship between sleep and cognitive functioning in older adults involves the interplay between cognition, sleep, and genetic factors. It is possible that certain genetic moderators underlie this complex relationship. For example, apolipoprotein E has been implicated in the development of both sleep apnea and dementing illnesses. It remains possible that such an underlying genetic factor could have somewhat independent effects on both sleep and cognition within the same individuals. Others, however, may not show such a relationship because of the lack of the presence of the genetic risk factor, highlighting individual differences in the relationship between sleep and cognition. At present, these models are highly speculative and there are likely many more potential mechanisms that will emerge with continued research. The discussion of such mechanisms, however, compels future studies to take a theory-driven approach when studying this complex relationship.

Summary

The goal of this line of research is eventually to identify modifiable sleep-related factors that can maximize functioning throughout the otherwise normal process of aging. Assuming that there is an established link between sleep and cognition, it may follow that to improve one would be also to improve the other. For example, if an individual's sleep habits are poor and their cognitive abilities are compromised, it may be possible to treat the sleep problems either behaviorally, psychologically, or pharmacologically. This could, theoretically, improve the individual's cognitive abilities. It seems clear that perceived poor sleep quality, sleep fragmentation, sleep deprivation, napping, and sleep disorders are related to cognitive dysfunction in older adults. Cognitive dysfunction has the ability functionally to compromise the quality of life in older adults. It is vital for future programs of research to create a concise model of the specific pathways of interaction between sleep and cognition in older adults.

References

[1] Ohayon MM, Vecchierini MF. Normative sleep data, cognitive function, and daily living activities in older adults in the community. Sleep 2005;28:981–9.

[2] Ohayon MM. Epidemiology of insomnia: what we know and what we still need to learn. Sleep Med Rev 2002;6:97–111.

[3] Ohayon MM, Zulley J, Guilleminault C, et al. How age and daytime activities are related to insomnia in the general population? Consequences for elderly people. J Am Geriatr Soc 2001;49:360–6.

[4] Maggi S, Langlois JA, Minicuci N, et al. Sleep complaints in community-dwelling older persons: prevalence, associated factors, and reported causes. J Am Geriatr Soc 1998;46:161–8.

[5] Brabbins CJ, Dewey ME, Copeland JRM, et al. Insomnia in the elderly: prevalence, gender differences and relationships with morbidity and mortality Int J Geriatr Psychiatry 1993; 8:473–80.

[6] Foley DJ, Monjan AA, Broen S, et al. Sleep complaints among elderly persons: an epidemiologic study of three communities. Sleep 1995; 18:425–32.

[7] Campbell SS, Gillin JC, Kripke D, et al. Gender differences in the circadian temperature rhythms of healthy older subjects: relationships to sleep quality. Sleep 1989;12:529–36.

[8] Morin CM, Azrin NH. Behavioral and cognitive treatments of geriatric insomnia. J Consult Clin Psychol 1988;56:748–53.

[9] Webb WB. Sleep in older persons: sleep structures of 50- to 60-year-old men and women. J Gerontol 1982;37:581–6.

[10] Ancoli Israel S. Sleep problems in older adults: putting myths to bed. Geriatrics 1997; 52:20–30.

[11] Ancoli Israel S. Sleep and aging: prevalence of disturbed sleep and treatment considerations in older adults. J Clin Psychiatry 2005;66: 24–30.

[12] Campbell SS, Murphy PJ, Stauble TN. Effects of a nap on nighttime sleep and waking functions in older subjects. J Am Geriatr Soc 2005; 53:48–53.

[13] Prinz PP, Vitiello MV, Raskind MA, et al. Geriatrics: sleep disorders and aging. N Engl J Med 1990;323:520–6.

[14] Pollak CP, Perlick D, Linsner JP, et al. Sleep problems in the community elderly as predictors of death and nursing home placement. J Community Health 1990;15:123–35.

[15] Vitiello MV. Sleep disorders and aging: understanding the causes. J Gerontol A Biol Sci Med Sci 1997;52:M189–91.

[16] Bliwise DL. Sleep in normal aging and dementia. Sleep 1993;16:40–81.

[17] Ancoli-Israel S, Kripke D. Prevalent sleep problems in the aged. Biofeedback Self Regul 1991; 16:349–59.

[18] Ohayon MM, Vecchierini MF. Daytime sleepiness and cognitive impairment in the elderly population. Arch Intern Med 2002;162:201–8.

[19] Cervilla JA, Prince M, Mann A. Smoking, drinking, and incident cognitive impairment: a cohort community based study included in the Gospel Oak Project. J Neurol Neurosurg Psychiatry 2000;68:622–6.

[20] Melzer D, McWilliams B, Brayne C, et al. Profile of disability in elderly people: estimates from a longitudinal population study. BMJ 1999; 318:1108–11.

[21] Worrall G, Moulton N. Cognitive function: survery of elderly persons living at home in rural Newfoundland. Can Fam Physician 1993; 39:772–7.

[22] Christensen H. What cognitive changes can be expected with normal aging? Aust N Z J Psychiatry 2001;35:768–75.

[23] Salthouse TA. Theoretical perspectives on cognitive aging. Hillsdale (NJ): Erlbaum; 1991.

[24] Schaie KW. Intellectual development in adulthood. The Seattle longitudinal study. Cambridge: Cambridge University Press; 1996.

[25] Hultsch DF, Hertzog C, Dixon RA, et al. Memory change in the aged. Cambridge: Cambridge University Press; 1998.

[26] Folstein M, Folstein S, McHugh PR. Mini-Mental State: a practical method for grading the cognitive state of patients for the clinician. Psychiatric Research 1975;12:189–98.

[27] Jacqmin-Gadda H, Fabriogoule C, Commenges D, et al. A 5-year longitudinal study of the Mini-Mental State Examination in normal aging. Am J Epidemiol 1997;145:498–506.

[28] Unger JM, vanBelle G, Heyman A. Cross-sectional versus longitudinal estimates of cognitive change in nondemented older people: a CERAD study. J Am Geriatr Soc 1999;47: 559–73.

[29] Zhu L, Viitanen M, Guo Z, et al. Blood pressure reduction, cardiovascular diseases, and cognitive declines in the mini-mental state examination in a community population of normal very old people: a three-year follow-up. J Clin Epidemiol 1998;51:385–91.

[30] Brayne C, Spiegelhalter DJ, Dufouil C, et al. Estimating the true extent of cognitive decline in the old old. J Am Geriatr Soc 1999; 47:1283–8.

[31] Scuteri A, Palmieri L, LoNoce C, et al. Age-related changes in cognitive domains: a population-based study. Aging Clin Exp Res 2005; 17:367–73.

[32] Royall DR, Palmer R, Chiodo LK, et al. Declining executive control in normal aging predicts change in functional status: the Freedom House study. J Am Geriatr Soc 2004;52:346–52.

[33] Grigsby J, Kaye K, Baxter J, et al. Executive cognitive abilities and functional status among community-dwelling older persons in the San Luis Valley Health and Aging study. J Am Geriatr Soc 1998;46:590–6.

[34] Lezak MD. Neuropsychological assessment. 3rd edition. New York: Oxford University Press; 1995.

[35] Zec R. The neuropsychology of aging. Exp Gerontol 1995;30:431–42.

[36] Wilkinson RT, Allison S. Age and simple reaction time: decade differences for 5325 subjects. J Gerontol 1989;44:29–35.

[37] Sliwinski M, Buschke H. Cross-sectional and longitudinal relationship among age, cognition, and processing speed. Psychol Aging 1999;14:18–33.

[38] Anstey KJ, Luszcz MA, Giles L, et al. Demographic, health, cognitive and sensory variables as predictors of mortality in very old adults. Psychol Aging 2001;16:3–11.

[39] Foley DJ, Monjan AA, Masaki KH, et al. Associations of symptoms of sleep apnea with cardiovascular disease, cognitive impairment, and mortality among older Japanese-American men. J Am Geriatr Soc 1999;47:524–8.

[40] Dealberto MJ, Pajot N, Courbon D, et al. Breathing disorders during sleep and cognitive performance in an older community sample: the EVA study. J Am Geriatr Soc 1996;44: 1287–94.

[41] Bonnet MH, Arand DL. Clinical effects of sleep fragmentation versus sleep deprivation. Sleep Med Rev 2003;7:297–310.

[42] Gooneratne NS, Weaver TE, Cater JR, et al. Functional outcomes of excessive daytime sleepiness in older adults. J Am Geriatr Soc 2003;51:642–9.

[43] Hoddes E, Dement W, Zarcone V. Quantification of sleepiness: a new approach. Psychophysiology 1973;10:431–6.

[44] Johns MW. A new method for measuring daytime sleepiness: the Epworth Sleepiness Scale. Sleep 1991;14:540–5.

[45] Chervin RD, Aldrich MS. The Epworth Sleepiness Scale may not reflect objective measures of sleepiness or sleep apnea. Neurology 1999; 52:125–31.

[46] Sauter C, Asenbaum S, Popovic R, et al. Excessive daytime sleepiness in patients suffering from different levels of obstructive sleep apnea syndrome. J Sleep Res 2000;9:293–301.

[47] Mitler MM, Gujavarty KS, Brownman CP. Maintenance of wakefulness test: a polysomnographic technique for evaluation treatment efficacy in patients with excessive somnolence. Electroencephalogr Clin Neurophysiol 1982; 53:658–61.

[48] Whitney CW, Enright P, Newman A, et al. Correlates of daytime sleepiness in 4578 elderly persons: the Cardiovascular Health Study. Sleep 1997;21:27–36.

[49] Foley DJ, Monjan AA, Masaki KH, et al. Daytime sleepiness is associated with 3-year incident dementia and cognitive decline in older Japanese-American men. J Am Geriatr Soc 2001;49:1628–32.

[50] Bonnet MH. The effect of sleep fragmentation on sleep and performance in younger and older subjects. Neurobiol Aging 1989;10:21–5.

[51] Bonnet MH, Arand DL. Sleep loss in aging. Clin Geriatr Med 1989;5:405–20.

[52] Brendel D, Reynolds CF III, Jennings J, et al. Sleep stage physiology, mood, and vigilance responses to total sleep deprivation in healthy 80-year-olds and 20-year-olds. Psychophysiology 1990;27:677–85.

[53] Smulders F, Kenemans J, Jonkman L, et al. The effects of sleep loss on task performance and the electroencephalogram in young and elderly subjects. Biol Psychol 1997;45:217–39.

[54] Durmer JS, Dinges D. Neurocognitive consequences of sleep deprivation. Semin Neurol 2005;25:117–29.

[55] Jewett ME, Dijk DJ, Kronauer RE, et al. Dose-response relationship between sleep duration and human psychomotor vigilance and subjective alertness. Sleep 1999;22:171–9.

[56] VanDongen HP, Maislin G, Mullington JM, et al. The cumulative cost of additional wakefulness: dose-response effects on neurobehavioral functions and sleep physiology from chronic sleep restriction and total sleep deprivation. Sleep 2003;26:117–26.

[57] Pilcher JJ, Huffcutt A. Effects of sleep deprivation on performance: a meta-analysis. Sleep 1996;19:318–26.

[58] Dinges D, Pack F, Williams K, et al. Cumulative sleepiness, mood disturbance, and psychomotor vigilance performance decrements during a week of sleep restricted to 4–5 hours per night. Sleep 1997;20:267–77.

[59] Davis CJ, Harding JW, Wright JW. REM sleep deprivation-induced deficits in the latency-to-peak induction and maintenance of long-term potentiation within the CA1 region of the hippocampus. Brain Res 2003; 973:293–7.

[60] Hornung OP, Regen F, Schredl M, et al. Manipulating REM sleep in older adults by selective REM sleep deprivation and physiological as well as pharmacological REM sleep augmentation methods. Exp Neurol 2006;197: 486–94.

[61] Pigeau R, Naitoh P, Buguet A, et al. Modafinil, d-amphetamine, and placebo during 64 hours of sustained mental work: effects on mood, fatigue, cognitive performance, and body temperature. J Sleep Res 1995;4:212–28.

[62] Stivalet P, Esquivie D, Barraud PA, et al. Effects of modafinil on attentional processes during 60 hours of sleep deprivation. Hum Psychopharmacol 1998;13:501–7.

[63] Wesensten NJ, Killgore WD, Balkin TJ. Performance and alertness effects of caffeine, dextroamphetamine, and modafinil during sleep deprivation. J Sleep Res 2005;14:255–66.

[64] Lee HJ, Kim L, Suh KY. Cognitive deterioration and changes of P300 during total sleep deprivation. Psychiatry Clin Neurosci 2003;57:490–6.

[65] Munch M, Knoblauch V, Blatter K, et al. The frontal predominance in human EEG delta activity after sleep loss decreases with age. Eur J Neurosci 2004;20:1402–10.

[66] Carskadon M, Dement W. Sleep loss in elderly volunteers. Sleep 1985;8:207–21.

[67] Philip P, Taillard J, Sagaspe P, et al. Age, performance, and sleep deprivation. J Sleep Res 2004; 13:105–10.

[68] Stenuit P, Kerkhofs M. Age modulates the effects of sleep restriction in women. Sleep 2005; 28:1283–8.

[69] Roge J, Pebayle T, El Hannachi S, et al. Effect of sleep deprivation and driving duration on the useful visual field in younger and older subjects during simulator driving. Vision Res 2003; 43:1465–72.

[70] Philip P, Taillard J, Quera-Salva M, et al. Simple reaction time, duration of driving and sleep deprivation in young versus old automobile drivers. J Sleep Res 1999;8:9–14.

[71] Takahashi M. The role of prescribed napping in sleep medicine. Sleep Med Rev 2003;7:227–35.

[72] Dinges D. Adult napping and its effects on ability to function. In: Stampi C, editor. Why we nap: evaluation, chronobiology, and functions of polyphasic and ultrashort sleep. Boston: Birkhauser; 1992. p. 118–34.

[73] Taub J. Effects of habitual variations in napping on psychomotor performance, memory, and subjective states. Int J Neurosci 1979; 9:97–112.

[74] Tietzel A, Lack L. The short-term benefits of brief and long naps following nocturnal sleep restriction. Sleep 2001;24:293–300.

[75] Monk T, Buysse D, Carrier J, et al. Effects of afternoon 'siesta' naps on sleep, alertness, performance, and circadian rhythms in the elderly. Sleep 2001;24:680–7.

[76] Bliwise D, Swan GE. Habitual napping and performance on the Trail Making Test. J Sleep Res 2005;14:209–10.

[77] Tamaki M, Shirota A, Tanaka H, et al. Effects of a daytime nap in the aged. Psychiatry Clin Neurosci 1999;53:273–5.

[78] Stepanski E, Wyatt J. Use of sleep hygiene in the treatment of insomnia. Sleep Med Rev 2003;7:215–25.

[79] Hayes J, Blazer D, Foley DJ. Risk of napping: excessive daytime sleepiness and mortality in an older community population. J Am Geriatr Soc 1996;44:693–8.

[80] Buysse D, Browman K, Monk T, et al. Napping and 24-hour sleep/wake patterns in healthy elderly and young adults. J Am Geriatr Soc 1992;40:779–86.

[81] Pilcher JJ, Michalowski K, Carrigan R. The prevalence of daytime napping and its relationship to nighttime sleep. Behav Med 2001;27:71–6.

[82] Avidan AY. Sleep changes and disorders in the elderly patient. Curr Neurol Neurosci Rep 2002;2:178–85.

[83] Piani A, Brotini S, Dolso P, et al. Sleep disturbances in elderly: a subjective evaluation over 65. Arch Gerontol Geriatr 2004;9:325–31.

[84] Vgontzas AN, Kales A. Sleep and its disorders. Annu Rev Med 1999;50:387–400.

[85] Dauvilliers Y, Gosselin A, Paquet J, et al. Effect of age on MSLT results in patients with narcolepsy-cataplexy. Neurology 2004;62:46–50.

[86] Schwartz JR, Nelson MT, Schwartz ER, et al. Effects of modafinil on wakefulness and executive function in patients with narcolepsy experiencing late-day sleepiness. Clin Neuropharmacol 2004;27:74–9.

[87] Hood B, Bruck D. Sleepiness and performance in narcolepsy. J Sleep Res 1996;5:128–34.

[88] Hood B, Bruck D. A comparison of sleep deprivation and narcolepsy in terms of complex cognitive performance and subjective sleepiness. Sleep Med 2002;3:259–66.

[89] Naumann A, Bierbrauer J, Przuntek H, et al. Attentive and preattentive processing in narcolepsy as revealed by event-related potentials (ERPs). Neuroreport 2001;12:2807–11.

[90] Fulda S, Schulz H. Cognitive dysfunction in sleep disorders. Sleep Med Rev 2001;5:423–45.

[91] Hood B, Bruck D. Metamemory in narcolepsy. J Sleep Res 1997;6:205–10.

[92] Naumann A, Daum I. Narcolepsy: pathophysiology and neuropsychological changes. Behav Neurol 2003;14:89–98.

[93] Youngstedt SD, Kripke D, Elliot JA, et al. Circadian abnormalities in older adults. J Pineal Res 2001;31:264–72.

[94] Yoon IY, Kripke D, Elliot JA, et al. Age-related changes of circadian rhythms and sleep-wake cycles. J Am Geriatr Soc 2003;51:1085–91.

[95] Dagan Y. Circadian rhythm sleep disorders (CRSD). Sleep Med Rev 2002;6:45–55.

[96] Dagan Y, Einstein M. Circadian rhythm sleep disorders: towards a more precise definition and diagnosis. Chronobiol Int 1999;6:213–22.

[97] May CP, Hasher L, Foong N. Implicit memory, age, and time of day. Psychol Sci 2005;16:96–100.

[98] Yasukouchi H, Wada S, Urasaki E, et al. Effects of night work on the cognitive function in young and elderly subjects with specific reference to the auditory P300. J UOEH 1995;17:229–46.

[99] Brown LN, Goddard KM, Lahar CJ, et al. Age-related deficits in cognitive functioning are not mediated by time of day. Exp Aging Res 1999;25:81–93.

[100] Bonnefond A, Rohmer O, Hoeft A, et al. Interaction of age with time of day and mental load in different cognitive tasks. Percept Mot Skills 2003;96(3 pt 2):1223–36.

[101] Kales A, Kales J. Evaluation and treatment of insomnia. New York: Oxford University Press; 1984.

[102] Kales A, Soldatos CR, Kales J. Sleep disorders: insomnia, sleepwalking, night terrors, nightmares, and enuresis. Ann Intern Med 1987;106:582–92.

[103] Ford DE, Kamerow DB. Epidemiologic study of sleep disturbances and psychiatric disorders. JAMA 1989;262:1479–84.

[104] Mellinger GD, Balter MB, Uhlenhuth EH. Insomnia and its treatment: prevalence and correlates. Arch Gen Psychiatry 1995;42:225–32.

[105] Morin CM, Gramling SE. Sleep patterns and aging: comparison of older adults with and without insomnia complaints. Psychol Aging 1989;4:290–4.

[106] Morin CM, Kowatch RA, Barry T, et al. Cognitive-behavior therapy for late-life insomnia. J Consult Clin Psychol 1993;61:137–46.

[107] Morin CM, Baillargeon L, Bastien CH. Treatment of late-life insomnia. Oakland: Sage Publications; 2000.

[108] Alapin I, Fichten CS, Libman E, et al. How is good and poor sleep in older adults and college students related to daytime sleepiness, fatigue, and ability to concentrate? J Psychosom Res 2000;49:381–90.

[109] Zammit GK. Subjective ratings of the characteristics and sequelae of good and poor sleep in normals. J Clin Psychol 1988;44:123–30.

[110] Broman JE, Lundh LG, Aleman K, et al. Subjective and objective performance in patients with

persistent insomnia. Scandanavian Journal of Behavior Therapy 1992;21:115–26.

[111] Bastien CH, Fortier-Brochu E, Rioux I, et al. Cognitive performance and sleep quality in the elderly suffering from chronic insomnia. J Psychosom Res 2003;54:39–49.

[112] Hauri P. Cognitive deficits in insomnia patients. Acta Neurol Belg 1997;97:113–7.

[113] Mendelson WB, Garnett D, Gillin JC, et al. The experience of insomnia and daytime and nighttime functioning. Psychiatr Res 1984;12:235–50.

[114] Vignola A, Lamoureux C, Bastien CH, et al. Effects of chronic insomnia and use of benzodiazepines on daytime performance in older adults. J Gerontol 2000;55B:54–62.

[115] Hart R, Morin CM, Best AM. Neuropsychological performance in elderly insomnia patients. Aging Cognition 1995;2:268–78.

[116] Cricco M, Simonsick EM, Foley DJ. The impact of insomnia on cognitive functioning in older adults. J Am Geriatr Soc 2001;49:1185–9.

[117] Stone J, Morin CM, Hart RP, et al. Neuropsychological functioning in older insomniacs with or without obstructive sleep apnea. Psychol Aging 1994;9:231–6.

[118] Glass J, Lanctot KL, Herrmann N, et al. Sedative hypnotics in older people with insomnia: meta-analysis of risks and benefits. BMJ 2005;331:1169.

[119] Aparasu RR, Mort JR, Brandt H. Psychotropic prescription use by community-dwelling adults in the United States. J Am Geriatr Soc 2003;51:671–7.

[120] Craig D, Passmore AP, Fullerton KJ, et al. Factors influencing prescription of CNS medications in different elderly populations. Pharmacoepidemiol Drug Saf 2003;12:383–7.

[121] Nau SD, McCrae CS, Cook KG, et al. Treatment of insomnia in older adults. Clin Psychol Rev 2005;25:645–72.

[122] Smith MT, Perlis ML, Park A, et al. Comparative meta-analysis of pharmacotherapy and behavior therapy for persistent insomnia. Am J Psychiatry 2002;159:5–11.

[123] Irwin MR, Cole JC, Nicassio PM. Comparative meta-analysis of behavioral interventions for insomnia and their efficacy in middle-aged adults and in older adults 55 + years of age. Health Psychol 2006;25:3–14.

[124] Greisberg S, McKay D. Neuropsychology of obsessive-compulsive disorder: a review and treatment implications. Clin Psychol Rev 2003;23:95–117.

[125] Shenal BV, Harrison DW, Demaree HA. The neuropsychology of depression: a literature review and preliminary model. Neuropsychol Rev 2003;13:33–42.

[126] Austin MP, Mitchell P, Goodwin GM. Cognitive deficits in depression. Br J Psychiatry 2001;178:200–6.

[127] Fossati P, Ergis AM, Allilaire JF. Executive functioning in unipolar depression: a review. Encephale 2002;28:97–107.

[128] Rogers MA, Kasai K, Koji M, et al. Executive and prefrontal dysfunction in unipolar depression: a review of neuropsychological and imaging evidence. Neurosci Res 2004;50:1–11.

[129] Young T, Palta M, Dempsey J, et al. The occurrence of sleep-disordered breathing among middle-aged adults. N Engl J Med 1993;328:1230–5.

[130] Ancoli-Israel S, Kripke DF, Klauber MR, et al. Sleep-disordered breathing in community dwelling elderly. Sleep 1991;14:486–95.

[131] Aloia MS, Arnedt JT, Davis JD, et al. Neuropsychological consequences of sleep apnea: a critical review. J Int Neuropsychol Soc 2004;10:772–85.

[132] Aloia MS, Arnedt JT, Smith L, et al. Examining the construct of depression in obstructive sleep apnea syndrome. Sleep Med 2005;6:115–21.

[133] Aikens JE, Caruana-Montaldo B, Vanable PA, et al. MMPI correlates of sleep and respiratory disturbance in obstructive sleep apnea. Sleep 1999;22:362–9.

[134] Engleman HM, Douglas NJ. Sleepiness, cognitive function, and quality of life in obstructive sleep apnoea/hypopnoea syndrome. Thorax 2004;59:618–22.

[135] Aldrich MS. Automobile accidents in patients with sleep disorders. Sleep 1989;12:487–94.

[136] George CF, Nickerson PW, Hanly PJ, et al. Sleep apnoea patients have more automobile accidents. Lancet 1987;8556:447.

[137] George CF, Smiley A. Sleep apnea and automobile crashes. Sleep 1999;22:790–5.

[138] Guilleminault C, Robinson A. Sleep-disordered breathing and hypertension: past lessons, future directions. Sleep 1997;20:806–11.

[139] Hudgel D, Devadatta P, Quadri M, et al. Mechanism of sleep-induced periodic breathing in convalescing stroke patients and healthy elderly subjects. Chest 1993;104:1503–10.

[140] Partinen M, Guilleminault C. Daytime sleepiness and vascular morbidity at seven-year follow-up in obstructive sleep apnea patients. Chest 1990;97:27–32.

[141] Schäfer H, Berner S, Ewig S, et al. Cardiovascular morbidity in patients with obstructive sleep apnea in relation to the severity of respiratory disorder. Deutsch Med Wochenschr 1998;123:1127–33.

[142] Nieto FJ, Young TB, Lind BK, et al. Association of sleep-disordered breathing, sleep apnea, and hypertension in a large community-based study. Sleep Heart Health Study. JAMA 2000;283:1829–36.

[143] Shahar E, Whitney CW, Redline S, et al. Sleep-disordered breathing and cardiovascular disease: cross-sectional results of the Sleep Heart Health Study. Am J Respir Crit Care Med 2001;163:19–25.

[144] Sateia MJ. Neuropsychological impairment and quality of life in obstructive sleep apnea. Clin Chest Med 2003;24:249–59.

[145] Beebe D, Gozal D. Obstructive sleep apnea and the prefrontal cortex: towards a comprehensive model linking nocturnal upper airway obstruction to daytime cognitive and behavioral deficits. J Sleep Res 2002;11:1–16.

[146] Verstraeten E, Cluydts R. Executive control of attention in sleep apnea patients: theoretical concepts and methodological considerations. Sleep Med Rev 2004;8:257–67.

[147] Feuerstein C, Naegele B, Pepin J, et al. Frontal lobe-related cognitive functions in patients with Sleep Apnea Syndrome before and after treatment. Acta Neurologica Belgica 1997; 97:96–107.

[148] Naegele B, Thouvard V, Pepin JL, et al. Deficits of cognitive executive functions in patients with sleep apnea syndrome. Sleep 1995;18: 43–52.

[149] Bédard M-A, Montplaisir J, Richer F, et al. Obstructive sleep apnea syndrome: pathogenesis of neuropsychological deficits. J Clin Exp Neuropsychol 1991;13:950–64.

[150] Bédard M-A, Montplaisir J, Malo J, et al. Persistent neuropsychological deficits and vigilance impairment in sleep apnea syndrome after treatment with continuous positive airways pressure (CPAP). J Clin Exp Neuropsychol 1993;15:330–41.

[151] Greenberg GD, Watson RK, Deptula D. Neuropsychological dysfunction in sleep apnea. Sleep 1987;10:254–62.

[152] Verstraeten E, Cluydts R, Verbraecken J, et al. Psychomotor and cognitive performance in nonapneic snorers: preliminary findings. Percept Mot Skills 1997;84:1211–22.

[153] Knight H, Millman RP, Gur RC, et al. Clinical significance of sleep apnea in the elderly. Am Rev Respir Dis 1987;136:845–50.

[154] Cohen-Zion M, Stepnowsky CJ Jr, Marler MR, et al. Changes in cognitive function associated with sleep disordered breathing in older people. J Am Geriatr Soc 2001;49:1622–7.

[155] Antonelli Incalzi R, Marra C, Salvigni BL, et al. Does cognitive dysfunction conform to a distinctive pattern in obstructive sleep apnea? J Sleep Res 2004;13:79–86.

[156] Keenan SP, Burt H, Ryan F, et al. Long-term survival of patients with obstructive sleep apnea treated by uvulopalatopharyngoplasty or nasal CPAP. Chest 1994;105:155–9.

[157] He J, Kryger MH, Zorick F, et al. Mortality and apnea index in obstructive sleep apnea: experience in 385 male patients. Chest 1988; 94:9–14.

[158] Campos-Rodriguez F, Pena-Grinan N, Reyes-Nunez N, et al. Mortality in obstructive sleep apnea-hypopnea patients treated with positive airway pressure. Chest 2005;128:624–33.

[159] Aloia MS, Ilniczky N, Di Dio P, et al. Neuropsychological changes and treatment compliance in older adults with sleep apnea. J Psychosom Res 2003;54:71–6.

[160] Aloia MS, Stanchina ML, Arnedt JT, et al. Treatment adherence and outcomes in flexible versus continuous positive airway pressure therapy. Chest 2005;127:2085–93.

[161] McArdle N, Devereux G, Heidarnejad H, et al. Long-term use of CPAP therapy for sleep apnea/hypopnea syndrome. Am J Respir Crit Care Med 1999;159:1108–14.

[162] Barbé F, Mayoralas LR, Duran J, et al. Treatment with continuous positive airway pressure is not effective in patients with sleep apnea but no daytime sleepiness. a randomized, controlled trial. Ann Intern Med 2001;134:1015–23.

[163] Karasek M. Melatonin, human aging, and age-related diseases. Exp Gerontol 2004;39:1723–9.

[164] Pandi-Perumal SR, Seils LK, Kayumov L, et al. Senescence, sleep, and circadian rhythms. Aging Research Reviews 2002;1:559–604.

[165] McKinney M, Jacksonville MC. Brain cholinergic vulnerability: relevance to behavior and disease. Biochem Pharmacol 2005;70:1115–24.

ELSEVIER
SAUNDERS

SLEEP
MEDICINE
CLINICS

Sleep Med Clin 1 (2006) 221–229

Insomnia in the Elderly

Kenneth L. Lichstein, PhD[a],*, Kristen C. Stone, MS[b],
Sidney D. Nau, PhD[a], Christina S. McCrae, PhD[c],
Kristen L. Payne, MA[a]

- Epidemiology
- Diagnosis
  Contributing factors
  Clinical features of late-life insomnia
  Daytime functioning in insomnia
- Assessment
- Pharmacologic treatments for insomnia
  Types of hypnotics
  Side effects

- Cognitive behavior therapy for insomnia
  *Cognitive behavioral therapy for primary
  insomnia*
  *Cognitive behavioral therapy for
  secondary or comorbid insomnia*
  *Cognitive behavioral therapy for
  hypnotic-dependent insomnia*
- Discussion
- References

Compared with other age groups, insomnia is more prevalent and more severe among older adults [1]. Insomnia can signal the presence of other sleep disorders (eg, sleep apnea, periodic limb movement disorder, and circadian rhythm disorders) and is a health risk factor for depression, anxiety, substance abuse, and suicide [2]. This article comprehensively examines older adults with insomnia (OAWI), emphasizing a behavioral sleep medicine perspective.

Epidemiology

A recent review of epidemiologic studies of insomnia by Ohayon [3] concluded that insomnia complaints are more common in women and prevalence increases with advancing age. The authors' randomized survey of people's sleep experience [1] is distinguished by the use of 2 weeks of sleep diaries; sampling across the entire range of the adult

lifespan; and using empirically derived, conservative criteria for insomnia. In general, the authors' data agree with the conclusions of Ohayon's [3] review.

The authors found the prevalence of insomnia among women is on average 40% greater than among men. As shown in Table 1, the sex difference is consistent across ages. The prevalence of insomnia is higher in women than in men in every decade except one, 30 to 39. Regarding change in insomnia across the adult life span, prevalence is relatively stable during the middle years and abruptly jumps in decades 70 to 79 and 80 to 89 to about double the mean rate during earlier years. The weighted point prevalence for chronic, clinically significant insomnia is 15.9%. The spike in insomnia in the later years is more pronounced in women than in men. Insomnia presence climaxes at 41% in women between the ages of 80 and 89.

This work was supported by Grant No. DA13574 from the National Institute on Drug Abuse
[a] Department of Psychology, The University of Alabama, 348 Gordon Palmer Hall, Box 870348, Tuscaloosa, AL 35487–0348, USA
[b] Department of Psychology, University of Memphis, 202 Psychology Building, Memphis, TN 38152, USA
[c] Department of Psychology, University of Florida, McCarty C, Room 502, Gainesville, FL 32611–5911, USA
* Corresponding author.
E-mail address: lichstein@ua.edu (K.L. Lichstein).

1556-407X/06/$ – see front matter © 2006 Elsevier Inc. All rights reserved.

doi:10.1016/j.jsmc.2006.04.009

Table 1: Prevalence of insomnia by age and gender

Age group	% Prevalence	
	Men	*Women*
20–29	6	12
30–39	22	12
40–49	11	20
50–59	10	21
60–69	9	17
70–79	23	26
80–89+	23	41

Data from Lichstein KL, Durrence HH, Riedel BW, et al. Epidemiology of sleep: age, gender, and ethnicity. Mahwah (NJ): Erlbaum; 2004.

There has been some interest in whether certain types of insomnia are more common at different ages. It is commonly asserted that onset insomnia predominates in younger adults and maintenance insomnia in older adults [4,5], although direct data supporting this view are not plentiful. This logic has implications for the type of treatment chosen for people with insomnia, because some psychologic and some pharmacologic interventions target onset or maintenance disturbance. The data show that there is some tendency for type of insomnia to correlate with age as suggested previously, but in general all types of insomnia are commonly observed in all age groups [1]. Similarly, Ohayon and colleagues [6] reported that in a survey of over 13,000 people between the ages of 15 and 100, type of insomnia was uncorrelated with age.

It should be noted that there may be ethnic differences in the epidemiology of insomnia. The sharp rise in prevalence in older adults is less likely to occur among African Americans [7]. A spike in insomnia among middle-aged African Americans has been observed [1], and this pattern has not been reported in white samples.

Diagnosis

Contributing factors

Six categories of contributing factors are often noted in people with insomnia: (1) circadian, (2) psychiatric, (3) pharmacologic, (4) medical or neurologic illness, (5) psychophysiologic reactivity, and (6) negative conditioning factors. OAWI are at increased risk for the first four types. The complexity of factors contributing to chronically disturbed sleep often necessitates a multicomponent treatment plan. This is especially true for older adults, who experience age-related changes in sleep and increased risk for various sleep-disruptive problems associated with physical health and psychologic adjustment. Presumably, this group also experiences at least average risk for psychophysiologic reactivity and negative conditioning factors [4].

The stereotypic primary insomnia disorder includes subclinical worry and somatic arousal characterized as psychophysiologic reactivity. This reactivity may predate mild to moderate stress precipitants and represent a vulnerability to insomnia. Alternatively, conditioned reactivity may arise in response to temporary sleeplessness resulting from moderate-severe stressors (eg, death of a spouse) and induce insomnia in individuals not otherwise disposed to sleep disturbance.

The psychophysiologic reactivity factors and conditioning factors include (1) psychologic characteristics (eg, subclinical anxiety and low mood); (2) physiologic tension or arousal; and (3) a history of negative conditioning (caused by frequent nights with excessive amounts of time spent lying awake). Negative conditioning is sometimes compounded by learning negative sleep habits (poor sleep hygiene), such as late afternoon naps, increasing caffeine intake to compensate for anticipated drowsiness, irregular bedtimes, and excessively extending the sleep period to obtain more sleep. The physiologic tension or arousal of insomnia varies across individuals and may include cognitive overarousal (eg, "mind racing," "thinking about all kinds of things," "thoughts jumping from topic to topic"); physiologic overarousal (eg, tense muscles, restlessness, "feel wide awake," and so forth); and arousability or sensitivity to stimuli (eg, environmental sounds, temperature, light, bedcovers).

Clinical features of late-life insomnia

Psychiatric disorders contribute to OAWI [8], but it is unclear if this factor is stronger in older than younger age groups. There is mounting evidence that physical illness (separate from normal aging processes) plays a stronger role in instigating insomnia in older adults compared with younger samples [6,9]. Further, such factors as bereavement, physical inactivity, and social isolation may way more heavily among OAWI. In addition, late-life insomnia includes sleep-related physiologic disorders (eg, sleep apnea); insomnia associated with medical and neurologic disorders; substance use disorders; and circadian rhythm disorders. Among the more than 30 adult sleep disorders that often present with an insomnia complaint, most are more common in older adults (eg, obstructive sleep apnea, periodic limb movement disorder, and restless legs syndrome [10]). Many of these disorders increase sharply after age 40; some first appear in late life. For example, insomnia associated with parkinsonism typically onsets around age 50 to 60 years.

Daytime functioning in insomnia

The perceived daytime consequences of insomnia generally concern adverse effects on psychosocial, occupational, and physical functioning [11], and include fatigue, negative affect, cognitive impairment, and excessive worries about sleep. Researchers have sought, with limited success, to operationalize the perceived consequences of chronic insomnia (for a review see, Riedel and Lichstein [12]). Investigations comparing daytime functioning in people with insomnia and people without insomnia usually do not find a significant difference between the two groups on objective measures (eg, reaction time, the Multiple Sleep Latency Test, digit symbol substitution, card sorting, logical reasoning). Subjective measures separate the groups more reliably (eg, Minnesota Multiphasic Personality Inventory depression and anxiety scales, Profile of Mood States, Beck Depression Inventory, State-Trait Anxiety Inventory, Dysfunctional Beliefs and Attitudes about Sleep scale, Insomnia Impairment Scale, fatigue ratings, and some subjective daytime sleepiness scales).

Young people with insomnia, OAWI, and normal-sleeping older adults exhibit disturbed nocturnal sleep without abnormal daytime sleepiness (measured by the Multiple Sleep Latency Test). Some have interpreted this finding as an indication for decreased sleep need in these groups [8], a hypothesis that departs from the more standard emphasis on insomnia as a disorder of unmet sleep need. Alternatively, there could be a 24-hour hyperarousal state in people with insomnia [13], or changes accompanying aging may obstruct sleep both at night and during the day. Consistent with the hyperarousal hypothesis is evidence of increased sensitivity to noise during sleep in older adults compared with younger adults, despite older adults' reduced hearing sensitivity [14].

There is little consensus about how to measure daytime functioning changes during treatment for OAWI. Only four daytime functioning measures were used more than one time in the clinical trials reviewed, and only the Beck Depression Inventory was used more than two times.

Assessment

Morgan [4] offers specific principles to guide the challenging assessment of older adults: (1) there is a need to separate treatable causes of insomnia complaints from normal aging-related changes in sleep; (2) the contributing factors for late-life insomnia are frequently multiple and interacting, so it is important to identify the most appropriate targets for psychologic intervention; and (3) some late-life insomnia problems begin years earlier, which highlights the importance of a carefully taken sleep history.

Studies of medical practice suggest that, even though most insomnia treatments are delivered by physicians, physicians are often unaware of severe insomnia in their patients [15,16]. Even when physicians prescribe medication for sleep, there is usually no documented evaluation of sleep [17]. The assessment approach for OAWI is similar to that used with other patients. Although the American Academy of Sleep Medicine's report on the indications for use of polysomnogram (PSG) [18] indicates that PSG is not routinely indicated in the evaluation of transient or chronic insomnia, the report also lists the two exceptions to this rule, which are prior treatment failure and diagnostic uncertainty (eg, suspected sleep-related breathing disorder or narcolepsy, and cases of strongly suspected periodic limb movement disorder). The potential benefits of PSG increase with age because covert sleep-related physiologic factors, such as sleep apnea and periodic limb movements, increase in prevalence with age, muddying the diagnostic process.

Interview assessment of other sleep disorders is often inadequate. In a sample of 100 people presenting with insomnia, apnea and periodic limb movements were more likely to be found by PSG among older individuals [19]. Only one of three sleep apnea cases was suspected by clinical interview. Similarly, among older individuals seeking insomnia treatment and screened for sleep apnea by interview, PSG revealed 29% of the sample had occult sleep apnea [20].

Pharmacologic treatments for insomnia

The ideal hypnotic induces sleep rapidly; sustains sleep; preserves normal sleep architecture; leaves the individual feeling well rested in the morning and unburdened by cognitive, psychomotor, or motivational defects during the day; maintains its therapeutic potency for months or years; and has low toxicity. This is a tall order, thus far undelivered, but since the era of barbiturates, tremendous progress has been made toward these goals [21].

Although hypnotics are the most common treatment for insomnia at all ages, usage is disproportionately high in older adults. Community use rates for hypnotics among adults over age 65 range from 3% to 21% for men and 7% to 29% for women [22] compared with only 2% to 4% for younger age groups [23].

Types of hypnotics

Nine drugs in two drug classes have received Food and Drug Administration approval for insomnia: benzodiazepine receptor agonists (eg, the older estazolam, flurazepam, quazepam, temazepam, and triazolam and the newer eszopiclone, zaleplon, and zolpidem), and a melatonin agonist (ramelteon).

A sizable literature suggests that the older benzodiazepine receptor agonists can be helpful for OAWI, but adverse effects may also occur. Most of the data were based on short-term trials [21]. Diminished rapid eye movement and slow wave sleep, anterograde amnesia, and residual sedation are not uncommon with these drugs. The newer nonbenzodiazepine agonists may be better tolerated by older adults [24,25]. Zaleplon, characterized by a very short half-life, may have a more favorable safety profile than other hypnotics [26]. A recent 1-year clinical trial, although open-label, showed that zaleplon maintained therapeutic effectiveness for a year with older adults [27]. Changes in pharmacodynamics and pharmacokinetics, such as slower absorption and elimination and heightened site sensitivity, may occur in the elderly [28]. Such changes often justify lower dosing regimens with the elderly [29].

Exogenous melatonin has been recommended for insomnia, particularly in the elderly, because lower levels of circulating melatonin have been observed in OAWI [30]. A recent meta-analysis concluded, however, that whereas melatonin has an acceptable safety profile, its efficacy is limited [31]. No significant therapeutic effects were found for wake time after sleep onset (WASO), total sleep time (TST), REM percentage, or rated sleep quality. The authors did find staistically significant, small magnitude improvement in sleep onset latency (SOL) of 11.7 minutes. Among individuals diagnosed with delayed sleep phase syndrome, melatonin was associated with clinically meaningful improvement, averaging 38.8 minutes reduction in SOL. Age-related effects did not occur for any of these variables. The only age effect occurred with sleep efficiency percent (SE). Significant improvement of 5.3% occurred only among older adults. Ramelteon, a melatonin agonist, has a stronger affinity for melatonin receptor sites than exogenous melatonin and may have stronger therapeutic effects [32]. Ramelteon has been approved by the Food and Drug Administration for treatment of sleep-onset insomnia in adults and in older adults.

Sedating antidepressants are in widespread use as hypnotics, but there are scant data to evaluate wanted and unwanted effects. Drowsiness and dizziness are common side effects of trazodone, occurring in greater than 20% of patients, and trazodone is not well-tolerated by about 20% to 30% of patients. Other side-effects reported with trazodone treatment include cardiovascular effects and priapism. Given that trazodone leads sales in sleep-inducing medications [33,34], more research with this and related drugs is highly warranted.

Over-the-counter sleep aids are mostly comprised of antihistamines, such as diphenhydramine. There are limited data supporting their efficacy. In addition, side effects, particularly in the elderly, may be serious including inattentiveness, disorganized speech, and agitation [35].

The recent National Institutes of Health State of the Science Conference on Insomnia [36] concluded that good evidence supports the short-term efficacy of benzodiazepine receptor agonists, particularly the newer ones, in the treatment of insomnia. Limited data preclude drawing inferences on long-term efficacy with most of these drugs. Concerns were raised about the efficacy or safety of sedating antidepressants and over-the-counter antihistamines, in part because of inadequate data and concerns about the risk/benefit ratio.

Side effects

Complications associated with hypnotic use in older adults should not be ignored. Older adults are more likely to be chronic hypnotic users [37] and are more vulnerable to the hazards associated with hypnotics, in part because of slower drug absorption and elimination. Because older adults consume more medications in general [38], there is a heightened risk of polypharmacy complications. Serious potential side effects of hypnotic use in the elderly are more closely related to long half-life benzodiazepines. Examples include increased automobile accidents [39], higher rate of falls producing hip fracture [40], and femur fracture [41]. Undiagnosed sleep apnea is routinely encountered in older adults. Administration of hypnotics, particularly the older benzodiazepines, to individuals with occult sleep apnea misdiagnosed as insomnia risks exacerbation of respiratory disturbance.

Cognitive behavior therapy for insomnia

The set of psychologic or behavioral interventions for insomnia have collectively come to be called cognitive behavior therapy (CBT) for insomnia, and there have been about 30 CBT clinical trials with OAWI. The most widely used CBT techniques for insomnia in older adults are relaxation (including progressive relaxation and passive relaxation [42]); stimulus control, which limits bedroom use to sleep [43]; sleep restriction, which prescribes abrupt reduction of time in bed [44]; sleep compression, which prescribes gradual reduction of time in bed [45]; cognitive therapy, which addresses self-defeating thinking [46]; sleep education and sleep hygiene, which promote sleep-enhancing and discourages sleep-obstructing behaviors [47]; and CBT treatment packages. Table 2 provides a more detailed description of standard CBT interventions.

A recent meta-analysis compared CBT for insomnia in middle-aged and older adults [48]. Stronger treatment effects were observed for SE and TST in younger adults. In the remaining three variables, rated sleep quality, SOL, and WASO, however, there was no significant difference in the therapeutic impact of CBT according to age.

Cognitive behavioral therapy for primary insomnia

Stimulus control, sleep restriction, sleep compression, and CBT packages typically obtain the strongest results on SOL, WASO, and SE. Relaxation therapies and sleep hygiene for OAWI attain less consistent, but still favorable results. Gains in TST are generally weaker than with other sleep variables, and PSG changes are usually weaker than self-reported change [45,49–51].

To facilitate a positive treatment response, interventions can be modified for older adults. Passive relaxation methods can be substituted for muscle tensing methods to avoid exacerbating pain [52,53]. Stimulus control instructions can be altered for older adults who have difficulties ambulating, by eliminating the requirement to leave the bedroom during long awakenings [54]. More flexible sleep schedules might improve tolerance to sleep restriction [52,55].

There is little consistency in the daytime functioning measures chosen for clinical trials with OAWI and the results have been inconsistent. Some examples of gains in daytime functioning associated with sleep improvement are self-efficacy [49], insomnia severity [56], and depression [49].

In recent times, only two studies of older adults with primary insomnia used a placebo control condition. One used a behavior therapy placebo [45] and one a placebo pill [50]. In both cases, CBT outperformed placebo.

Relaxation treatment
In two studies with OAWI, the therapeutic response to progressive relaxation has been mild-moderate [43,46], but two others have shown progressive relaxation to be ineffective [57,58]. Passive forms of relaxation have been more consistently effective than progressive relaxation for OAWI [45,53,59].

Stimulus control
Five studies of stimulus control with older adults show moderate to strong sleep effects on both SOL and WASO [49,54,58–60].

Sleep restriction and sleep compression
The five studies that have examined sleep restriction or sleep compression [45,52,55,61,62] have shown consistent, strong sleep effects.

Sleep hygiene
Three clinical trials have tested sleep hygiene as a stand-alone treatment. Sleep hygiene has consistently shown improvement, although less improvement than more standard treatments with which it has been compared [49,55,62].

Cognitive behavior therapy packages
Three CBT studies have used similar treatment combinations, typically comprising stimulus control, sleep restriction, cognitive therapy, and sleep education, for maintenance and mixed insomnia and have obtained uniformly positive results [50,51,57]. Cognitive therapy as a unitary treatment has not been tested.

Cognitive behavioral therapy for secondary or comorbid insomnia

Because of the gradual decline of general health with age, and increasing prescription drug use, older adults are more at risk for secondary or comorbid insomnia than younger adults. For insomnia to be correctly classified as secondary insomnia, there must be a persistent causal relationship between another condition and the insomnia [63]. Such determination is difficult to make and may shift over time within an individual. The authors subscribe to the recent National Institutes of Health State-of-the-Science Panel's 2005 recommendation that secondary insomnia is poorly understood and comorbid insomnia is a more appropriate term [36].

There is a wealth of data on CBT for secondary insomnia reviewed elsewhere [64]. Four randomized controlled trials with secondary insomnia in older adults have been published. Lichstein and coworkers [65] randomly assigned 44 secondary insomnia participants either to four sessions of a CBT package or to a wait-list control condition . Sleep improvements found with the treated group exceeded those in the wait-list group at posttreatment and follow-up. There was no outcome differences between the two types of secondary insomnia studied, psychiatric and medical. Rybarczyk and coworkers [66] also studied secondary insomnia related to medical conditions, but not psychiatric disorders. Thirty-eight patients were randomly assigned to one of three conditions: (1) eight sessions of group CBT, (2) home-based audio relaxation, or (3) wait list. Again, strong sleep gains were achieved only by the CBT group. Using part of the data from their first study, Rybarczyk and coworkers [67]

Table 2:   **Common methods of cognitive behavior therapy for insomnia**

Method	Rationale and description
Relaxation	This is a collection of methods of quiescent self-inquiry that promote both physiologic and cognitive reductions in arousal. Common types of relaxation include biofeedback, progressive muscle relaxation, passive relaxation, guided imagery, and varieties of meditation.
Stimulus control	This set of instructions is designed to limit the bedroom to sleep with the goal of conditioning the patient to become sleepy when approaching bedtime. The instructions are 1. Enter bed only when you have a strong urge to sleep. 2. Do not use the bed or bedroom for anything but sleep (and sex). Activities, such as television, reading, paperwork, and so forth, should be removed from the bedroom. 3. If you do not fall asleep within about 15 min, exit the bedroom. 4. Return to the bedroom only when you have a strong urge to sleep. 5. Repeat instructions 2–4 throughout the night. 6. Set a fixed morning wake time. 7. Reduce napping.
Sleep restriction	This procedure is designed to reduce fragmented sleep and wake time in bed by matching the sleep period to actual sleep time. The goal is a long block of continuous sleep characteristic of normal sleepers. 1. Determine mean TST from 2 wk of diaries. 2. Phone answering machine daily report on TIB and TST. 3. If mean SE $\geq$ 90% for previous 5 d, increase TIB 15 min for at least next 5 d. 4. If mean SE $\geq$ 85% for previous 5 d, decrease TIB to match mean TST of previous 5 d for at least next 10 d. 5. If mean SE >85% and <90% for previous 5 d, no change in TIB. 6. No napping.
Sleep compression	This intervention has the same rationale and goals as sleep restriction and is procedurally similar. 1. Determine mean TST and mean TIB from 2 wk of diaries. 2. Divide TIB – TST difference by the number of treatment sessions (usually about eight – one to calculate weekly TIB part reductions. 3. In each treatment session, fix bedtime and awake time for the coming week to compress TIB by one part each week. 4. Try to keep morning wake time stable.
Cognitive therapy	This procedure is more difficult to encapsulate neatly than the other interventions. An exaggerated worrisome response to poor sleep may contribute to the initiation and maintenance of chronic insomnia. Similarly, exaggerated worry about the daytime impact of insomnia and dysfunctional beliefs about sleep may promote maladaptive habits, such as napping and excessive time in bed. Treatment consists of adapting the cognitive therapy method developed for depression: identify specific dysfunctional sleep cognitions, challenge their validity, substitute more rational, and moderate attitudes.
Sleep education and sleep hygiene	Sleep education is a didactic procedure designed to educate individuals about reasonable, age-appropriate sleep goals. Sleep hygiene refers to promoting daytime habits that are sleep friendly and discouraging daytime practices that are sleep disruptive. Following are typical sleep hygiene rules. 1. Exercise regularly early or midday 2. Regularize bedtime 3. Regularize wake time 4. Minimize caffeine 5. Minimize naps 6. Minimize exercise within 2 h of bedtime 7. Avoid smoking within 2 h of bedtime 8. Avoid alcohol within 2 h of bedtime 9. Avoid heavy meals within 2 h of bedtime

Abbreviations: SE, sleep efficiency percent; TIB, time in bed; TST, total sleep time.

recently reported that a self-administered, home-based video version was as effective as the therapist-delivered CBT treatment. A third study by the Rybarczyk group is the first in this area to use a placebo condition [68]. A CBT package applied to medical comorbid insomnia attained significantly greater gains than a credible placebo wellness program on a number of quantitative and qualitative variables including SE, SOL, WASO, napping, Pittsburgh Sleep Quality Index, and Dysfunctional Beliefs and Attitudes About Sleep.

Cognitive behavioral therapy for hypnotic-dependent insomnia

Chronic use of hypnotic or sedative medication can produce hypnotic-dependent insomnia, a disorder characterized by dependence on sleep medication, continued insomnia, and rebound insomnia and anxiety when sleep medication is abruptly discontinued. Focusing on studies of older adults with hypnotic-dependent insomnia, two studies treated hypnotic-dependent insomnia individuals with CBT without supplementation of a specific withdrawal plan [53,59]. Positive sleep change was obtained along with reduced medication consumption. More recent studies with older adults have shown that a gradual hypnotic withdrawal plan is not likely to lead to worsening sleep, and when supplemented with CBT, sleep improvement can be expected [56,69–71].

Discussion

Insomnia in the elderly exhibits high prevalence, but is amenable to intervention. Available assessment or differential diagnosis procedures are satisfactory. Both pharmacologic and behavioral interventions have proven use. Hypnotics are conveniently available and require little effort in administration, features that pose an obstacle in the use of CBT. In contrast, whereas the safety profile of CBT for OAWI has never been questioned, long-term safety of hypnotics still needs to be evaluated. Health care providers must weigh efficacy, convenience, adherence, and safety when considering the clinical management of insomnia among the elderly.

Although behavioral scientists were slow to address insomnia aggressively in this age group, great progress has been made in the past 15 years. Once studied systematically and earnestly, the early negative biases (that older adults would be refractory to treatment, that comorbidity would erode the therapeutic response, and that the complexities of managing the untoward effects of pharmacotherapy would be an insurmountable obstacle to CBT) proved unwarranted.

The differential diagnosis of insomnia and sleep apnea by interview alone is inadequate. Given the escalating rate of both these disorders in older adults, compounded by the potential for hypnotics to exacerbate undetected sleep apnea or daytime impairment [72,73], this is a matter of serious concern. Although routine PSG assessment is not recommended in the clinic [18], it may have a more important clinical role with OAWI. If insomnia studies, particularly with older adults, wish to ensure that they are not mistakenly studying people with sleep apnea, routine PSG for screening purposes may be justified in the research setting.

Insomnia in the elderly, an area that once had great difficulty attracting the interest of clinicians and scientists, is now thriving in both arenas. Current domains of fertile inquiry include expanding the availability and dissemination of CBT services, effectiveness trials that bridge the gap between carefully controlled clinical efficacy trials and routine care, and more clearly articulating the connection between sleep and daytime functioning.

References

[1] Lichstein KL, Durrence HH, Riedel BW, et al. Epidemiology of sleep: age, gender, and ethnicity. Mahwah (NJ): Erlbaum; 2004.

[2] Taylor DJ, Lichstein KL, Durrence HH. Insomnia as a health risk factor. Behav Sleep Med 2003; 1:227–47.

[3] Ohayon MM. Epidemiology of insomnia: what we know and what we still need to learn. Sleep Med Rev 2002;6:97–111.

[4] Morgan K. Sleep and aging. In: Lichstein KL, Morin CM, editors. Treatment of late-life insomnia. Thousand Oaks (CA): Sage; 2000. p. 3–36.

[5] Morin CM. Insomnia: psychological assessment and management. New York: Guilford; 1993.

[6] Ohayon MM, Zulley J, Guilleminault C, et al. How age and daytime activities are related to insomnia in the general population: consequences for older people. J Am Geriatr Soc 2001; 49:360–6.

[7] Durrence HH, Lichstein KL. The sleep of African Americans: a comparative review. Behav Sleep Med 2006;4:29–44.

[8] Chambers MJ, Keller B. Alert insomniacs: are they really sleep deprived? Clin Psychol Rev 1993;13:649–66.

[9] Bastien CH, Vallieres A, Morin CM. Precipitating factors of insomnia. Behav Sleep Med 2004; 2:50–62.

[10] Ancoli-Israel S, Cooke JR. Prevalence and comorbidity of insomnia and effect on functioning in elderly populations. J Am Geriatr Soc 2005; 53:S264–71.

[11] Morin CM, Gramling SE. Sleep patterns and aging: comparison of older adults with and

without insomnia complaints. Psychol Aging 1989;4:290–4.

[12] Riedel BW, Lichstein KL. Insomnia and daytime functioning. Sleep Med Rev 2000;4:277–98.

[13] Bonnet MH, Arand DL. 24-hour metabolic rate in insomniacs and matched normal sleepers. Sleep 1995;18:581–8.

[14] Zepelin H, McDonald CS, Zammit GK. Effects of age on auditory awakening thresholds. J Gerontol 1984;39:294–300.

[15] Hohagen F, Rink K, Kappler C, et al. Prevalence and treatment of insomnia in general practice: a longitudinal study. Eur Arch Psychiatry 1993; 242:329–36.

[16] Schramm E, Hohagen F, Kappler C, et al. Mental comorbidity of chronic insomnia in general practice attenders using DSM-III-R. Acta Psychiatr Scand 1995;91:7–10.

[17] Shorr R, Bauwens S. Diagnosis and treatment of outpatient insomnia by psychiatric and non-psychiatric physicians. Am J Med 1992; 93:78–82.

[18] Littner M, Hirshkowitz M, Kramer M, et al. Practice parameters for using polysomnography to evaluate insomnia: an update. Sleep 2003; 26:754–60.

[19] Edinger JD, Hoelscher TJ, Webb MD, et al. Polysomnographic assessment of DIMS: empirical evaluation of its diagnostic value. Sleep 1989; 12:315–22.

[20] Lichstein KL, Riedel BW, Lester KW, et al. Occult sleep apnea in a recruited sample of older adults with insomnia. J Consult Clin Psychol 1999; 67:405–10.

[21] Buysse DJ, Reynolds CF III. Pharmacologic treatment. In: Lichstein KL, Morin CM, editors. Treatment of late-life insomnia. Thousand Oaks (CA): Sage; 2000. p. 231–67.

[22] Ohayon MM, Caulet M, Priest RG, et al. Psychotropic medication consumption patterns in the UK general population. J Clin Epidemiol 1998; 51:273–83.

[23] Maggi S, Langlois JA, Minicuci N, et al. Sleep complaints in community-dwelling older persons: prevalence, associated factors, and reported causes. J Am Geriatr Soc 1998;46:161–8.

[24] Hedner J, Yaeche R, Emilien G, et al. Zaleplon shortens subjective sleep latency and improves subjective sleep quality in elderly patients with insomnia. Int J Geriatr Psychiatry 2000; 15:704–12.

[25] Scott MA, Stigleman S. What is the best hypnotic for use in the elderly? J Fam Pract 2003;52:976–8.

[26] Israel AG, Kramer JA. Safety of zaleplon in the treatment of insomnia. Ann Pharmacother 2002;36:852–9.

[27] Ancoli-Israel S, Richardson GS, Mangano RM, et al. Long-term use of sedative hypnotics in older patients with insomnia. Sleep Med 2005; 6:107–13.

[28] Olubodun JO, Ochs HR, von Moltke LL, et al. Pharmacokinetic properties of zolpidem in elderly and young adults: possible modulation by testosterone in men. Br J Clin Pharmacol 2003;56:297–304.

[29] Albrecht S, Ihmsen H, Hering W, et al. The effect of age on the pharmokinetics and pharmacodynamics of midazolam. Clin Pharmacol Ther 1999;65:630–9.

[30] Haimov I, Lavie P, Laudon M, et al. Melatonin replacement therapy of elderly insomniacs. Sleep 1995;18:598–603.

[31] Buscemi N, Vandermeer B, Hooton N, et al. The efficacy and safety of exogenous melatonin for primary sleep disorders: a meta-analysis. J Gen Intern Med 2005;20:1151–8.

[32] Erman M, Seidan D, Zammit G, et al. An efficacy, safety, and dose-response study of ramelteon in patients with chronic primary insomnia. Sleep Med 2006;7:17–24.

[33] Mendelson WB. A review of the evidence for the efficacy and safety of trazodone in insomnia. J Clin Psychiatry 2005;66:469–76.

[34] Walsh JK. Drugs used to treat insomnia in 2002: regulatory-based rather than evidence-based medicine. Sleep 2004;27:1441–2.

[35] Ancoli-Israel S. Sleep and aging: prevalence of disturbed sleep and treatment considerations in older adults. J Clin Psychiatry 2005;66:24–30.

[36] State-of-the-Science Panel. National Institutes of Health State of the Science Conference Statement: manifestations and management of chronic insomnia in adults, June 13–15, 2005. Sleep 2005;28:1049–57.

[37] Morgan K, Clarke D. Longitudinal trends in late-life insomnia: implications for prescribing. Age Ageing 1997;26:179–84.

[38] Lebowitz BD, Niederehe G. Concepts and issues in mental health and aging. In: Birren JE, Sloane RB, Cohen GD, editors. Handbook of mental health and aging. 2nd edition. San Diego: Academic Press; 1992. p. 3–26.

[39] Neutel CI. Risk of traffic accident injury after a prescription for a benzodiazepine. Ann Epidemiol 1995;5:239–44.

[40] Ray WA, Griffin MR, Downey W. Benzodiazepines of long and short elimination half-life and the risk of hip fracture. JAMA 1989;262:3303–7.

[41] Herings RMC, Stricker BHC, de Boer A, et al. Benzodiazepines and the risk of falling leading to femur fractures: dosage more important than elimination half-life. Arch Intern Med 1995; 155:1801–7.

[42] Lichstein KL. Clinical relaxation strategies. New York: Wiley; 1988.

[43] Bootzin RR, Epstein DR. Stimulus control. In: Lichstein KL, Morin CM, editors. Treatment of late-life insomnia. Thousand Oaks (CA): Sage; 2000. p. 167–84.

[44] Spielman AJ, Saskin P, Thorpy MJ. Treatment of chronic insomnia by restriction of time in bed. Sleep 1987;10:45–56.

[45] Lichstein KL, Riedel BW, Wilson NM, et al. Relaxation and sleep compression for late-life

insomnia: a placebo-controlled trial. J Consult Clin Psychol 2001;69:227–39.

[46] Bélanger L, Morin CM, Savard J., Clinical management of insomnia using cognitive therapy. Behav Sleep Med, in press.

[47] Riedel BW. Sleep hygiene. In: Lichstein KL, Morin CM, editors. Treatment of late-life insomnia. Thousand Oaks (CA): Sage; 2000. p. 125–46.

[48] Irwin MR, Cole JC, Nicassio PM. Comparative meta-analysis of behavioral interventions for insomnia and their efficacy in middle-aged adults and in older adults 55 + years of age. Health Psychol 2006;25:3–14.

[49] Engle-Friedman M, Bootzin RR, Hazlewood L, et al. An evaluation of behavioral treatments for insomnia in the older adult. J Clin Psychol 1992;4:77–90.

[50] Morin CM, Colecchi C, Stone J, et al. Behavioral and pharmacological therapies for late-life insomnia: a randomized controlled trial. JAMA 1999;281:991–9.

[51] Morin CM, Kowatch RA, Barry T, et al. Cognitive-behavior therapy for late-life insomnia. J Consult Clin Psychol 1993;61:137–46.

[52] Friedman L, Bliwise DL, Yesavage JA, et al. A preliminary study comparing sleep restriction and relaxation treatments for insomnia in older adults. J Gerontol 1991;46:1–8.

[53] Lichstein KL, Johnson RS. Relaxation for insomnia and hypnotic medication use in older women. Psychol Aging 1993;8:103–11.

[54] Davies R, Lacks P, Storandt M, et al. Countercontrol treatment of sleep-maintenance insomnia in relation to age. Psychol Aging 1986; 3:233–8.

[55] Friedman L, Benson K, Noda A, et al. An actigraphic comparison of sleep restrictions and sleep hygiene treatments for insomnia in older adults. J Geriatr Psychiatry Neurol 2000; 13:17–27.

[56] Morin CM, Bastien C, Guay B, et al. Insomnia and chronic use of benzodiazepines: a randomized clinical trial of supervised tapering, cognitive-behavioral therapy, and a combined approach to facilitate benzodiazepine discontinuation. Am J Psychiatry 2004;161:332–42.

[57] Edinger JD, Hoelscher TJ, Marsh GR, et al. A cognitive-behavioral therapy for sleep-maintenance insomnia in older adults. Psychol Aging 1992; 7:282–9.

[58] Pallesen S, Nordhus IH, Kvale G, et al. Behavioral treatment of insomnia in older adults: an open clinical trial comparing two interventions. Behav Res Ther 2003;41:31–48.

[59] Morin CM, Azrin NH. Behavioral and cognitive treatments of geriatric insomnia. J Consult Clin Psychol 1988;56:748–53.

[60] Puder R, Lacks P, Bertelson AD, et al. Short-term stimulus control treatment of insomnia in older adults. Behav Ther 1983;14:424–9.

[61] McCurry SM, Logsdon RG, Vitiello MV, et al. Successful behavioral treatment for reported sleep problems in elderly caregivers of dementia patients: a controlled study. J Gerontol 1998;53B:P122–9.

[62] Riedel BW, Lichstein KL, Dwyer WO. Sleep compression and sleep education for older insomniacs: self-help vs. therapist guidance. Psychol Aging 1995;10:54–63.

[63] Lichstein KL, McCrae CS, Wilson NM. Secondary insomnia: diagnostic issues, cognitive-behavioral treatment, and future directions. In: Perlis ML, Lichstein KL, editors. Treating sleep disorders. Hoboken (NJ): Wiley; 2003. p. 286–304.

[64] Lichstein KL, Nau SD, McCrae CS, et al. Psychological and behavioral treatments for secondary insomnias. In: Kryger MH, Roth T, Dement WC, editors. Principles and practice of sleep medicine. 4th edition. Philadelphia: WB Saunders; 2005. p. 738–48.

[65] Lichstein KL, Wilson NM, Johnson CT. Psychological treatment of secondary insomnia. Psychol Aging 2000;15:232–40.

[66] Rybarczyk B, Lopez M, Benson R, et al. Efficacy of two behavioral treatment programs for comorbid geriatric insomnia. Psychol Aging 2002; 17:288–98.

[67] Rybarczyk B, Lopez M, Schelble K, et al. Home-based video CBT for comorbid geriatric insomnia: a pilot study using secondary data analyses. Behav Sleep Med 2005;3:158–75.

[68] Rybarczyk B, Stepanski E, Fogg L, et al. A placebo-controlled test of cognitive-behavioral therapy for comorbid insomnia in older adults. J Consult Clin Psychol 2005;73:1164–74.

[69] Baillargeon L, Landreville P, Verreault R, et al. Discontinuation of benzodiazepines among older insomnia adults treated with cognitive-behavioural therapy combined with gradual tapering: a randomized trial. Can Med Assoc J 2003;169:1015–20.

[70] Lichstein KL, Nau S, Wilson NM, et al. Behavioral management of hypnotic dependent insomnia in older adults. Sleep 2005;28:A248.

[71] Morgan K, Dixon S, Mathers N, et al. Psychological treatment for insomnia in the management of long-term hypnotic drug use: a pragmatic randomized controlled trial. Br J Gen Pract 2003; 53:923–8.

[72] George CFP. Perspectives on the management of insomnia in patients with chronic respiratory disorders. Sleep 2000;23(Suppl 1):31–5.

[73] Lu B, Budhiraja R, Parthasarathy S. Sedating medications and undiagnosed obstructive sleep apnea: physician determinants and patient consequences. J Clin Sleep Med 2005;1:367–71.

SLEEP
MEDICINE
CLINICS

Sleep Med Clin 1 (2006) 231–245

ELSEVIER
SAUNDERS

Comorbidities: Psychiatric, Medical, Medications, and Substances

Steven R. Barczi, MD[a,b,*], Timothy M. Juergens, MD[c,d]

- Psychiatric conditions that disturb sleep
  Depressive disorders
  Bipolar affective disorder
  Caregiving and bereavement
  Anxiety disorders
- Substance abuse
  Alcohol dependence
  Caffeine
  Tobacco and nicotine
  *Neurotransmitter overlap between
    psychiatric illness, substance use, and
    sleep*
- Medical conditions that disturb sleep
  Pain
  Arthritis
  *Acid reflux and gastroesophageal reflux
    disease*

  Heart disease
  Chronic lung disease
  Diabetes and endocrine disorders
  Renal and urologic diseases
  Cancer
- Medications that disturb sleep
  *Medications that promote daytime
    sleepiness*
  *Medications that activate or stimulate the
    central nervous system*
  *Medications that affect sleep by
    worsening other conditions*
  *Medications that can exacerbate primary
    sleep disorders*
  *Medications that affect sleep architecture
    by other mechanisms*
- Summary
- References

Sleep is a highly regulated and essential behavior across the lifespan. It is susceptible to the influence of many endogenous and exogenous factors. A number of studies have investigated the risk factors and correlates of sleep disturbances in older adults. Results support that these sleep difficulties are more strongly associated with psychosocial and health

factors rather than aging [1–3]. These findings have important implications when one considers the disease prevalence in populations over age 60 (Fig. 1) and the frequency of comorbid medical and psychiatric conditions in this group. These health problems seem to have additive effects when considering the likelihood of concomitant sleep

This work was supported by the Madison VA GRECC and Middleton VA Hospital
[a] Section of Geriatrics, University of Wisconsin School of Medicine and Public Health, 2870 University Ave., Suite 106, Madison, WI 53705, USA
[b] Madison VA Geriatrics, Research, Education and Clinical Center, Wm. S. Middleton Veterans Hospital, 2500 Overlook Terrace, Madison, WI 53705, USA
[c] Department of Psychiatry, Wisconsin Psychiatric Institute & Clinics, 6001 Research Park Blvd., Madison, WI 53719, USA
[d] Clinical Sleep Laboratory, Geriatric Psychiatry, Wm. S. Middleton Veterans Hospital, 2500 Overlook Terrace, Madison, WI 53705, USA
* Corresponding author. Madison VA GRECC, 2500 Overlook Terrace, Madison, WI 53705.
E-mail address: steven.barczi@va.gov (S.R. Barczi).

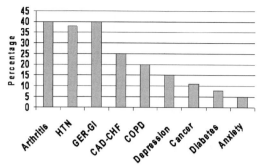

Fig. 1. Disease prevalence in adults 65 years and older. (*Data from* Guralnik JM. Assessing the impact of co-morbidity in the older population. Ann Epidemiol 1996;6:376–80; and Boult C, Kane RL, Louis TA, et al. Chronic conditions that lead to functional limitation in the elderly. J Gerontol 1994;49:M28–36.) CAD-CHF, coronary artery disease–congestive heart failure; COPD, chronic obstructive pulmonary disease; HTN, hypertension; GER-GI, gastroesophageal reflux–gastrointestinal.

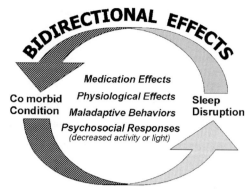

Fig. 2. Bidirectional effects between illness, sleep, and medications.

complaints. The 2003 "Sleep in America" survey found that 36% of people age 65 years and older without comorbid illnesses had sleep problems, 52% with one to three comorbidities had sleep disturbances, and 69% of those with four or more comorbidities had disturbed sleep [3]. The self-perceived quality of these respondents' sleep was also inversely proportional to the number of their comorbidities [3].

Secondary insomnia is frequently used to describe the sleep changes associated with medical or psychiatric diagnoses. It implies a causal relationship between the illness and the accompanying sleep disruption. The International Classification of Sleep Disorders, the nosologic hierarchy used by sleep clinicians, was recently revised with substantive changes made in areas relevant to secondary insomnia [4]. The new International Classification of Sleep Disorders-2 includes two categories that encompass the breadth of secondary insomnia: Other Insomnia Due to Mental Disorder, and Other Insomnia Due to a Known Physiological Condition. Given the inconsistency of scientific evidence for many of these associations, expert consensus recommends that the term "comorbid insomnia" be used rather than "secondary insomnia." The 2005 National Institutes of Health State-of-the-Science Conference on Insomnia proposed using the diagnosis of comorbid insomnia when an illness coexists with sleep changes but the dynamics of cause and effect are not proved [5]. This complex interplay between illness, sleep, and medications is depicted in Fig. 2 with increasing evidence that poor sleep also influences disease status and outcomes. Because comorbid disease

and medication use are so common in older persons, multiple factors may contribute to complaints in this group. This multifactorial and bidirectional relationship is important to recognize and address as clinicians evaluate sleep disturbances in older adults.

The specific relationship between an illness and the neuropsychologic, biochemical, and hormonal sequelae that contribute to sleep decay remains speculative in many cases. Frequently, health conditions produce symptoms of discomfort or emotional distress that may lead to a sympathetic response, hypothalamic-pituitary-adrenal activity, and ultimately activation of neural systems to produce arousal [6,7]. Psychologic factors of hyperarousal, stress response, predisposing personality traits, and maladaptive attitudes can perpetuate sleep changes seen during illness in later life [8]. Acute pathophysiologic changes, such as hypoxemia, metabolic derangements, fever, or systemic inflammatory responses, can also lead to characteristic alterations in sleep-wake patterns [9].

The viewpoint on the management of comorbid insomnia is evolving. Historically, if a sleep problem was attributed to an associated mental or physical illness, then the primary focus was on optimizing treatment of that underlying health concern. This placed an emphasis on correcting metabolic, neurochemical, and physiologic derangement in illness with the hope that sleep improves. The role for cognitive-behavioral therapies and hypnotics was de-emphasized in this situation because pathophysiologic mechanisms were believed to be different than those seen in primary insomnia. Many sleep authorities believe that this led to undertreatment of the accompanying insomnia. More recently, a series of controlled trials have demonstrated the efficacy of cognitive behavior therapy in managing insomnia complaints in a variety of different illnesses. On these grounds, some argue that all comorbid or secondary insomnia should be treated the same as primary insomnia with cognitive behavior therapy and, when indicated, adjunctive hypnotic therapy [10]. Although the most efficacious approach remains to be determined, it seems prudent that a multifaceted intervention that equally emphasizes optimizing comorbid health issues using cognitive behavior therapy and hypnotics is justified.

Psychiatric conditions that disturb sleep

People with psychiatric illness commonly complain of sleep problems, and sleep disruption is a part of the diagnostic criteria of many psychiatric disorders. These mental health conditions are prevalent in the geriatric population as shown in Table 1. Psychiatric and somatic symptoms, and the level of physical activity, can significantly and independently increase the risk of insomnia in older clinical patients [11]. Sleep electroencephalogram (EEG) findings in acutely ill psychiatric patients show reduced sleep efficiency, prolonged sleep latency, decreased total night sleep, and increased arousals [12]. Conversely, people in the general population with sleep difficulties demonstrate a higher prevalence of psychiatric disorders and symptoms compared with those without sleep complaints [13,14]. In clinic and hospital practice, this

Table 1: **Prevalence of psychiatric diagnoses in the elderly**

Mood disorder	Major depressive disorder	1%–2% **(10%)**
	Dysthymia	3%
	Minor depression	15% **(30%–37%)**
	Bipolar affective disorder	1%
Anxiety disorder	Generalized anxiety disorder	4%–6%
	Panic disorder Posttraumatic stress disorder	<1%
Schizophrenia		1%
Alcohol use disorder		1%–2% **(5%–44%)**
Nicotine use disorder		12%

% indicates community population.
(BOLD), general clinic population.
Women greater than men for all disorders except alcohol or drug abuse.
Data from Coffey CE, Cummings JL, editors. Textbook of geriatric neuropsychiatry. 2nd edition. Washington: American Psychiatric Press; 2000.

correlation of psychiatric conditions in people with insomnia is even stronger, where 50% to 69% of patients with insomnia in primary care settings had a psychiatric disorder [15,16]. Part of this strong clinical correlation may reflect the high overlap of medical conditions with psychiatric conditions, especially in later life.

Depressive disorders

Depression is associated with sleep disturbances in the elderly general and clinical populations [1], with insomnia in the primary care setting showing a stronger association to depression than any other medical condition [17]. In the geriatric population, sleep difficulties increase the risk for comorbid depression [18]. Sleep complaints also foreshadow the onset of depression in older adults, with insomnia a strong risk factor for future depression in elderly patients not currently depressed [19]. Insomnia at baseline and 1 year later increased the risk of depression onset by eight times [20] in one elderly cohort.

Between 63% and 80% of depressed adults and older adults complain of difficulty falling or staying asleep, or being tired in the day [21,22]. These subjective sleep complaints can persist beyond the resolution of depressive symptoms [23]. Prevalence of symptoms is comparable between genders [24]. Furthermore, about 8% of persons in the general population complain of hypersomnia, which is also predictive of onset of depression, particularly for bipolar affective disorder or seasonal affective disorder [13]. Older adults endorsing daytime sleepiness are also more likely to report depressive symptoms [25].

Objective sleep findings in older adults with depression include prolonged time to sleep onset, decreased sleep efficiency, poor sleep continuity, and increased early morning awakening. Additionally, total sleep time drops with relative increases in stage 1 and 2 sleep in the setting of decreased slow wave sleep (SWS). There is also shortened rapid eye movement (REM) latency, a longer first REM period, and increased total REM sleep and REM density [12,26]. Although these patterns of sleep change are well described in depressed persons, there is no single sleep variable that is currently specific enough to distinguish depression from other psychiatric disorders by polysomnography [12]. Further, longitudinal studies of EEG sleep profiles in depression show state and trait characteristics, meaning some of these characteristics can change over time [27]. Such differentiation may play a role in identifying those at high risk for depression, predicting future episodes of depression, and assessing the response to pharmacologic and behavioral treatments.

Bipolar affective disorder

A distinguishing feature of bipolar affective disorder is a manic episode, which involves a prolonged time of increased activity with minimal sleep. Insomnia can precede manic episodes as a first symptom in up to 77% of cases [28]. Although first-onset mania can occur in the elderly, this warrants suspicion of medical illness or drug effects as contributors. Of those with first onset of mania in later life, many have a history of previous depression [29]. Moreover, sleep loss may trigger manic episodes, emphasizing a need clinically to monitor sleep changes, and address sleep-disrupting factors to decrease such exacerbations [28].

Caregiving and bereavement

Caregivers of persons with dementia or disability have an increased risk for depressive disorders, and the sleep problems that accompany that depression. Spouses of patients with Alzheimer's disease objectively slept less than older noncaregivers, and subjectively reported more sleep problems and functional impairment as a result of poor sleep [30]. There are also situational needs that the caregiver must respond to, such as nocturnal wandering in a demented spouse, which may fragment sleep. This situation puts the caregiver at risk for long-term partial sleep deprivation that may explain why one of the strongest factors in deciding to institutionalize a spouse or family member with dementia is poor overnight sleep of the affected individual [31]. Baseline complicated grief scores of recently widowed elderly individuals were significantly associated with sleep difficulties at 18-month follow-up [32]. It is also important to assess sleep in caregivers during bereavement, because disrupted sleep may be predictive of current and future depression and offer a potential target of treatment.

Anxiety disorders

Common anxiety conditions in older adults include generalized anxiety disorder and panic disorder. Most anxiety conditions in the elderly are continued disorders from earlier in their life, with the exception of some increased agoraphobia. Although not a specific anxiety disorder, many older adults can have increased anxiety when faced with chronic health conditions; functional limitations; or concerns about issues, such as safety or finances. Certain health problems and the medications used to treat them may contribute to neurochemical changes or increased adrenergic drive. In Parkinson's disease, for example, increased anxiety may be partly caused by the neurodegenerative process and also related to the patient's response to medications and their fear of falling.

Generalized anxiety disorder, a condition of persistent hyperarousal, is the most prevalent condition of subjects complaining of insomnia who have a mental health diagnosis in the adult population [33]. Sleep disturbance is a core symptom in the diagnosis of generalized anxiety disorder, and is endorsed in about two thirds of patients with this diagnosis [34]. Objective findings include increased time until sleep onset, frequent awakenings, decreased sleep efficiency, and reduced total sleep time, with less consistent findings of more stage 2, and decreased SWS [12,35]. In the elderly, about 80% of people with generalized anxiety disorder also have a depressive disorder, making specific objective sleep findings difficult to interpret.

Sleep complaints are also common in people with panic disorder, including trouble falling asleep, disturbed and restless sleep, and nocturnal panic attacks. Although complaints are high, objective studies are not as strongly supportive of the subjective complaints and are not consistent between studies [12,36,37]. Nocturnal panic attacks occur at least weekly in 18% to 45% of panic disorder patients [34,38]. These attacks are characterized by similar symptom severity and duration of daytime panic attacks and occur usually in transition from stage 2 to SWS [39]. Accordingly, a clinical history may detail an occurrence usually in the first few hours of sleep, and not necessarily associated with dreams. People with nocturnal panic attacks have higher rates of insomnia and depression than people with panic disorder without nighttime episodes [40]. Sleep panic attacks can present with a clinical history similar to sleep apnea, parasomnias, gastroesophageal reflux disease, and posttraumatic stress disorder (PTSD), a consideration during the workup of sleep complaints.

Sleep disturbance commonly occurs in PTSD with rates from 44% to 91%, including insomnia, nonrestorative sleep, and nightmares [41]. Frequent nightmares are reported in about two thirds of patients with PTSD with REM and non-REM arousals [42]. The most specific findings in PTSD are middle insomnia, recurrent awakenings, and excessive body movement [43]. Objective studies, however, have not been consistent with each other or with the subjective reporting regarding awakenings, continuity, hyperalertness, or nocturnal movements.

PTSD has shown an increased overlap with some primary sleep conditions, including sleep apnea. People with PTSD were more likely to have sleep apnea [44]. Importantly, treatment of sleep apnea in people with PTSD has been shown to improve PTSD symptoms. In older adults with PTSD, many have had symptoms for years with this condition continuing in later life. They may also be more predisposed to exacerbations or new onset of symptoms in the context of worsening health conditions, confronted with death of friends or spouses, and their own mortality. Further, previous mechanisms for coping may be limited, such as a man who works himself to fatigue, or runs to relieve tension, but now has retired or has pain that limits his exercise ability. Cognitive impairment, which is more likely to occur with increased age, also may impair coping mechanisms in a person at risk for PTSD.

Substance abuse

Common substances of abuse that are legal (alcohol, nicotine, caffeine) and illicit (stimulants, marijuana, opiates) can disrupt sleep. There is a high amount of substance use in older adults with comorbid psychiatric conditions and health problems, with rates of some of the overlap shown in Fig. 3. This use likely further contributes and complicates sleep disturbances, and warrants clinical assessment and treatment as a potential route of improving sleep complaints. Among those with a mental disorder, the lifetime prevalence of an addictive disorder not including nicotine or caffeine dependence is 29%, mostly accounted for by alcohol [45].

Alcohol dependence

Although the overall use of alcohol declines with age, there are many older adults with alcohol problems. Community rates of alcohol dependence in the geriatric population are 2% to 3% of men and 1% of women [46]. Rates are much higher at 4% to 23% in older patients in the clinic and hospital

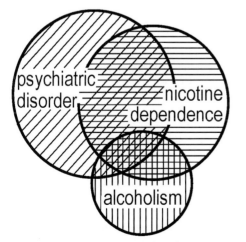

Fig. 3. Substance abuse with comorbid psychiatric conditions. (*Data from* Atkinson R. Substance abuse. In: Coffey C, Cummings J, editors. Textbook of geriatric neuropsychiatry. 2nd edition. Washington: American Psychiatry Press; 2000. p. 367–400.)

setting, likely caused by the increased comorbid medical disorders that accompany alcohol dependence [47]. Elderly alcoholics are quite likely to have other substance-related comorbidities, which may further impair their sleep, including nicotine dependence (50%–70%) and dependence on prescribed sedatives, anxiolytics, and opioid analgesic (2%–14%) [47]. Although most older persons who abuse alcohol had onset of drinking problems earlier in life, about one third of patients with alcohol use disorders have onset after middle life. Compared with earlier-onset alcoholics, those with later onset tend to have less family history, less psychiatric comorbidity, and higher socioeconomic status [48].

Alcoholics report high rates of insomnia with ranges from 36% to 72% in inpatient and outpatient studies. In a recent Canadian study of clinic subjects with subjective sleep disturbance, 24% had alcohol problems, with 13% meeting dependence, compared with 2.2% in the general population [49]. There is a paucity of data on the sleep of geriatric patients with alcohol use disorders, with much of the information discussed in the following paragraphs coming from adult population studies that may or may not have had older adults enrolled.

After excluding those with other psychiatric disorders, subjects with insomnia had a significantly increased likelihood (odds ratio, 2.3) of developing alcohol abuse compared with adults without insomnia [50]. The direction of sleep disruption and alcohol dependence seems bidirectional, because a number of alcoholics report, at least retrospectively, that their sleep difficulty preceded their alcohol problems. Fifty percent of alcoholics reported sleep problems before the onset of alcohol dependence [51]. During drinking, there are the acute affects of alcohol, and the chronic effects seen with habitual use. Although sleep complaints vary, difficulty falling asleep is reported as the most significant factor associated with substance use [52]. Alcoholics over the age of 55 had higher sleep latency, lower sleep efficiency, and lower SWS when compared with younger alcoholics and with nonalcoholics of both age groups [53]. In acute withdrawal, polysomnogram findings include increased sleep latency, decreased total sleep time, and increased REM percentage.

Although many people describe that alcohol helps them to fall asleep, alcohol-induced sleep may be of poorer quality and shorter duration. Increased arousals occur as the blood-alcohol level falls in the hours after alcohol intake, with resultant middle insomnia [54]. Acute alcohol intake also disrupts the circadian cycle and body temperature, stimulating the release of cortisol and interfering with nocturnal release of growth hormone. Acute alcohol intake affects multiple neurotransmitter systems, including acetylcholine, glutamate, γ-aminobutyric acid, norepinephrine, dopamine, and adenosine. Chronic consumption results in long-term alterations and adaptation of the neurotransmitter systems affected by alcohol. All these factors may contribute to disrupted sleep. Alcohol is speculated to decrease tone in upper airway musculature and lowers the arousal threshold, putting those who drink at higher risk of apneas and more severe oxygen desaturation during apneas after acute intake.

Sleep disruption commonly continues in alcoholics long after they stop drinking, and may predict relapse. Alcoholics who have been abstinent for 3 to 6 weeks have worse sleep than nonalcoholics by polysomnographic assessment [55]. Even after 2.5 years of abstinence, sleep abnormalities can persist [56]. During abstinence, sleep problems may increase the risk of relapse. The presence of insomnia and sleep architecture changes are significant factors predicting alcohol relapse [53]. In abstinent male alcoholics, 3% of men under age 40 years had sleep-disordered breathing compared with 25% of men between ages 40 and 59 and 75% of those above age 60 [57]. Abstinent alcoholics also have higher rates of periodic limb movements of sleep [58].

Alcoholics experience disrupted sleep before becoming alcoholics, during periods of drinking, in withdrawal, and in periods of acute and extended abstinence. Evidence suggests a bidirectional nature between alcohol dependence and insomnia. Clinical implications include that an older person with alcohol dependence is likely to still have disrupted sleep even after quitting alcohol and having sustained abstinence. Additionally, sleep problems may increase the risk of an older adult developing alcohol problems [59,60]. The higher alcohol use patterns among older patients with sleep complaints, compared with the general population, warrants appropriate screening and close tracking of sleep and comorbid sleep disorders in people during substance use and recovery.

Caffeine

The consumption of caffeine in coffee, tea, sodas, and medications is common in the elderly and may contribute to sleep disruption. Caffeine has stimulatory effects on the cerebral cortex and medullary centers, with blood levels peaking 15 to 45 minutes after intake and a half life of 3 to 7.5 hours. It is an adenosine antagonist and interferes with the role of adenosine on sleep promotion and maintenance. In adult populations, daytime sleepiness and insomnia were associated with high daily caffeine consumption [61]. Intake within 2 hours before

bedtime has been shown to disrupt sleep in adults on objective and subjective measures [62,63]. Adults over 67 years old on caffeine-containing medications report significantly more trouble falling asleep after controlling for multiple factors [64]. Hospital-dwelling elderly with a higher serum caffeine concentration reported sleep problems more than those with lower levels [65].

Tobacco and nicotine

Tobacco use is a chronic disease with multiple relapses, especially in older adults. Although the prevalence of smoking among older adults is lower than among younger persons, nearly 11% of Americans aged 65 and older smoke [66]. Several studies have suggested that insomnia and sleep apnea are more common in smokers, but establishing a causal relationship has been difficult [67]. Nicotine enhances acetylcholine neurotransmission in the basal forebrain and also dopamine release, thereby potentially shifting sleep-wake control mechanisms toward wakefulness [68]. Nicotine is associated with a dose-dependent reduction in REM and SWS, along with an increase in wakefulness and total sleep time [69]. In persons 50 to 84 years old, smokers endorsed more difficulty with sleep onset, staying asleep, and daytime sleep than nonsmokers. Those who smoked were much more likely to score high on depression scales than nonsmokers. In all age groups, smokers drank more caffeine and were more likely to be depressed [70]. The overlap of nicotine dependence in people with psychiatric conditions is an important issue. In clinic and community populations of depressed patients, 40% to 60% smoke, with even higher rates in PTSD and schizophrenia [71]. Quit rates are also much less in people with psychiatric disorders. Nevertheless, smoking cessation may be a viable intervention to improve sleep quality in older adults. When offered the tools they need, older smokers quit smoking at rates comparable with those of younger smokers.

Neurotransmitter overlap between psychiatric illness, substance use, and sleep

With these strong correlations, it is still not certain how psychiatric conditions and substance use disorders specifically relate to sleep disruption. One potential explanation is that sleep disruption and mood, anxiety, and substance disorders may be caused by a similar underlying process, including anatomic and neurotransmitter overlap. The high amount of overlap in brain areas and neurotransmitters involved in sleep, mood, anxiety, and substance disorders further supports this idea. Neuropeptides, such as corticotrophin-releasing factor, may disrupt both REM and non-REM sleep with subsequent arousals. Subjective stress is associated with insomnia and activation of the hypothalamic axis with increased corticotrophin-releasing factor and cortisol [7]. These neurotransmitters tend to inhibit sleep and increase alertness [72]. Elevated corticotrophin-releasing factor in anxiety conditions and in depression and substance use may be a common underlying mechanism. Serotonin plays an important role in sleep onset and maintenance. The greatest density of delta waves in sleep is observed in areas of the prefrontal cortex that are serotoninergically innervated [73]. Serotonergic neurons prevent cholinergic neurons from firing, which may delay REM. If a person has a decrease in serotonin in depression, such may explain some findings like decreased REM latency in depression. Ascending norepinephrine and dopamine tracts likely increase arousal, and subsequently disrupt sleep. Such may inhibit REM by keeping the normal sleep cycle from getting through the stages to REM. The potential roles and interactions of common neurotransmitters in sleep and some psychiatric conditions are demonstrated in Table 2.

Medical conditions that disturb sleep

There are many examples of how medical illness negatively influences sleep quantity and quality. Furthermore, a single illness may have several mechanisms that interfere with sleep and it may have different effects on sleep architecture in its acute versus chronic state. The immediate physiologic derangements or distress of an illness may produce transient sleep disruption. This sleep change can be perpetuated by maladaptive or learned responses to become a more protracted sleep difficulty that mirrors the profile of primary insomnia. Indirect support for this mechanism arises from recent randomized controlled trials demonstrating the efficacy for cognitive-behavioral therapies in the treatment of insomnia in a variety of medical illnesses [74]. Likewise, sleep disturbance may worsen symptoms in these disorders or even worsen the prognosis.

Pain

Pain is speculated as being one of the most common mechanisms for comorbid insomnia. Studies suggest that 25% to 50% of community-dwelling older persons have important pain problems [75]. In a general population of adults aged 55 to 84, 19% reported that pain disrupted their sleep at least a few nights per week and 12% reported almost nightly sleep fragmentation because of pain [3]. Among referral populations of patients with chronic pain, prevalence rates of insomnia can range between 50% and 70% [76]. Painful conditions are frequently associated with reduced total sleep time, reduced REM sleep, frequent brief arousals, and increased wakefulness after sleep onset [77]. There is a paucity of data reviewing pain and objective sleep parameters in older adults. The relationship between pain and sleep is complex; pain can disrupt sleep, and poor sleep may increase perceived pain intensity [78].

Arthritis

Osteoarthritis is a disabling disease that affects 50% to 80% of the elderly population [79]. Nearly 60% of those with arthritis experience pain during the night. Adults over age 65 with knee arthritis have been observed to have problems initiating sleep (31%); problems maintaining sleep (81%); and a tendency to awaken early in the morning (51%) [80]. Patients with rheumatoid arthritis have a 25% prevalence of restless legs syndrome [81]. Poor sleep in patients with osteoarthritis correlates with increased perceived pain, decreased self-rated health, poor functional status, and depression [80]. Furthermore, individuals with self-reported arthritis-related sleep disruption are more likely than those without sleep disturbance to pursue multiple sources of self-care and medical care [82]. A recent randomized clinical trial involving older adults with arthritis and comorbid insomnia demonstrated efficacy for cognitive-behavioral approaches in improving self-reported measures of sleep [83].

Table 2: Neurotransmitters in sleep, psychiatric disease, and substance abuse

	Normal REM sleep	Normal SWS sleep	Acute alcohol	Chronic alcohol	Depression or anxiety
Acetycholine	⬆	⬇	⬇	⬆	
GABA	⬇	⬆	⬆	⬇	⬇
Glutamate	⬆	⬇	⬇	⬆	⬆
Norepinephrine	⬇	⬇	⬆	⬆	⬇⬆
Dopamine	⬇	⬇	⬆	⬇	⬇
Adenosine	⬇	⬆	⬆	⬇	⬇

Abbreviations: GABA, γ-aminobutyric acid; REM, rapid eye movement; SWS, slow wave sleep.

Acid reflux and gastroesophageal reflux disease

Gastroesophageal reflux disease affects over 44% of the general population with monthly symptoms, and about 7% with daily symptoms [84]. These symptoms increase with aging with a prevalence of 10% for daily reflux symptoms for those older than 50 years [85]. In population surveys, between 50% and 70% of individuals with gastroesophageal reflux disease report nighttime symptoms and reduced sleep quality [86]. The relationship between disturbed sleep and gastroesophageal reflux disease is bidirectional: sleeping increases the likelihood of reflux, and reflux episodes often awaken the patient [87].

Patients with nighttime acid reflux may underestimate the degree of sleep disruption that occurs when objective measurements of pH and EEG arousal are compared with patient recollection the next morning [87]. Reviewing the patient history for nocturnal cough or wheezing as a surrogate for reflux is also important, because not all patients with overnight reflux experience classic chest pain, but their sleep may be disrupted nevertheless. Acid-suppression therapy for gastroesophageal reflux disease reduces nighttime heartburn symptoms, reduces gastroesophageal reflux disease–associated sleep disturbances, and improves subjective sleep quality and next day's work performance [88]. Finally, a mechanical link between the phrenoesophageal ligament and the lower esophageal sphincter may explain the coexistence of sleep apnea and reflux [89].

Heart disease

Coronary artery disease and congestive heart failure are a leading cause of morbidity and mortality in older adults. Many relationships exist between cardiac disease and sleep. Nocturnal ischemia, nighttime arrhythmias, and sleep-disordered breathing are all linked to altered sleep in underlying heart disease. A well-described circadian pattern of myocardial ischemia or infarction occurs early to midmorning and is ascribed to the catecholamine surge that accompanies awakening and upright status. In a retrospective analysis of 3309 adults presenting with acute coronary syndrome, however, 26% of the individuals were awakened from sleep [90]. On multivariate analysis only older age and lower left ventricular ejection fraction were independent predictors of a nocturnal acute coronary syndrome in this cohort. Chronic problems with sleep initiation correlate with an increased risk of death from coronary artery disease in male patients [91]. Finally, coronary artery bypass surgery is associated with protracted sleep disturbance up to 2 years

following the procedure [92]. The mechanism for this is unclear with occult heart failure, secondary mood issues, or brain microvascular ischemic changes as possibilities.

With increasing average life span and improvements in the management of acute coronary ischemia, it is projected that the incidence and prevalence of congestive heart failure will continue to rise. The classic sleep maintenance disturbance associated with congestive heart failure includes orthopnea, paroxysmal nocturnal dyspnea, nocturia, and sleep-disordered breathing. Increasingly, concomitant depression is also identified as a factor that contributes to sleep disturbance in elderly patients with congestive heart failure [93]. More than 50% of patients with moderate-to-severe congestive heart failure experience a form of periodic breathing called Cheyne-Stokes respiration. This may lead to increased sleep fragmentation, and an increase in daytime sleepiness [94]. When reviewing risk factors for central sleep apnea and obstructive sleep apnea in men and women with congestive heart failure, age over 60 years is an independent predictor for obstructive sleep apnea in both genders and for central sleep apnea in women [95]. More severe nighttime periodic breathing occurring in heart failure correlates with worse prognosis and increased cardiac death [94]. It is also suggested that sleep apnea exposes the failing heart to adverse adrenergic and hemodynamic loads, which may further worsen heart failure. Small trials that treat obstructive sleep apnea with continuous positive airway pressure have shown improvement in blood pressure and left ventricular systolic function in those with clinical heart failure [96].

Chronic lung disease

Chronic lung disease in the form of chronic obstructive pulmonary disease contributes to poor sleep continuity, and increased daytime sleepiness [97]. Approximately 25% of patients with chronic obstructive pulmonary disease complain of excessive sleepiness. The mean age of subjects in these studies was typically greater than 60 years consistent with the prevalence of chronic obstructive pulmonary disease in older adults. Coexistent obstructive sleep apnea and chronic obstructive pulmonary disease is termed "overlap syndrome." By retrospective analysis, the prevalence of overlap syndrome in chronic obstructive pulmonary disease was 12% and 41% in obstructive sleep apnea patients in an older Veterans Administration population [98]. Hypoxemia, which is common in chronic obstructive pulmonary disease during REM sleep, correlates with an increase in arousal and excessive daytime sleepiness. Although the use of oxygen therapy frequently corrects the underlying hypoxemia, it does not seem to improve sleep quality [99]. This suggests that other mechanisms, such as cough, impaired airflow, excessive respiratory secretions, or dyspnea, may be contributing to the observed sleep disruption. The use of ipratropium bromide inhaler improves sleep quality and duration presumably by improved airflow [100]. A small observational study of lung volume reduction surgery in older adults, mean age 63 years, also demonstrates improved polysomnographic sleep quality and nocturnal oxygenation [101].

Diabetes and endocrine disorders

Endocrine disorders, such as diabetes, and menopause are age-related with characteristic sleep difficulties. Thirty percent of diabetic patients demonstrate sleep maintenance disturbances, with the severity of disruption correlating with the degree of hyperglycemia [102]. Causes for this include nocturia, leg cramps, leg pain, and cough. Likewise, patients with diabetes have an increased prevalence of both restless legs syndrome and periodic limb movements of sleep [103]. A growing body of epidemiologic and experimental evidence links sleep apnea and disorders of glucose metabolism; however, the cause and effect relationship remains to be determined [104]. Recent work has demonstrated an independent association between sleep-disordered breathing and insulin resistance but treatment of sleep apnea has produced mixed results on insulin sensitivity and glycemic control [104]. In menopause, an estimated 40% to 50% of women report sleep difficulties following cessation of menstruation. Although some of this is transient during the time of acute hormonal changes, others have persisting symptoms for years later. Hormone-replacement therapy has been shown to improve subjective but not objective sleep measures [105].

Renal and urologic diseases

Sleep disruption is common in urologic and kidney diseases. Benign prostatic hyperplasia and prostate cancer are typically diseases of the aging male, steeply increasing with age. Urinary obstructive symptoms, including nocturia, are hallmarks for these conditions. Overactive bladder is characterized by urinary urgency, frequency, nocturia, and sometimes incontinence. It increases markedly with advancing age in both men and women [106]. Nocturia is a well-recognized etiology for sleep maintenance disturbance in later life and nighttime urination is often associated with poor quality of sleep and increased fatigue in the daytime [107].

Chronic kidney disease and end-stage renal disease have a steady increase over age 60 with a striking rise in prevalence beyond age 75 [108]. Overall prevalence of insomnia in hemodialysis patients ranges between 45% and 86% [109]. Fifty-seven percent of patients with end-stage renal disease report sleep maintenance problems, and 55% report early morning awakening. There are marked abnormalities seen in the sleep EEGs of patients with chronic kidney disease with overall reduction in total sleep time, decreased sleep efficiency caused by wakefulness after sleep onset, and reduced total REM [110]. This may reflect the impact of uremia and other metabolic derangements on brain function during sleep. Patients on hemodialysis have a higher prevalence of obstructive sleep apnea (which improves following dialysis); restless legs syndrome; periodic limb movements; early insomnia; and excessive daytime sleepiness [111–113]. In a study involving hemodialysis patients with a mean age of 65 years, the treatment of anemia of kidney disease with erythropoietin improved sleep quality by polysomnographic and subjective measures [114]. This seems to correspond to reduced numbers of periodic limb movements. Over 50% of hemodialysis patients endorse chronic pain and this is believed to be significantly associated with insomnia and depression in this condition [115].

Cancer

Cancer is primarily a disease of older persons insofar that 60% of all cancers are diagnosed after age 65 [116]. The prevalence of sleep problems in individuals with cancer is difficult to determine with wide variance based on type and stage of cancer. Large epidemiologic studies suggest that sleep problems are very common involving 55% to 87% of patients [117,118]. Cancer-related fatigue is a well-known symptom but its relationship to impaired sleep continues to be elucidated. It may be difficult for patients to distinguish fatigue from daytime sleepiness. Persons with cancer may have a baseline history of insomnia or a primary sleep disorder; or they may have sleep effects from the cancer, its treatment, or the psychologic response to the diagnosis [118]. Most of the studies reported in the literature report on sleep changes in early stage cancer [119]. Forty-four percent of hospitalized cancer patients are prescribed hypnotic therapy [120]. Sleep difficulties may be undertreated in persons with cancer because of underdiagnosis, minimization of importance in the context of the cancer diagnosis, concerns about drug-drug interactions, or reluctance to take more medication [121]. No controlled hypnotic trials have been conducted to date in this population. Trials using cognitive-behavioral therapy in cancer patients, although limited in number and size, suggest significant improvement in their sleep [117].

Medications that disturb sleep

The use of prescription drugs and over-the-counter drugs is common in older adults. Results of several population-based surveys suggest that between 89% and 94% of those over 65 years take prescription medication with nearly 46% taking over five medications and 12% taking over 10 medications [122]. Polypharmacy, frequently defined as taking over five medications, increases incrementally with prevalence rates of 39% for those over age 75 [123]. A multitude of over-the-counter and prescription medications are known to influence the sleep-wake cycle and produce comorbid insomnia. Their adverse effects are diverse but can be broadly categorized as those that produce drowsiness or daytime somnolence, those that are activating or stimulating to the brain, those that interfere with sleep by indirect mechanisms, those that may directly exacerbate primary sleep disorders, and those that influence sleep architecture by other affects. The practitioner should be sensitized to consider how adverse side effects, drug-drug, or drug-disease interactions are more likely to occur in older adults and can include central nervous system depressing or excitatory sequelae. These effects can then lead to direct or indirect effects on overnight sleep quality and quantity. Many of these drugs can alter patterns of sleep and wakefulness both during periods of administration and during periods of withdrawal. It is especially important to avoid using hypnotics as agents to manage the adverse sleep effects of other medications unless all other attempts at medication adjustment have been considered.

Medications that promote daytime sleepiness

Drowsiness is an extremely common side effect of medications, with over 584 medications being cited as causing drowsiness in the side effects index of the *Physician's Desk Reference* [124]. Excessive daytime sleepiness is a frequent sleep complaint in the elderly with a baseline tendency for older adults to have shorter sleep latency during the day [125]. Many medications have the capacity to interfere with acetylcholine or histamine, both regulatory neurotransmitters for wakefulness. These anticholinergic agents are known to have somnogenic effects; waking drowsiness; and negative cognitive, affective, and quality of life outcomes in older adults [126]. Antihistaminergic drugs seem to have variable central nervous system penetration and binding with H1 antagonists like diphenhydramine have much greater likelihood for sedation and cognitive impairment than do tertiary antihistamines [127]. General classes of agents with these effects include antihistamines, antispasmodics, antipsychotics, antiemetics, and antiparkinsonian drugs. Notable specific examples include tricyclic antidepressants, such as amitriptyline, imipramine, cimetidine, mirtazapine, and oxybutynin. A comprehensive review of all of these agents is published elsewhere [128].

Medications can also produce sleepiness by other mechanisms. In those individuals taking levodopa or dopamine agonists, there is an increased prevalence of excessive daytime sleepiness and sleep attacks [129]. Anticonvulsant agents, such as gabapentin, lamotrigine, tiagabine, and levetiracetam, frequently produce sleepiness in older adults. Opiate analgesics can contribute to daytime somnolence and decreased alertness and disrupt overnight sleep efficiency and architecture.

Medications that activate or stimulate the central nervous system

A large number of medications disturb sleep by excitation or activation of the central nervous system. Sleep quality may be affected if these agents are taken before the patient's bedtime or have a sustained half-life that extends into the typical sleep period. Commonly prescribed over-the-counter therapies for cold and flu containing pseudoephedrine, ephedrine, or other sympathomimetics can have this effect. Over-the-counter analgesics with caffeine used for headache therapy are also a concern. Agents used to manage chronic lung disease, such as β-agonist inhalants or oral formulations, corticosteroids, and theophylline can all contribute to sleep disruption. Activating antidepressants can sometimes adversely affect sleep initiation and maintenance. These can include desipramine, bupropion, venlafaxine, reboxetine, and most selective serotonin reuptake inhibitors. Insomnia has been reported as a frequent side effect with selective serotonin reuptake inhibitor use with prevalence of 16.4% with sertraline, 15% with fluoxetine, and 14% with paroxetine [130]. With selective serotonin reuptake inhibitors, although individuals may appreciate an improvement in subjective sleep quality, objective sleep often worsens [131]. Other activating medications, such as methylphenidate, selegiline, and modafinil, are often seen on geriatric medication lists. Accordingly, it is reasonable for such medications, if needed, to be taken far from the desired sleep period when possible, and stopped if not needed.

Medications that affect sleep by worsening other conditions

Medications can sometimes interfere with sleep by worsening an underlying medical or psychiatric condition that then impacts sleep. Medications that worsen heart failure, such as nonsteroidal anti-inflammatory drugs, have the potential to cause central sleep apnea, nocturia, or other sleep problems seen in this condition. Medications including nitrates and calcium channel blockers can decrease lower esophageal sphincter tone with resultant nocturnal gastroesophageal reflux. Amitriptyline and other anticholinergic medications, although potentially helpful with sleep because of sedation, can also contribute to confusion and urinary retention, with subsequent arousals from delirium or nocturia. Late afternoon or evening diuretic treatment may cause nocturia and sleep fragmentation. Many antipsychotic medications, while being used for various symptoms in the elderly, have the potential to produce parkinsonian features, with the sleep difficulties commonly associated with these conditions. Quetiapine may be one of the least common offenders in this category of medications. Hypoglycemic agents, if they produce nocturnal hypoglycemia, can increase nocturnal arousals.

Medications that can exacerbate primary sleep disorders

A number of medications have been reported to exacerbate primary sleep disorders. Nocturnal movement disorders, such as restless legs syndrome and periodic limb movements of sleep, can worsen in the setting of a number of antidepressant medications. In looking at 274 consecutive patients on antidepressants, and 69 control subjects not on antidepressants, those taking selective serotonin reuptake inhibitors or venlafaxine had an odds ratio over 5 that they would have periodic limb movement index >20, compared with the control group [132]. Bupropion was similar to controls. Tricyclic antidepressants and lithium are also associated with a greater prevalence of nocturnal movement disorders. Caffeine, antihistamines, alcohol, and benzodiazepine withdrawal can all worsen restless legs syndrome. Antipsychotic therapies are associated with greater periodic limb movements of sleep prevalence.

Based on a series of small studies and case reports, opiate analgesia use, especially sustained-release or long half-life formulations, is associated with increased central apneas, sustained hypoxemia, and prolonged duration of the abnormal breathing events [133]. These changes occur in the context of the well-established acute respiratory depressant effects. Hypnotics, such as benzodiazepines, may also worsen sleep-disordered breathing by lowering the arousal threshold.

Medications that affect sleep architecture by other mechanisms

Certain medications are associated with worsening of sleep architecture by other influences. β-Blockers are frequently prescribed in older adults in the context of hypertension and heart disease. The more lipophilic agents, such as propranolol, and some of the newer generation β-blockers have been shown to suppress melatonin, increase sleep fragmentation, and increase nightmares in some people [134]. Other agents, such as lithium, benzodiazepine withdrawal, benzodiazepine receptor agonists, and gaba-hydroxy-butyrate are associated with a worsening of disorders of non-REM parasomnias. Tricyclic antidepressants, monoamine oxidase inhibitors, venlafaxine, and mirtazapine have all been documented to induce REM sleep behavior disorder, a parasomnia very specific to older adults.

Summary

As the field of medicine continues to advance, people are living longer with more comorbid medical and psychiatric conditions. This higher burden of illness and the numbers of medications used to treat these conditions plays an important role in the quality and quantity of sleep in older adults. In approaching sleep complaints in geriatric patients, it is essential that practitioners recognize the multidimensional mechanisms by which illness impacts sleep. Equally important, a balanced management approach that includes optimizing the underlying illness, adjusting medications, using cognitive-behavioral approaches, and using judicious hypnotic therapy seems justified based on the current evidence.

References

[1] Foley DJ, Monjan AA, Brown SL, et al. Sleep complaints among elderly persons: an epidemiologic study of three communities. Sleep 1995; 18:425–32.

[2] Roberts RE, Shema SJ, Kaplan GA. Prospective data on sleep complaints and associated risk factors in an older cohort. Psychosom Med 1999;61:188–96.

[3] Foley D, Ancoli-Israel S, Britz P, et al. Sleep disturbances and chronic disease in older adults: results of the 2003 National Sleep Foundation Sleep in America Survey. J Psychosom Res 2004;56:497–502.

[4] American Academy of Sleep Medicine. International classification of sleep disorders. Diagnostic and coding manual. 2nd edition. Westchester (IL): American Academy of Sleep Medicine; 2005.

[5] State-of-the Science Panel. National Institutes of Health State of the Science Conference Statement: manifestations and management of chronic insomnia in adults, June 13–15. Sleep 2005;28:1049–57.

[6] Rodenbeck A, Huether G, Ruther E, et al. Interactions between evening and nocturnal cortisol

secretion and sleep parameters in patients with severe chronic primary insomnia. Neurosci Lett 2002;324:159–63.

[7] Vgontzas AN, Bixler EO, Lin HM, et al. Chronic insomnia is associated with nyctohemeral activation of the hypothalamic-pituitary-adrenal axis: clinical implications. J Clin Endocrinol Metab 2001;86:3787–94.

[8] Alapin I, Libman E, Bailes S, et al. Role of nocturnal cognitive arousal in the complaint of insomnia among older adults. Behav Sleep Med 2003;1:155–70.

[9] Peter R, Peter T, Brigitta B, et al. From psychophysiological insomnia to organic sleep disturbances: a continuum in late onset insomnia with special concerns relating to its treatment. Med Hypotheses 2005;65:1165–71.

[10] Stepanski E, Rybarczyk B. Emerging research on the treatment and etiology of secondary or comorbid insomnia. Sleep Med Rev 2006;10:7–18.

[11] Morgan K, Clarke D. Risk factors for late-life insomnia in a representative general practice sample. Br J Gen Pract 1997;47:166–9.

[12] Benca RM, Obermeyer WH, Thisted RA, et al. Sleep and psychiatric disorders: a meta-analysis. Arch Gen Psychiatry 1992;49:651–68 [discussion: 669–70].

[13] Breslau N, Roth T, Rosenthal L, et al. Sleep disturbance and psychiatric disorders: a longitudinal epidemiological study of young adults. Biol Psychiatry 1996;39:411–8.

[14] Ford DE, Kamerow DB. Epidemiologic study of sleep disturbances and psychiatric disorders: an opportunity for prevention? JAMA 1989;262:1479–84.

[15] Katz DA, McHorney CA. Clinical correlates of insomnia in patients with chronic illness. Arch Intern Med 1998;158:1099–107.

[16] Shochat T, Umphress J, Israel AG, et al. Insomnia in primary care patients. Sleep 1999;22(Suppl 2):S359–65.

[17] Katz DA, McHorney CA. The relationship between insomnia and health-related quality of life in patients with chronic illness. J Fam Pract 2002;51:229–35.

[18] Almeida OP, Pfaff JJ. Sleep complaints among older general practice patients: association with depression. Br J Gen Pract 2005;55:864–6.

[19] Livingston G, Blizard B, Mann A. Does sleep disturbance predict depression in elderly people? A study in inner London. Br J Gen Pract 1993;43:445–8.

[20] Roberts RE, Shema SJ, Kaplan GA, et al. Sleep complaints and depression in an aging cohort: a prospective perspective. Am J Psychiatry 2000;157:81–8.

[21] Thase ME. Antidepressant treatment of the depressed patient with insomnia. J Clin Psychiatry 1999;60(Suppl 17):28–31. [discussion: 46].

[22] Hamilton M. Frequency of symptoms in melancholia (depressive illness). Br J Psychiatry 1989;154:201–6.

[23] Reynolds CF III, Hoch CC, Buysse DJ, et al. Sleep in late-life recurrent depression: changes during early continuation therapy with nortriptyline. Neuropsychopharmacology 1991;5:85–96.

[24] Lepine JP, Gastpar M, Mendlewicz J, et al. Depression in the community: the first pan-European study DEPRES (Depression Research in European Society). Int Clin Psychopharmacol 1997;12:19–29.

[25] Whitney CW, Enright PL, Newman AB, et al. Correlates of daytime sleepiness in 4578 elderly persons: the Cardiovascular Health Study. Sleep 1998;21:27–36.

[26] Thase ME. Depression, sleep, and antidepressants. J Clin Psychiatry 1998;59(Suppl 4):55–65.

[27] Kupfer DJ, Ehlers CL. Two roads to rapid eye movement latency. Arch Gen Psychiatry 1989;46:945–8.

[28] Jackson A, Cavanagh J, Scott J. A systematic review of manic and depressive prodromes. J Affect Disord 2003;74:209–17.

[29] Young RC, Klerman GL. Mania in late life: focus on age at onset. Am J Psychiatry 1992;149:867–76.

[30] McKibbin CL, Ancoli-Israel S, Dimsdale J, et al. Sleep in spousal caregivers of people with Alzheimer's disease. Sleep 2005;28:1245–50.

[31] Hope T, Keene J, Gedling K, et al. Predictors of institutionalization for people with dementia living at home with a carer. Int J Geriatr Psychiatry 1998;13:682–90.

[32] Prigerson HG, Frank E, Kasl SV, et al. Complicated grief and bereavement-related depression as distinct disorders: preliminary empirical validation in elderly bereaved spouses. Am J Psychiatry 1995;152:22–30.

[33] Monti JM, Monti D. Sleep disturbance in generalized anxiety disorder and its treatment. Sleep Med Rev 2000;4:263–76.

[34] Uhde T. Anxiety disorders. In: Kryger M, Roth T, Dement W, editors. Principles and practice of sleep medicine. 3rd edition. Philadelphia: WB Saunders; 2000. p. 1123–39.

[35] Fuller KH, Waters WF, Binks PG, et al. Generalized anxiety and sleep architecture: a polysomnographic investigation. Sleep 1997;20:370–6.

[36] Saletu-Zyhlarz GM, Anderer P, Berger P, et al. Nonorganic insomnia in panic disorder: comparative sleep laboratory studies with normal controls and placebo-controlled trials with alprazolam. Hum Psychopharmacol 2000;15:241–54.

[37] Arriaga F, Paiva T, Matos-Pires A, et al. The sleep of non-depressed patients with panic disorder: a comparison with normal controls. Acta Psychiatr Scand 1996;93:191–4.

[38] Stein MB, Enns MW, Kryger MH. Sleep in non-depressed patients with panic disorder: II. Polysomnographic assessment of sleep architecture and sleep continuity. J Affect Disord 1993;28:1–6.

[39] Shapiro CM, Sloan EP. Nocturnal panic: an underrecognized entity. J Psychosom Res 1998; 44:21–3.

[40] Mellman TA, Uhde TW. Sleep panic attacks: new clinical findings and theoretical implications. Am J Psychiatry 1989;146:1204–7.

[41] Ohayon MM, Shapiro CM. Sleep disturbances and psychiatric disorders associated with posttraumatic stress disorder in the general population. Compr Psychiatry 2000;41:469–78.

[42] Ross RJ, Ball WA, Sullivan KA, et al. Sleep disturbance as the hallmark of posttraumatic stress disorder. Am J Psychiatry 1989;146:697–707.

[43] Mellman TA, Kulick-Bell R, Ashlock LE, et al. Sleep events among veterans with combat-related posttraumatic stress disorder. Am J Psychiatry 1995;152:110–5.

[44] Krakow B, Haynes PL, Warner TD, et al. Nightmares, insomnia, and sleep-disordered breathing in fire evacuees seeking treatment for posttraumatic sleep disturbance. J Trauma Stress 2004;17:257–68.

[45] Regier DA, Farmer ME, Rae DS, et al. Comorbidity of mental disorders with alcohol and other drug abuse: results from the Epidemiologic Catchment Area (ECA) Study. JAMA 1990;264:2511–8.

[46] Grant BF. Prevalence and correlates of alcohol use and DSM-IV alcohol dependence in the United States: results of the National Longitudinal Alcohol Epidemiologic Survey. J Stud Alcohol 1997;58:464–73.

[47] Atkinson R. Substance abuse. In: Coffee C, Cummings J, editors. Textbook of geriatric neuropsychiatry. 2nd edition. Washington: American Psychiatry Press; 2000. p. 367–400.

[48] Liberto JG, Oslin DW. Early versus late onset of alcoholism in the elderly. Int J Addict 1995; 30:1799–818.

[49] Teplin D, Raz B, Daiter J, et al. Screening for substance use patterns among patients referred for a variety of sleep complaints. Am J Drug Alcohol Abuse 2006;32:111–20.

[50] Weissman MM, Greenwald S, Nino-Murcia G, et al. The morbidity of insomnia uncomplicated by psychiatric disorders. Gen Hosp Psychiatry 1997;19:245–50.

[51] Currie SR, Clark S, Rimac S, et al. Comprehensive assessment of insomnia in recovering alcoholics using daily sleep diaries and ambulatory monitoring. Alcohol Clin Exp Res 2003; 27:1262–9.

[52] Johnson EO, Roehrs T, Roth T, et al. Epidemiology of alcohol and medication as aids to sleep in early adulthood. Sleep 1998;21:178–86.

[53] Brower KJ, Aldrich MS, Hall JM. Polysomnographic and subjective sleep predictors of alcoholic relapse. Alcohol Clin Exp Res 1998;22: 1864–71.

[54] Walsh JK, Humm T, Muehlbach MJ, et al. Sedative effects of ethanol at night. J Stud Alcohol 1991;52:597–600.

[55] Le Bon O, Verbanck P, Hoffmann G, et al. Sleep in detoxified alcoholics: impairment of most standard sleep parameters and increased risk for sleep apnea, but not for myoclonias: a controlled study. J Stud Alcohol 1997;58:30–6.

[56] Williams HL, Rundell OH Jr. Altered sleep physiology in chronic alcoholics: reversal with abstinence. Alcohol Clin Exp Res 1981;5:318–25.

[57] Aldrich MS, Shipley JE, Tandon R, et al. Sleep-disordered breathing in alcoholics: association with age. Alcohol Clin Exp Res 1993;17: 1179–83.

[58] Brower KJ. Alcohol's effects on sleep in alcoholics. Alcohol Res Health 2001;25:110–25.

[59] Crum RM, Storr CL, Chan YF, et al. Sleep disturbance and risk for alcohol-related problems. Am J Psychiatry 2004;161:1197–203.

[60] Wong MM, Brower KJ, Fitzgerald HE, et al. Sleep problems in early childhood and early onset of alcohol and other drug use in adolescence. Alcohol Clin Exp Res 2004;28: 578–87.

[61] Shirlow MJ, Mathers CD. A study of caffeine consumption and symptoms; indigestion, palpitations, tremor, headache and insomnia. Int J Epidemiol 1985;14:239–48.

[62] Curatolo PW, Robertson D. The health consequences of caffeine. Ann Intern Med 1983; 98(5 Pt 1):641–53.

[63] Landolt HP, Dijk DJ, Gaus SE, et al. Caffeine reduces low-frequency delta activity in the human sleep EEG. Neuropsychopharmacology 1995; 12:229–38.

[64] Brown SL, Salive ME, Pahor M, et al. Occult caffeine as a source of sleep problems in an older population. J Am Geriatr Soc 1995;43:860–4.

[65] Curless R, French JM, James OF, et al. Is caffeine a factor in subjective insomnia of elderly people? Age Ageing 1993;22:41–5.

[66] LaCroix AZ, Lang J, Scherr P, et al. Smoking and mortality among older men and women in three communities. N Engl J Med 1991; 324:1619–25.

[67] Wetter DW, Young TB. The relation between cigarette smoking and sleep disturbance. Prev Med 1994;23:328–34.

[68] Boutrel B, Koob GF. What keeps us awake: the neuropharmacology of stimulants and wakefulness-promoting medications. Sleep 2004;27: 1181–94.

[69] Davila D, Hurt R, Offord K, et al. Acute effects of transdermal nicotine on sleep architecture, snoring, and sleep-disordered breathing in nonsmokers. Am J Respir Crit Care Med 1994; 150:469–74.

[70] Phillips BA, Danner FJ. Cigarette smoking and sleep disturbance. Arch Intern Med 1995; 155:734–7.

[71] Kalman D, Morissette SB, George TP. Co-morbidity of smoking in patients with psychiatric and substance use disorders. Am J Addict 2005;14:106–23.

[72] Tsuchiyama Y, Uchimura N, Sakamoto T, et al. Effects of hCRH on sleep and body temperature rhythms. Psychiatry Clin Neurosci 1995; 49:299–304.

[73] Horne J. Human slow wave sleep: a review and appraisal of recent findings, with implications for sleep functions, and psychiatric illness. Experientia 1992;48:941–54.

[74] Lichstein KL, Wilson NM, Johnson CT. Psychological treatment of secondary insomnia. Psychol Aging 2000;15:232–40.

[75] Helme RD, Katz B, Gibson SJ, et al. Multidisciplinary pain clinics for older people. Do they have a role? Clin Geriatr Med 1996;12:563–82.

[76] Latham J, Davis BD. The socioeconomic impact of chronic pain. Disabil Rehabil 1994; 16:39–44.

[77] Ellis BW, Dudley HA. Some aspects of sleep research in surgical stress. J Psychosom Res 1976; 20:303–8.

[78] Roehrs T, Hyde M, Blaisdell B, et al. Sleep loss and REM sleep loss are hyperalgesic. Sleep 2006;29:145–51.

[79] MacLean CH. Quality indicators for the management of osteoarthritis in vulnerable elders. Ann Intern Med 2001;135(8 Pt 2):711–21.

[80] Wilcox S, Brenes GA, Levine D, et al. Factors related to sleep disturbance in older adults experiencing knee pain or knee pain with radiographic evidence of knee osteoarthritis. J Am Geriatr Soc 2000;48:1241–51.

[81] Salih AM, Gray RE, Mills KR, et al. A clinical, serological and neurophysiological study of restless legs syndrome in rheumatoid arthritis. Br J Rheumatol 1994;33:60–3.

[82] Jordan JM, Bernard SL, Callahan LF, et al. Self-reported arthritis-related disruptions in sleep and daily life and the use of medical, complementary, and self-care strategies for arthritis: the National Survey of Self-care and Aging. Arch Fam Med 2000;9:143–9.

[83] Rybarczyk B, Stepanski E, Fogg L, et al. A placebo-controlled test of cognitive-behavioral therapy for comorbid insomnia in older adults. J Consult Clin Psychol 2005;73:1164–74.

[84] Locke GR III, Talley NJ, Fett SL, et al. Prevalence and clinical spectrum of gastroesophageal reflux: a population-based study in Olmsted County, Minnesota. Gastroenterology 1997; 112:1448–56.

[85] Bretagne JF, Richard-Molard B, Honnorat C, et al. Gastroesophageal reflux in the French general population: national survey of 8000 adults. Presse Med 2006;35(1 Pt 1):23–31.

[86] Farup C, Kleinman L, Sloan S, et al. The impact of nocturnal symptoms associated with gastroesophageal reflux disease on health-related quality of life. Arch Intern Med 2001; 161:45–52.

[87] Orr WC. Sleep and gastroesophageal reflux disease: a wake-up call. Rev Gastroenterol Disord 2004;4(Suppl 4):S25–32.

[88] Johnson DA, Orr WC, Crawley JA, et al. Effect of esomeprazole on nighttime heartburn and sleep quality in patients with GERD: a randomized, placebo-controlled trial. Am J Gastroenterol 2005;100:1914–22.

[89] Herr J. Chronic cough, sleep apnea, and gastroesophageal reflux disease. Chest 2001; 120:1036–7.

[90] Peters RW, Zoble RG, Brooks MM. Onset of acute myocardial infarction during sleep. Clin Cardiol 2002;25:237–41.

[91] Mallon L, Broman JE, Hetta J. Sleep complaints predict coronary artery disease mortality in males: a 12-year follow-up study of a middle-aged Swedish population. J Intern Med 2002; 251:207–16.

[92] Chocron S, Tatou E, Schjoth B, et al. Perceived health status in patients over 70 before and after open-heart operations. Age Ageing 2000; 29:329–34.

[93] Lesman-Leegte I, Jaarsma T, Sanderman R, et al. Depressive symptoms are prominent among elderly hospitalised heart failure patients. Eur J Heart Fail, in press.

[94] Lanfranchi PA, Braghiroli A, Bosimini E, et al. Prognostic value of nocturnal Cheyne-Stokes respiration in chronic heart failure. Circulation 1999;99:1435–40.

[95] Sin DD, Fitzgerald F, Parker JD, et al. Risk factors for central and obstructive sleep apnea in 450 men and women with congestive heart failure. Am J Respir Crit Care Med 1999;160:1101–6.

[96] Kaneko Y, Floras JS, Usui K, et al. Cardiovascular effects of continuous positive airway pressure in patients with heart failure and obstructive sleep apnea. N Engl J Med 2003; 348:1233–41.

[97] Klink M, Quan SF. Prevalence of reported sleep disturbances in a general adult population and their relationship to obstructive airways diseases. Chest 1987;91:540–6.

[98] O'Brien A, Whitman K. Lack of benefit of continuous positive airway pressure on lung function in patients with overlap syndrome. Lung 2005;183:389–404.

[99] Fleetham J, West P, Mezon B, et al. Sleep, arousals, and oxygen desaturation in chronic obstructive pulmonary disease: the effect of oxygen therapy. Am Rev Respir Dis 1982; 126:429–33.

[100] Martin RJ, Bartelson BL, Smith P, et al. Effect of ipratropium bromide treatment on oxygen saturation and sleep quality in COPD. Chest 1999;115:1338–45.

[101] Krachman SL, Chatila W, Martin UJ, et al. Effects of lung volume reduction surgery on sleep quality and nocturnal gas exchange in patients with severe emphysema. Chest 2005; 128:3221–8.

[102] Lamond N, Tiggemann M, Dawson D. Factors predicting sleep disruption in type II diabetes. Sleep 2000;23:415–6.

[103] Rijsman RM, de Weerd AW. Secondary periodic limb movement disorder and restless legs syndrome. Sleep Med Rev 1999;3:147–58.

[104] Punjabi NM, Polotsky VY. Disorders of glucose metabolism in sleep apnea. J Appl Physiol 2005;99:1998–2007.

[105] Purdie DW, Empson JA, Crichton C, et al. Hormone replacement therapy, sleep quality and psychological wellbeing. Br J Obstet Gynaecol 1995;102:735–9.

[106] Milsom I, Abrams P, Cardozo L, et al. How widespread are the symptoms of an overactive bladder and how are they managed? A population-based prevalence study. BJU Int 2001; 87:760–6.

[107] Donahue JL, Lowenthal DT. Nocturnal polyuria in the elderly person. Am J Med Sci 1997; 314:232–8.

[108] Stolzmann KL, Camponeschi JL, Remington PL. The increasing incidence of end-stage renal disease in Wisconsin from 1982–2003: an analysis by age, race, and primary diagnosis. Wis Med J 2005;104:66–71.

[109] Sabbatini M, Minale B, Crispo A, et al. Insomnia in maintenance haemodialysis patients. Nephrol Dial Transplant 2002;17:852–6.

[110] Parker KP, Bliwise DL, Bailey JL, et al. Polysomnographic measures of nocturnal sleep in patients on chronic, intermittent daytime haemodialysis vs those with chronic kidney disease. Nephrol Dial Transplant 2005;20:1422–8.

[111] Williams SW, Tell GS, Zheng B, et al. Correlates of sleep behavior among hemodialysis patients. The Kidney Outcomes Prediction and Evaluation (KOPE) Study. Am J Nephrol 2002; 22:18–28.

[112] Parker KP. Sleep disturbances in dialysis patients. Sleep Med Rev 2003;7:131–43.

[113] Hanly PJ, Pierratos A. Improvement of sleep apnea in patients with chronic renal failure who undergo nocturnal hemodialysis. N Engl J Med 2001;344:102–7.

[114] Benz RL, Pressman MR, Hovick ET, et al. A preliminary study of the effects of correction of anemia with recombinant human erythropoietin therapy on sleep, sleep disorders, and daytime sleepiness in hemodialysis patients (The SLEEPO study). Am J Kidney Dis 1999; 34:1089–95.

[115] Davison SN, Jhangri GS. The impact of chronic pain on depression, sleep, and the desire to withdraw from dialysis in hemodialysis patients. J Pain Symptom Manage 2005;30:465–73.

[116] Ries LAG, Eisner M, Kosary C, et al. SEER Cancer Statistics Review, 1973–2002. Available at: http://seer.cancer.gov/csr/1975–2003/. Accessed June 2006.

[117] Davidson JR, Waisberg JL, Brundage MD, et al. Nonpharmacologic group treatment of insomnia: a preliminary study with cancer survivors. Psychooncology 2001;10:389–97.

[118] Savard J, Morin CM. Insomnia in the context of cancer: a review of a neglected problem. J Clin Oncol 2001;19:895–908.

[119] Davidson JR, MacLean AW, Brundage MD, et al. Sleep disturbance in cancer patients. Soc Sci Med 2002;54:1309–21.

[120] Stiefel FC, Kornblith AB, Holland JC. Changes in the prescription patterns of psychotropic drugs for cancer patients during a 10-year period. Cancer 1990;65:1048–53.

[121] Lee K, Cho M, Miaskowski C, et al. Impaired sleep and rhythms in persons with cancer. Sleep Med Rev 2004;8:199–212.

[122] Kaufman DW, Kelly JP, Rosenberg L, et al. Recent patterns of medication use in the ambulatory adult population of the United States: the Slone survey. JAMA 2002;287:337–44.

[123] Linjakumpu T, Hartikainen S, Klaukka T, et al. Use of medications and polypharmacy are increasing among the elderly. J Clin Epidemiol 2002;55:809–17.

[124] Pagel JF. Medications and their effects on sleep. Prim Care 2005;32:491–509.

[125] Richardson GS, Carskadon MA, Orav EJ, et al. Circadian variation of sleep tendency in elderly and young adult subjects. Sleep 1982; 5(Suppl 2):S82–94.

[126] Mintzer J, Burns A. Anticholinergic side-effects of drugs in elderly people. J R Soc Med 2000; 93:457–62.

[127] Nicholson AN, Stone BM. Antihistamines: impaired performance and the tendency to sleep. Eur J Clin Pharmacol 1986;30:27–32.

[128] Rudd KM, Raehl CL, Bond CA, et al. Methods for assessing drug-related anticholinergic activity. Pharmacotherapy 2005;25:1592–601.

[129] Larsen JP, Tandberg E. Sleep disorders in patients with Parkinson's disease: epidemiology and management. CNS Drugs 2001;15:267–75.

[130] Grimsley SR, Jann MW. Paroxetine, sertraline, and fluvoxamine: new selective serotonin reuptake inhibitors. Clinical Pharmacy 1992; 11:930–57.

[131] Argyropoulos SV, Hicks JA, Nash JR, et al. Correlation of subjective and objective sleep measurements at different stages of the treatment of depression. Psychiatry Res 2003; 120:179–90.

[132] Yang C, White DP, Winkelman JW. Antidepressants and periodic limb movements of sleep. Biol Psychiatry 2005;58(6):510–4.

[133] Wang D, Teichtahl H, Drummer O, et al. Central sleep apnea in stable methadone maintenance treatment patients. Chest 2005; 128:1348–56.

[134] Brzezinski A. Melatonin in humans. N Engl J Med 1997;336:186–95.

SLEEP
MEDICINE
CLINICS

Sleep Med Clin 1 (2006) 247–262

ELSEVIER
SAUNDERS

Sleep-Related Breathing Disorders in the Elderly

Katie L. Stone, PhD[a],*, Susan Redline, MD[b]

Sleep disorders are extremely common, yet frequently undiagnosed and untreated [1–3]. Prevalence of most sleep disorders increases with advancing age. Among adults over the age of 65, more than 50% complain of difficulty sleeping [2]. Sleep disturbance in older adults may be attributable to a variety of factors, including underlying medical or psychiatric conditions; medication use; or specific sleep disorders, such as insomnia, periodic leg movement disorder, or sleep-disordered breathing (SDB).

The estimated prevalence of SDB is much higher in older adults as compared with younger populations, ranging from about 5% to 80% depending on the definition that is applied, and the specific population being studied [4–9]. In general, the definition of SDB is based on the number of apnea and hypopnea episodes per hour of sleep (apnea-hypopnea index [AHI]). Apneas are typically defined as the complete cessation of airflow of duration lasting 10 seconds or more. A typical definition of hypopnea is a reduction of airflow for duration of 10 seconds or longer, accompanied by a 3% to 4% or more oxygen desaturation. Presence of SDB is then defined using various AHI cutpoints (eg, AHI ≥ 5, ≥ 10, ≥ 15 episodes per hour). Commonly recognized manifestations of SDB include snoring, daytime sleepiness, and fatigue. Accordingly, sleep apnea hypopnea syndrome has been defined as a condition where an increased number of sleep-related respiratory disturbances is accompanied by daytime symptoms, such as sleepiness or impaired quality of life unexplained by other findings [10]. Prevalence of SDB in middle-aged populations has been estimated to be between 2% and 4% [11]. Optimal definitions for the syndrome in the elderly do not exist, however, and prevalence has been more difficult to quantify. Furthermore, many studies report prevalence in select populations, such as demented or institutionalized elders, and

[a] San Francisco Coordinating Center/CPMC Research Institute, 185 Berry Street, Suite 5700, San Francisco, CA 94107, USA
[b] Case Western Reserve University, 11100 Euclid Avenue, Cleveland, OH 44106–6003, USA
* Corresponding author.
E-mail address: kstone@sfcc-cpmc.net (K.L. Stone).

1556-407X/06/$ – see front matter © 2006 Elsevier Inc. All rights reserved.
sleep.theclinics.com

doi:10.1016/j.jsmc.2006.04.003

these results cannot be generalized to populations of community-dwelling healthy older adults.

SDB is associated with a wide range of comorbidities, ranging from functional deficits to cardiovascular disease (CVD). In middle-aged adults SDB has been linked to impaired cognitive ability, decreased work ability, and higher risk for motor vehicle accidents [12–14]. More recent research has also suggested that SDB may influence the risk of chronic diseases, such as hypertension [15,16], diabetes [17], and CVD [18], and overall and cardiovascular-specific mortality [19]. There have been relatively few studies that have examined the sequelae of SDB specifically among older populations. Because elderly populations often suffer high rates of comorbidities, it is often difficult to attribute adverse health outcomes to any single condition, such as SDB. Studies performed on elderly cohorts also may selectively report data from subgroups that represent a survival cohort. As with many other conditions, the evidence that links SDB with health outcomes may not be as strong as in younger populations.

Physiologic features

Most epidemiologic studies have used the AHI obtained from polysomnography as the primary metric to quantify SDB. This index combines apneas (complete cessations of breathing) with hypopneas (incomplete airflow limitation), and obstructive (associated with respiratory effort) with central (no evidence of respiratory effort) events. This approach is supported by the greater scoring reliability of collapsing all event subtypes into a single index rather than identifying event subtypes [20]. In addition, most polysomnography-measured respiratory events in middle-aged community-based populations consist of hypopnea, and attempts to separate out unique associations that may be attributable to event subtypes (eg, apneas, central events, and so forth) generally have been unsuccessful [18,21]. Sleep-related respiration in older populations may differ than that in younger populations, however, and these differences may justify consideration of alternative indices to characterize SDB best in older populations. For example, underlying cardiovascular and neurologic disorders [22] or diabetes [23] in older individuals may increase the prevalence of Cheyne-Stokes breathing, which is associated with an increased frequency of central apnea. Quantification of central apnea by calculating a distinct central apnea index may facilitate identification of subgroups of the elderly with SDB whose disorder is substantively influenced by underlying medical problems, and whose primary breathing disturbances may have differing physiologic effects

than individuals with predominantly obstructive events (ie, by high levels of obstructive apnea and hypopnea and few central events). For example, central events may cause relatively large arousal responses, but perhaps lesser degrees of oxygen desaturation or mechanical changes in the chest, causing a different series of cardiovascular reflex activation than do obstructive events.

Clinical features

The most prominent symptoms of SDB described in middle-aged populations are snoring and excessive daytime sleepiness (EDS). The snoring associated with SDB (caused by airflow turbulence from upper airway collapse) may be loud enough to disrupt the bed partner. Overall, it has been reported that approximately 50% of individuals with habitual snoring have some degree of SDB, and snoring has been identified as an early predictor of SDB [24]. It should also be noted, however, that not all patients who snore have SDB, and most but not all patients with SDB snore. Furthermore, because many elderly live alone, this symptom may be difficult to identify and may be responsible for relative underreporting of snoring in the elderly.

The relationship between SDB and snoring may differ in elderly compared with younger populations. One study of a large cohort of men and women aged 65 years and older found that self-reported snoring was inversely related to age [25]. This finding, which shows an age relationship opposite of that observed for the rising AHI with increasing age, may be explained by reporting biases in the elderly caused by the unavailability of bed partners who often report this behavior. Alternatively, it is possible that elderly groups who may have a lower body mass index (BMI) than other samples, or who have more centrally mediated apneas, may indeed have fewer obstructive events that are typically associated with turbulent airflow that causes snoring noises. Finally, it is possible that relative weakness of respiratory neuromuscular forces in the elderly may prevent the generation of sufficient airflow turbulence to cause loud or disruptive snoring. Differences in the association of SDB with snoring may account for some of the differences in the presentation and outcomes of SDB in the elderly.

Few studies have examined the correlates and functional outcomes of snoring in elderly populations. In a large observational study of adults aged 65 and older, loud snoring was independently associated with BMI, diabetes, and arthritis in older women, but not men [25], whereas alcohol use, which can act as a respiratory depressant, was associated with snoring in older men. An association with arthritis had not been reported for younger populations. In the Sleep Heart Health Study, comprised of individuals greater than age 40 years, snoring was independently associated with EDS, even after accounting for presence of SDB [26], suggesting that snoring even in the absence of SDB may cause problems with daytime functioning in the elderly. The consequences of snoring apart from those explained by SDB in the elderly have not been well described.

EDS is common in older adults, and has been associated with a variety of factors including poor health and comorbidities, frequent nighttime awakenings, snoring, non-white race, use of medications, and depression [27–29]. Healthy older adults, however, may not experience more sleepiness than younger adults [30,31]. Few studies have examined whether severity of SDB predicts increased EDS in the elderly, and whether this relationship is similar to that observed in younger adults. Using the large sample studied as part of the Sleep Heart Health Study, Gottlieb and coworkers [32] confirmed a positive relationship between SDB and EDS, with no evidence of effect modification by age or gender. Among 461 older women participating in the Study of Osteoporotic Fractures (mean age 82.9 years), there was a modest association between AHI and EDS [33]: each SD increase in AHI (1 SD = approximately 15 points) was associated with an increase in EDS score of 0.44 points. This relationship was further attenuated and not statistically significant after adjusting for total sleep time, however, indicating that in this cohort of very elderly women, the relationship between AHI and EDS is at least partially explained by short sleep. Difficulties in delineating the relationships of EDS and SDB in the elderly may relate the high prevalence of other disorders that contribute to EDS in this population. Assessing EDS also may be difficult because of underlying daytime cognitive impairments and short-term memory loss [34].

Epidemiology

Prevalence and incidence of sleep-disordered breathing in the elderly

The prevalence of SDB increases with age [5,35], and is more common in men than women [35]. Young and coworkers [36] reported the estimated prevalence of SDB among middle-aged American adults 30 to 60 years of age, defined by an AHI ≥5 and the presence of EDS, to be 4% of men and 2% of women. Studies in middle-aged Korean [37] and Hong Kong [37] adults reported similar prevalence rates, which is somewhat surprising

given that obesity, a major risk factor for SDB, is less common in Asian populations.

Fewer studies have examined the prevalence rates among elderly subjects. Estimates vary broadly, however, from 5% to >80%, depending on the specific population being studied, the methods, and definitions used to assess and classify SDB.

In a large population of community-dwelling elderly aged 65 to 95 years, Ancoli-Israel and coworkers [4] reported that 24% had an apnea index ≥5 with an average apnea index of 13. In addition, 81% of the study subjects had an AHI ≥ 5, with an average AHI of 38. Using more stringent criteria, the prevalence rates were 62% for an AHI ≥ 10, 44% for an AHI ≥20, and 24% for an AHI ≥40. These rates were higher than had previously been reported, most likely because objective sleep recordings were used rather than subjective measurements, such as self-reported snoring with observed apneas [25].

The Sleep Heart Health Study, a study of a community-based cohort of over 6400 individuals (mean age 63.5 years with an age range of 40–98 years), reported prevalence rates of SDB by 10-year age groups [38]. When SDB was defined as AHI ≥15, prevalence increased steadily across age groups, but seemed to flatten out after about age 60 (Fig. 1): prevalence estimates were 19%, 21%, and 20% among those aged 60 to 69, 70 to 79, and 80 plus, respectively. The prevalence of AHI 5 to 14 was also similar across the older age groups (32%, 33%, and 36% among those aged 60–69, 70–79, and 80 plus, respectively). Sampling in this study was not random, however, and snorers were oversampled among the younger cohorts, limiting the generalizability of these relationships.

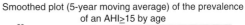
Smoothed plot (5-year moving average) of the prevalence of an AHI≥15 by age

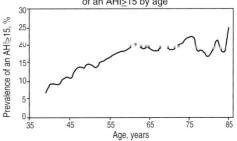

Fig. 1. An increase in SDB prevalence with increasing 10-year age groups in those with AHI ≥15. AHI, apnea-hypopnea index. (*From* Young T, Shahar E, Nieto J, et al. Predictors of sleep disordered breathing in community-dwelling adults. Arch Intern Med 2002; 162:895; with permission.)

Elderly nursing home patients have been shown to have higher prevalence rates of SDB than those who live independently [1,39]. For example, Ancoli-Israel and coworkers [1] studied 235 nursing home patients and found that 70% to 90% had an AHI ≥5 and 50% had an AHI ≥20. Hoch and Reynolds [40] reported that over 40% of Alzheimer disease patients had SDB, significantly higher than age-matched depressed or healthy elderly subjects. Other studies have reported similar results [41,42]. In a review of seven different studies examining the prevalence in those elderly versus those elderly without dementia, Ancoli-Israel [8] reported prevalence rates of SDB ranging from 33% to 70% in demented subjects, compared with the reported 5.6% to 45% rate found in the nondemented elderly. A few studies found that the severity of the dementia was positively correlated with the severity of the SDB [1,40].

Assessing the association between age, gender, and SDB from cross-sectional studies may be problematic given cohort effects and survival biases. There have been only limited longitudinal studies that have addressed, within individuals, the overall progression or regression of SDB with aging, and whether age-related effects vary in men and women and with menopause. The incidence of SDB has been evaluated in the Wisconsin Sleep Cohort [43], the Cleveland Family Study [44,45], and the Sleep Heart Health Study [46]. The first two studies included predominantly middle-aged individuals, whereas the latter study included a predominance of older subjects. These studies consistently have shown that weight gain is associated with increased severity of SDB; a 1% increase in weight was estimated to be associated with a 3% increase in SDB severity [43]. Overall, the 5-year incidence of SDB (ie, "new" SDB, as defined by an AHI >10, in individuals who's "baseline" AHI was <5) was estimated to be 11% in men and 4% in women [46]. Notable differences in progression of SDB, however, have been observed among individuals, and according to age, sex, and baseline weight. The highest rates of progression of SDB have been observed among older and heavier men [44,46], suggesting the potential vulnerability of older men to age- or weight-associated susceptibility to SDB.

Risk factors

Obesity is the most predictive physical finding of SDB in younger adults [47]. One study found that approximately 40% of those with a BMI over 40, and 50% of those with a BMI over 50, have SDB [48]. In middle-aged adults, visceral obesity, which is related to insulin resistance and hypercytokinemia, was shown to be a more important determinant of SDB than total body fat or subcutaneous

fat [49]. It is unclear if the association between obesity and SDB is as strong in older adults as compared with middle-aged adults, although several studies have demonstrated that obesity and an elevated BMI are still strong predictors of the presence of SDB in the elderly [4,47,48]. Unintentional weight loss and sarcopenia, however, are common manifestations of frailty in older adults [50,51]. Of interest, in the Sleep Hearth Health Study, men who lost large amounts of weight over a 5-year period had a relatively high incidence of SDB [46]. It may be important to account for interactions of obesity and body weight and health status or frailty in examining the relationship of obesity and SDB in older adults. It is plausible that indices of frailty may prove to be useful in refining risk estimates for SDB in older populations.

Other well-known risk factors for SDB include increasing age; male gender; and symptomatic status (eg, presence of snoring and EDS). In addition, the use of sedating medications, alcohol consumption, family history, race, smoking, and upper airway configuration have all been associated with risk of SDB [4,52,53]. In general, few studies have explored the association between race and SDB. There is some evidence to suggest that SDB may be more severe but not more prevalent in older African Americans than in older whites [6,54].

Estrogen and other hormonal factors may be protective for the development of SDB. Data from the Wisconsin Cohort Study suggest that menopause, independent of age, is associated with an increased level of SDB in women [55]. In the Sleep Heart Health Study, among predominantly postmenopausal women, hormone-replacement therapy use also was shown to be associated with a lower relative AHI [56]. In addition, Bixler and coworkers [57] found that premenopausal women and postmenopausal women on hormone-replacement therapy had a similar prevalence of SDB (0.6% and 0.5%, respectively), whereas the prevalence was considerably higher (2.7%) among postmenopausal women not taking hormone-replacement therapy. In this study, SDB was defined as an AHI ≥10 in combination with EDS. Overall, the evidence suggests that sex hormones may influence the severity of SDB, and that changes in sex hormones after menopause likely contribute to the higher prevalence of SDB in older compared with younger women.

Morbidity and mortality associated with sleep-disordered breathing

Cardiovascular consequences

Cross-sectional relationships have been reported between SDB and SDB symptoms (eg, snoring, daytime drowsiness) with hypertension, CVD, CVD risk factors, diabetes, or biochemical changes related to CVD risk [18,58,59].

SDB is an established risk factor for hypertension in younger adults [15,60]. Lavie and coworkers [61] demonstrated a dose-response relationship between apnea severity and elevations in blood pressure with each additional apneic event per hour of sleep increasing the odds of hypertension by 1%, and each oxygen desaturation of 10% increasing the odds by 13%. Even minimal amounts of SDB (AHI 0.1–4.9), considered by most to be nonpathologic, has been shown to increase the risk of developing hypertension compared with an AHI of zero [16]. A recent review also provides evidence that treatment of SDB with continuous positive airway pressure (CPAP) may be effective in reducing blood pressure, with effects most marked among individuals with severe SDB or concomitant sleepiness [62].

Several studies, however, indicate weaker associations between SDB and hypertension in the elderly. One potential explanation is that isolated systolic hypertension increases with aging because of generalized atherosclerosis, and studies that included systolic hypertension as an outcome may have underestimated the influence of SDB on blood pressure, which may be mediated by sympathetic nervous system overactivity. A recent analysis from the Sleep Heart Health Study that examined both systolic hypertension and essential hypertension (thought to reflect sympathetic overactivity), however, showed that a stronger association between SDB was observed in those aged <60 years compared with older cohort members using either definition of hypertension [63]. Although earlier studies reported an association between hypertension and SDB in the older adult [64,65], it is unclear the extent to which SDB contributes to hypertension in elderly populations among whom the risk for hypertension is so high. A further understanding of how arousal responses to respiratory stimuli vary across the age spectrum may shed further light on the apparent differences in hypertension susceptibility to SDB in elderly compared with younger populations.

In middle-aged individuals, modest levels of SDB have been estimated to increase risk of CVD (defined as coronary artery disease, congestive heart failure, or stroke) by 30% to 40%. These data, however, derived from a cross-sectional evaluation of CVD in the Sleep Heart Health Study, also showed somewhat stronger associations in younger than older individuals [18]. Such patterns are typical for other CVD risk relationships, where competing risks and comorbidities may reduce the strength of observed relationships among risk factors and outcomes.

A number of studies have found a high prevalence of SDB specifically among patients with congestive heart failure [66,67]. Although it is possible that there is a bidirectional causal relationship between SDB and congestive heart failure [68], it is likely that SDB and congestive heart failure are an adverse combination in which SDB causes or exacerbates the heart failure. Central and obstructive sleep apnea and Cheyne-Stokes respiration are all recognized as occurring commonly in patients with heart failure. These conditions represent a spectrum of severity from intermittent periodic respiration without apneas to cycles of hyperventilation and apneas during sleep. The hyperventilation that occurs postapnea is recognized clinically as paroxysmal nocturnal dyspnea. Javaheri and coworkers [66] reported that 40% to 50% of outpatients, predominantly male, with stable, mild, medically treated congestive heart failure had SDB, and AHI has been shown to be a powerful predictor of poor prognosis in this group of patients [69]. The Sleep Heart Health Study found that the severity of SDB was positively associated with the development of congestive heart failure and like ischemic disease, even mild to moderate SDB was associated with its development [18]. The increasing frequency of congestive heart failure in the population, and its frequency in the elderly, underscores the need to understand better the role of SDB, and its treatment, in this condition.

Studies have found an independent association between self-reported snoring and stroke, an association similar in strength to traditional risk factors for stroke, such as hypertension, smoking, and hyperlipidemia [70,71]. A number of studies, generally case-control and descriptive in design, have reported a high prevalence of SDB in patients who have suffered a cerebrovascular accident when compared with age- and gender-matched controls [71,72]. Furthermore, the SDB persisted despite resolution of many of the stroke-related symptoms, strengthening the argument that the SDB preceded the development of cerebrovascular disease [71]. For those patients who have suffered an acute ischemic stroke, the presence of SDB has been found to be an independent prognostic factor related to mortality [73].

Some of the strongest epidemiologic evidence to date of the association between cerebrovascular accidents and SDB again comes from the Sleep Heart Health Study [18]. This study has found an association between the severity of SDB and the risk of prevalent cerebrovascular disease and has also reported that even mild to moderate SDB increases this risk. Prospective studies are needed to determine if SDB precedes the development of stroke, in which case treatment of SDB may be effective in preventing stroke [71]. Martinez-Garcia and co-workers [74] showed that 18-month treatment with CPAP among poststroke patients with AHI ≥ 20 reduced the risk of subsequent vascular events.

New results from the Sleep Heart Health Study demonstrate strong relationships between SDB and cardiac arrhythmias [75]. After adjusting for age, sex, BMI, and prevalent coronary heart disease, individuals with SDB (defined as AHI ≥ 30) had four times the odds of atrial fibrillation (odds ratio [OR] 4.02; 95% confidence interval [CI] 1.03–15.74), three times the odds of nonsustained ventricular tachycardia (OR 3.40; 95% CI 1.03–11.20), and almost twice the odds of complex ventricular ectopy (OR 1.74; 95% CI 1.11–2.74) as compared with those without SDB. For complex ventricular ectopy, a significant interaction was found between SDB and age, such that the OR fell from 9.3 in those aged 50 years old, to 2 among those aged 70 years old. This latter result adds to the body of literature suggesting that cardiovascular consequences associated with SDB may be weaker in the elderly as compared with middle-aged adults. An intriguing possibility is that changes of the autonomic nervous system with aging may actually be protective in blunting adverse cardiovascular responses to SDB-associated physiologic perturbations. Large prospective studies in older adult populations are needed to understand better the age differences in CVD risk associated with SDB.

Endothelial function, as measured by changes in brachial artery flow and diameter after occluding blood flow for several minutes (flow-mediated brachial reactivity), has been used as an intermediate marker of CVD. Evidence of impaired endothelial function with increasing severity of SDB was demonstrated among the elderly participants (mean age approximately 80 years) of the Cardiovascular Health Study, with effects possibly strongest among hypertensive individuals and women [76]. These observations suggest that SDB may mediate adverse cardiovascular outcomes in elderly individuals, as has been described in a study of younger subjects [77].

Associations between CVD and SDB may be mediated through a number of pathways, including associations caused by common known CVD risk factors that are also related to SDB, or specific effects of SDB. Obesity and physical activity levels, major determinants of CVD risk, are also related to risk for SDB [78–80]. Large prospective studies are underway in middle-aged and older adults to test whether SDB is associated with incident CVD.

Metabolic consequences

There is also growing interest in SDB as a risk factor for metabolic syndrome, which has been defined as a cluster of risk factors for CVD and diabetes [81]. Factors commonly included in this definition include hypertension, obesity, dyslipidemia, and glucose intolerance. Metabolic syndrome is commonly observed in women and men with SDB [82–85]. It is uncertain whether these two conditions reflect a common underlying pathology, however, or whether SDB contributes toward development of metabolic syndrome. It is also not known whether similar associations are present in older individuals.

In laboratory studies among younger adult men it has been shown more generally that short-term sleep deprivation induces changes in glucose tolerance [86]. Both SDB and chronic sleep deprivation have been associated with increased inflammatory response [87,88], which may play a role in the development of metabolic syndrome [89]. Individuals with SDB or sleepiness have been shown to have increased levels of inflammatory markers, including C-reactive protein [88], and hypercytokinemia [90,91]. Furthermore, these levels may increase in proportion to overnight hypoxic stress. Results from the Sleep Heart Health Study indicate that average level of oxygen saturation predicts insulin resistance in nondiabetic participants [17]. Other studies indicate an elevation of antibodies to oxidized low-density lipoproteins in SDB patients compared with controls [92].

Evidence from a few large cohort studies have linked SDB or snoring to risk of diabetes. In an analysis of the Wisconsin Sleep Cohort, Reichmuth and coworkers [93] found significantly elevated prevalence of type II diabetes among those with AHI ≥ 15 compared with those with AHI < 5 (14.7% versus 2.8%, respectively). This finding remained significant in models adjusted for age, gender, and BMI. There was also an elevated but nonsignificant association between SDB and incident diabetes during a 4-year follow-up period. Al-Delaimy and colleagues [94] examined the association of self-reported snoring and incident diabetes among women aged 40 to 65 participating in the Nurses Health Study, and found a significant 50% increase in risk for developing type II diabetes among those who reported occasional snoring compared with nonsnorers, after adjustment for several diabetes risk factors and sleep-related factors. Results from the Sleep Heart Health Study, however, did not confirm these findings [23]. Resnick and coworkers [23] found that SDB was more frequent in diabetics compared with nondiabetics, but this association was explained by the higher BMI in the diabetic groups. In contrast, independent of BMI, diabetics had a higher prevalence of Cheyne-Stokes respiration, whether individuals with known heart disease were included or excluded in the analyses.

Some of the best evidence linking SDB to impaired glucose homeostasis and insulin sensitivity is from trials testing the short- and long-term effects of CPAP use among diabetics with SDB. Babu and coworkers [95] studied 25 patients undergoing CPAP treatment for a mean of 83 days ($\pm$50 days) and found days of treatment to be significantly inversely associated with reductions in hemoglobin A_{1c} levels, suggesting a direct link of SDB with impaired glucose homeostasis. In another study, Harsch and coworkers [96] tested the effects of both short-term (2 day) and long-term (3 month) treatment with CPAP on insulin sensitivity index (determined by euglycemic hyperinsulinemic clamp tests at baseline and after treatment). In this study, only long-term treatment resulted in significant improvements in insulin sensitivity. Effects, however, were strongest among nonobese individuals. Although the compendium of research seems to indicate that SDB may contribute to metabolic abnormalities, there have been no studies conducted in elderly subjects to determine if relationships are similar to those found in younger adults. Furthermore, the mechanisms remain unclear. Short sleep has also been related to risk for diabetes in observational studies [97], and laboratory-based studies in young healthy adults have linked sleep deprivation to impaired glucose tolerance [86]. Decreased sleep duration associated with SDB is one of several potential pathways linking SDB and risk of metabolic abnormalities.

Cognitive impairment and dementia

Cognitive impairment is another potentially harmful consequence of SDB. The most consistent findings are with regards to impairments in attention and concentration [98]. In a review of studies of SDB and cognition, Aloia and colleagues [98] reported that most studies examining cognitive changes associated with treatment of SDB found the strongest effects for attention and vigilance. In a large observational study of very elderly (ages 79–97) Japanese men residing in Hawaii, however, Foley and coworkers [99] showed that objectively measured SDB was associated with EDS, but not with cognitive functioning, including measures of memory function, concentration, and attention.

There are two proposed explanations for the cognitive deficits found in patients with SDB. The first theory is that hypoxia resulting from SDB causes impairment in cognitive functioning. A few studies have found that for patients with continuous hypoxia, there is a correlation between the severity of cognitive dysfunction and nocturnal oxygen saturation [100,101]. As the oxygen saturation decreases, performance on various neuropsychologic testing worsens. This relationship becomes less clear when

patients have more intermittent hypoxia. One important consideration, however, is the variability in the severity of SDB from night to night. It remains unclear whether these possible hypoxia-related cognitive deficits are reversible with treatment.

The second possible reason cited for the cognitive impairment found in patients with SDB is EDS. EDS has been shown to interfere with attention and concentration abilities and to cause inconsistent performances on neuropsychologic tests [102]. Cohen-Zion and coworkers [103] prospectively studied 48 adults aged 65 who were at high risk for SDB. During a 2-year follow-up period, changes in cognitive function (assessed using a global test) were related to changes in AHI, daytime sleepiness, and oxygen saturation. In multivariate analyses, only increases in daytime sleepiness (but not AHI or oxygen desaturation) predicted cognitive decline. It is plausible that the effect of SDB on cognitive functioning is predominantly mediated by sleepiness and associated attentional deficits.

In institutionalized elderly, it has been found that those with severe dementia based on the Dementia Rating Scale had more severe SDB compared with those with mild-moderate or no dementia [1]. Furthermore, those with more severe SDB performed worse on the Dementia Rating Scale, suggesting that more severe SDB was associated with more severe dementia [1]. Another study estimated that an AHI of 15 is equivalent to the decrement of psychomotor efficiency associated with an additional 5 years of age [104]. In addition, some researchers speculate that SDB could actually be a cause of vascular dementia [105], because there are data to suggest that the hypertension, arrhythmias, decreased cardiac output, stroke volume, and cerebral perfusion associated with SDB may lead to a greater likelihood of cerebral ischemia or localized infarcts [106].

Among both institutionalized and community-dwelling populations with Alzheimer's disease, SDB has been shown to be related to cognitive impairment [1,107–109]. In the institutionalized Alzheimer's disease patients, as AHI increased, cognitive functioning worsened, even when controlling for age [1]. There is also evidence to suggest that the severity of sleep disruptions in Alzheimer's disease parallels the decline in cognitive functioning. Anatomically, the brainstem regions and neuronal pathways that regulate sleep-wake patterns are affected by the degenerative changes in Alzheimer's disease [110].

Patients with Parkinson's disease have also been reported to have a higher prevalence of SDB when compared with age-matched controls [111,112]. In addition, most Parkinson's disease patients have some subtle changes in cognition, and some 40% progress to Parkinson's disease dementia [113]. Because Parkinson's disease patients commonly experience alterations in respiratory function while awake, there are compelling reasons to think that patients with Parkinson's disease may be at risk of nocturnal hypoxemia and SDB. Anatomically, there is degeneration of the neurons in the reticular activating system and degeneration of the pathways arising from the dorsal raphe and locus coeruleus in Parkinson's disease, all of which likely contribute to sleep disturbances and daytime sleepiness in these patients [114]. The role that SDB plays in the cognitive dysfunction and eventual development of dementia experienced by most Parkinson's disease patients remains unknown.

Mortality

Several studies have reported an association between SDB and decreased survival [7,115–117]. One study followed a cohort of noninstitutionalized older subjects (mean age 66) for 12 years and reported a mortality ratio of 2.7 for those with an AHI ≥ 10 [118]. Similarly, Hoch and coworkers [119] reported that SDB was associated with an excess mortality rate of 450% in elderly patients with depression and cognitive impairment. Ancoli-Israel and coworkers [7] found that community-dwelling elderly with more severe SDB (defined as an AHI ≥ 30) had significantly shorter survivals than those with mild-moderate or no SDB.

Results from several studies suggest, however, that the increased risk of mortality among those with SDB is indirect. For example, in studies of community-dwelling elderly, AHI was not found to be an independent predictor of mortality after accounting for cardiovascular and pulmonary conditions, including hypertension [7,120]. There is growing evidence to suggest that SDB represents a predisposing factor for cardiopulmonary disease, however, which in turn leads to increased mortality. Marin and coworkers [19] studied older men with severe SDB and a population-based sample of healthy men (matched for age and BMI). Over a 10-year follow-up period, patients with untreated severe disease had a higher incidence of fatal cardiovascular events (1.06 per 100 person-years) and nonfatal cardiovascular events (2.13 per 100 person-years) than did untreated patients with mild-moderate disease (0.55, $P = .02$; 0.89, $P < .0001$); simple snorers (0.34, $P = .0006$; 0.58, $P < .0001$); patients treated with CPAP (0.35, $P = .0008$; 0.64, $P < .0001$); and healthy participants (0.3, $P = .0012$; 0.45, $P < .0001$). The results from this observational study suggest that SDB increases risk of fatal and nonfatal cardiovascular events in older men, and that treatment of SDB with CPAP

reduces this risk. In another study, Ancoli-Israel and coworkers [121] showed that elderly men with congestive heart failure had more severe SDB than those with no heart disease, whereas men with both conditions (heart failure and SDB) had shortened life spans compared with those with congestive heart failure or SDB alone.

Daytime sleepiness, a major symptom of SDB, has also been associated with increased total and CVD mortality [122]. Using self-reported information on sleep quality among older men and women participating in the Cardiovascular Health Study, Newman and colleagues [122] showed that daytime sleepiness was associated with more than double the risk of mortality in older women (hazard ratio = 2.12; 95% CI 1.66–1.72), and a significant although somewhat weaker association in men (hazard ratio = 1.40; 95% CI 1.12–1.73).

In general, the risk of sudden death from cardiac causes is highest from 6:00 AM to noon and lowest from midnight to 6:00 AM [123]. This pattern, however, has been shown to differ among those with SDB [124]. Gami and coworkers [124] examined the time intervals of sudden cardiac death among patients who had undergone polysomnography, and compared those with SDB with those without SDB, and with those in the general population. The authors found that those who had died from midnight to 6:00 AM had a significantly higher AHI than those who died during other time intervals during the day. This study reported that for patients with SDB, the relative risk of sudden death from cardiac causes from midnight to 6:00 AM was 2.57. The peak in risk of sudden cardiac death during the sleeping hours among those with SDB contrasts with the typical nadir for this interval observed in the general population.

More studies need to be undertaken to elicit further the exact nature of the relationship of SDB and mortality in the elderly, specifically in older women because most of the studies completed in this age category have involved predominantly men.

Falls and fractures

Falls pose a major health risk among older adults and are a leading cause of mortality, morbidity, and premature nursing home placement [125,126]. The propensity for injury caused by a fall is also drastically increased in older persons, many of whom suffer from osteoporosis and are more prone to hip and other types of fractures. It is estimated that falls occur in approximately a third of persons over the age of 65 each year [127].

There is new evidence linking SDB to increased risk of falls in older men. Based on preliminary analysis of data from the multicenter study Outcomes of Sleep Disorders in Older Men, Stone and coworkers [128] found that among 2865 men aged 67 and older, each SD increase in AHI is associated with a 16% increased odds of falling (OR = 1.16; 95% CI 1.02–1.33). Each SD increase in the percentage of sleep time <90% oxygen saturation increased odds of falls by 27% (OR = 1.27; 95% CI 1.13–1.43). Among the 10% of men with any sleep time spent in <80% arterial oxygen saturation, the risk of falls was more than double (OR = 2.14; 95% CI 1.40–3.26) compared with men with no such episodes. These findings were unexplained by age, race, BMI, comorbidities, or medication use.

There are no comparative data directly linking SDB with risk of falls in older women or younger subjects. New findings based on the Study of Osteoporotic Fractures, however, indicate a strong relationship between self-reported napping and risk of falls and hip fractures among older women [129]. In particular, among 8101 primarily white women aged 69 and older, those who reported napping daily had a significantly increased odds of falling two or more times during the subsequent year as compared with those who did not report daily napping (OR = 1.32; 95% CI 1.03–1.69). These results were independent of age, BMI, comorbidities, health habits, medication use, and urinary incontinence. Those who reported daily napping also had a 33% increase in risk of hip fracture (relative hazard = 1.33; 95% CI 0.99–1.78). Further studies are needed to elucidate the mechanisms for these associations. At least in some women, however, daytime napping may be indicative of EDS as a result of disrupted nighttime sleep caused by SDB.

Clinical assessment and management of sleep-disordered breathing

Presentation and diagnosis

EDS and snoring are the two main clinical features of SDB. EDS may be a less useful specific marker of SDB in elderly compared with younger populations, however, given it's high prevalence in the elderly and association with a myriad of conditions (eg, Parkinson's disease, abnormal thyroid function, malignancies, depression, nocturia related to benign prostatic hypertrophy); its association with medications frequently used in the elderly (eg, hypnotics, antidepressants, antihistamines, dopaminergics); or its association with sleep deprivation from any number of causes. Elderly individuals tend to nap more frequently than younger adults, and regular napping has been reported to be common in the elderly [130]. In contrast, snoring may be a less sensitive marker of SDB in the elderly compared with other populations because of the frequent unavailability of a bed partner to report such symptoms. The absence of a positive snoring

history should not be used to exclude a possible diagnosis of SDB. As in younger populations, elderly individuals with unrefreshed sleep should be evaluated for sleep disorders. SDB should be considered especially among those who are also overweight, hypertensive, or diabetic.

As the prior discussion of clinical findings and cardiovascular, metabolic, neurocognitive outcomes suggest, there is growing evidence to support the importance of appropriately diagnosing and treating elderly individuals with sleep disorders. The notion that elderly subjects normally experience sleepiness or difficulty sleeping should be disbanded in favor of systematic attempts to identify reversible causes of these conditions, which directly or indirectly may be disabling. Although many symptoms of sleep disorders may lack specificity, further evaluation is needed when the elderly patient experiences difficulty maintaining wakefulness during daily activities, such as holding conversations or driving, or experiences unintentional napping or unexplained problems with concentration, attention, and memory. Nocturnal symptoms, such as fragmented or restless sleep, also should alert the clinician to the possibility of nocturnal awakenings related to the SDB, such as obstructive apneas with efforts made to breathe, or Cheyne-Stokes breathing, which is often associated with increased arousals. SDB also may present as nocturnal confusion.

Assessment of SDB should begin with a complete sleep history, including symptoms of SDB; symptoms of other sleep disorders (ie, restless leg syndrome); and sleep-related habits and routines. When possible, the history should include input from a bed partner, roommate, or caregiver. The patient's medical history, including psychiatric and medical records, should be thoroughly reviewed, paying particular attention to associated medical conditions (eg, heart failure, stroke) and medications, the use of alcohol, and evidence of cognitive impairment. The physical examination should include careful evaluation of cardiovascular, respiratory, and neurologic systems. Upper airway examination may reveal evidence of a high arched palate or "crowded" airway caused by macroglossia, redundant soft tissue, or a swollen uvular, all signs of a vulnerable or traumatized pharynx.

As with younger adults, the diagnosis of SDB in the elderly requires an overnight sleep recording where both breathing and sleep architecture can be characterized and other sleep problems, such as periodic leg movements, can be identified. Performing overnight sleep monitoring in a sleep laboratory may be challenging for an older person who may not adapt well to sleeping in an unfamiliar setting. Ensuring that the sleep laboratory is patient friendly and having the staff and amenities that meet the needs of older individuals often enhances both the patient's experience and the quality of the sleep test. Alternative technology is available to perform sleep studies in the homes of patients. As more experience is developed with these techniques, they may provide useful testing alternatives that are more acceptable to older patients.

Treatment of sleep-disordered breathing in the elderly

Older patients who present with symptoms of SDB or evidence of comorbidities that may be attributed to SDB should be considered for treatment. There are currently insufficient data, however, to establish specific criteria for initiating treatment. In younger populations, there is clear evidence that moderate to severe SDB, identified by an AHI ≥ 30 and daytime sleepiness, is associated with increased morbidity, mortality [19], and responsiveness to therapy [131]. Individuals with lesser levels of SDB but with symptoms or comorbidities unexplained by other factors, however, may warrant further study. Because successful treatment of SDB may markedly enhance quality of life, and because treatment adherence is difficult to predict, advanced age should not be used as a reason to withhold treatment.

Treatment of SDB in the elderly is similar to that in younger adults. All patients should be provided education and support to optimize nutrition, weight, physical activity, and as appropriate be advised to stop smoking (which can contribute to disturbed sleep and cause upper airway irritation). Alcohol, even in small amounts, can exacerbate SDB, and elderly patients with SDB should be encouraged to abstain completely from its consumption. Treatment of nasal congestion or nasal obstruction (medically or surgically) may also ameliorate symptoms of SDB. Because many patients experience more severe SDB in the supine position, avoidance of this position and attempting to sleep in the lateral decubitus position may be beneficial. Insufficient or irregular sleep may also exacerbate SDB and all efforts should be made for the patient to maintain regular sleep patterns (bedtimes and wake times), attempting to get at least 7.5 hours of sleep per night. Among older individuals with an advanced circadian rhythm (sleepiness occurring in the early evening), there may be benefit to adjusting sleep times to coincide with times of maximal sleepiness. Long-acting sedating benzodiazepines, which may have respiratory-depressant effects, potentially exacerbating SDB should generally be avoided in the elderly with SDB. Treatment and optimization of underlying medical problems that may contribute to SDB, such as heart failure and airway reactivity, and treatment of pain syndromes, which may contribute to disrupted or short sleep, are also of critical importance.

The gold standard for treatment is CPAP, a device that provides continuous positive pressure by way of the nasal passages or oral airway, creating a pneumatic splint to keep the airway open during inspiration. If used appropriately, CPAP has been shown safely and effectively to manage SDB at night with minimal side effects [132]. It also has been shown to have some beneficial effects on both Cheyne-Stokes breathing and heart function in patients with impaired cardiac function [133].

For those patients who are able to tolerate CPAP, beneficial effects have been shown in older adults, including decreased nocturia and daytime somnolence, and improved depression ratings and quality of life scores [134]. Other studies suggest treatment of SDB is associated with improvements in cognition, particularly in the areas of attention, psychomotor speed, executive functioning, and nonverbal delayed recall [135].

There are special challenges associated with use of CPAP in dementia. There is evidence, however, that adequate CPAP compliance may be achieved even in this population [136] and that not only is AHI reduced, but the amount of daytime sleepiness is also significantly reduced [137]. Depression is another condition in which adherence with treatment may be difficult, and special care and support of these patients may be required [136].

For patients who have difficulty adhering to CPAP, there are two alternative treatments that should be considered: oral appliances and surgery. Oral appliances, worn during sleep to increase airway dimensions (often by advancing the position of the jaw) should generally be reserved for those individuals who are not obese [138]. Effectiveness ranges from 50% to 100%. Patients with dentures, however, are generally not candidates for this device, although newer models can be fitted with dentures.

Surgical treatment includes procedures that reduce or eliminate excessive soft or lymphoid tissue in the airway, or that alter the bony configuration of the airway. Such treatments often are not recommended in the elderly given the risks of general surgery in conjunction with overall response rates that may be <50% [139].

Oxygen supplementation has been considered in the elderly with significant oxyhemoglobin desaturation in whom other therapies cannot be tolerated or were ineffective. Studies showing clinical objective improvement in SDB with the use of chronic supplemental oxygen administration are inconclusive. Furthermore, use of oxygen in this setting should be carefully monitored to ensure that its administration does not result in a prolongation of apneas or the occurrence of respiratory acidosis [140]. Patients who meet these criteria should undergo a full attended polysomnogram with oxygen supplementation to ensure that there is are no adverse physiologic sequelae, including increases in apnea duration, before being prescribed oxygen for home use.

Discussion

Clinical features of SDB in older adults, including snoring and EDS, partly mirror those observed in their younger counterparts. There is some evidence, however, that snoring may be less predominant in older populations with SDB [25]. Furthermore, in addition to SDB, a variety of other factors may contribute to EDS in the elderly. The specific contribution of SDB to EDS may be more difficult to distinguish.

The natural history of SDB in the elderly remains largely unknown. Furthermore, the natural history of any disease in the elderly is complicated by issues of competing risks and multiple comorbidities [36]. Although studies have consistently shown that the prevalence of SDB increases with age [5,35], it is unclear whether the severity and clinical significance of SDB are also increasing. For example, Bixler and coworkers [141] reported that the prevalence of SDB increased in a sample of older men but that after controlling for BMI, the severity based on number of events and oxygen saturation actually decreased with age. Ancoli-Israel and coworkers [142] showed in an 18-year follow-up study of elderly patients with SDB that AHI did not continue to increase with age. Rather, if the patient's BMI remained stable, so did the AHI.

In addition, controversy exists regarding the effect of SDB on morbidity and mortality in the elderly. Despite the growing body of literature exploring SDB in the elderly, more evidence is needed to determine if SDB in the elderly is a distinct pathologic condition from SDB in younger adults. For example, it remains inconclusive as to whether or not the traditional risk factors for SDB observed in middle-aged populations, including obesity and gender, are as strongly related to SDB risk in older adults.

Furthermore, the associations of SDB with such outcomes as CVD, metabolic abnormalities, and cognitive impairments may differ in older adults as compared with their younger counterparts given possible age-related differences in end-organ response. For example, underlying coronary artery disease in older adults may increase vulnerability to ischemia related to intermittent hypoxia and sympathetic effects. Some studies, however, have reported considerably weaker relationships between SDB and cardiac outcomes. For example, in an analysis of data from the Sleep Heart Health Study, Mehra and coworkers [75] reported more than fourfold higher odds of complex ventricular ectopy associated with SDB among adults aged 50 years as compared with 70 years. It has been speculated that changes in autonomic nervous system with aging may be protective in blunting adverse cardiovascular responses to SDB-related physiologic perturbations.

Despite the lack of clear guidance in terms of optimal definition of SDB in relation to functional outcomes, morbidity, and mortality in older adults, older patients who present with symptoms of SDB or evidence of comorbidities that may be attributed to SDB should be further evaluated and considered for treatment.

References

[1] Ancoli-Israel S, Klauber MR, Butters N, et al. Dementia in institutionalized elderly: relation to sleep apnea. J Am Geriatr Soc 1991;39:258–63.
[2] Foley DJ, Monjan AA, Brown SL, et al. Sleep complaints among elderly persons: an epidemiologic study of three communities. Sleep 1995; 18:425–32.
[3] Prinz PN, Vitiello MV, Raskind MA, et al. Geriatrics: sleep disorders and aging. [see comments]. N Engl J Med 1990;323:520–6.
[4] Ancoli-Israel S, Kripke DF, Klauber MR, et al. Sleep-disordered breathing in community-dwelling elderly. Sleep 1991;14:486–95.
[5] Ancoli-Israel S, Kripke DF, Klauber MR, et al. Natural history of sleep disordered breathing in community dwelling elderly. Sleep 1993; 16(8 Suppl):S25–9.
[6] Ancoli-Israel S, Klauber MR, Stepnowsky C, et al. Sleep-disordered breathing in African-American elderly. Am J Respir Crit Care Med 1995;152(6 Pt 1):1946–9.
[7] Ancoli-Israel S, Kripke DF, Klauber MR, et al. Morbidity, mortality and sleep-disordered breathing in community dwelling elderly. Sleep 1996;19:277–82.
[8] Ancoli-Israel S. Epidemiology of sleep disorders. Clin Geriatr Med 1989;5:347–62.
[9] Boehlecke BA. Epidemiology and pathogenesis of sleep-disordered breathing. Curr Opin Pulm Med 2000;6:471–8.
[10] Flemons WW. Measuring health related quality of life in sleep apnea. Sleep 2000;23(Suppl 4): S109–14.
[11] Young T, Palta M, Dempsey J, et al. The occurrence of sleep-disordered breathing among middle-aged adults. N Engl J Med 1993;328: 1230–5.
[12] Findley L, Unverzagt M, Guchu R, et al. Vigilance and automobile accidents in patients with

sleep apnea or narcolepsy. Chest 1995; 108:619–24.

[13] Bedard MA, Montplaisir J, Richer F, et al. Nocturnal hypoxemia as a determinant of vigilance impairment in sleep apnea syndrome. Chest 1991;100:367–70.

[14] Ingram F, Henke KG, Levin HS, et al. Sleep apnea and vigilance performance in a community-dwelling older sample. Sleep 1994;17: 248–52.

[15] Nieto FJ, Young TB, Lind BK, et al. Association of sleep-disordered breathing, sleep apnea, and hypertension in a large community-based study. Sleep Heart Health Study. JAMA 2000; 283:1829–36.

[16] Peppard PE, Young T, Palta M, et al. Prospective study of the association between sleep-disordered breathing and hypertension. N Engl J Med 2000;342:1378–84.

[17] Punjabi NM, Shahar E, Redline S, et al. Sleep-disordered breathing, glucose intolerance, and insulin resistance: the Sleep Heart Health Study. Am J Epidemiol 2004;160:521–30.

[18] Shahar E, Whitney CW, Redline S, et al. Sleep-disordered breathing and cardiovascular disease: cross-sectional results of the Sleep Heart Health Study. Am J Respir Crit Care Med 2001;163:19–25.

[19] Marin JM, Carrizo SJ, Vicente E, et al. Long-term cardiovascular outcomes in men with obstructive sleep apnoea-hypopnoea with or without treatment with continuous positive airway pressure: an observational study. Lancet 2005; 365:1046–53.

[20] Bliwise D, Bliwise NG, Kraemer HC, et al. Measurement error in visually scored electrophysiological data: respiration during sleep. J Neurosci Methods 1984;12:49–56.

[21] Redline S, Min NI, Shahar E, et al. Polysomnographic predictors of blood pressure and hypertension: is one index best? Sleep 2005; 28:1122–30.

[22] Bradley TD, Floras JS. Pathophysiologic and therapeutic implications of sleep apnea in congestive heart failure. J Card Fail 1996; 2:223–40.

[23] Resnick HE, Redline S, Shahar E, et al. Diabetes and sleep disturbances: findings from the Sleep Heart Health Study. Diabetes Care 2003; 26:702–9.

[24] Collop NA, Cassel DK. Snoring and sleep-disordered breathing. In: Lee-Chiong TL, Sateia MJ, Carskadon MA, editors. Sleep medicine. Philadelphia: Hanley & Belfus; 2002. p. 349–55.

[25] Enright PL, Newman AB, Wahl PW, et al. Prevalence and correlates of snoring and observed apneas in 5,201 older adults. Sleep 1996; 19:531–8.

[26] Gottlieb DJ, Yao Q, Redline S, et al. Does snoring predict sleepiness independently of apnea and hypopnea frequency? Am J Respir Crit Care Med 2000;162(4 Pt 1):1512–7.

[27] Asplund R. Daytime sleepiness and napping amongst the elderly in relation to somatic health and medical treatment. J Intern Med 1996;239:261–7.

[28] Schmitt FA, Phillips BA, Cook YR, et al. Self report on sleep symptoms in older adults: correlates of daytime sleepiness and health. Sleep 1996;19:59–64.

[29] Whitney CW, Enright PL, Newman AB, et al. Correlates of daytime sleepiness in 4578 elderly persons: the Cardiovascular Health Study. Sleep 1998;21:27–36.

[30] Reynolds CF III, Jennings JR, Hoch CC, et al. Daytime sleepiness in the healthy "old old": a comparison with young adults. J Am Geriatr Soc 1991;39:957–62.

[31] Hoch CC, Reynolds CF III, Jennings JR, et al. Daytime sleepiness and performance among healthy 80 and 20 year olds. Neurobiol Aging 1992;13:353–6.

[32] Gottlieb DJ, Whitney CW, Bonekat WH, et al. Relation of sleepiness to respiratory disturbance index: the Sleep Heart Health Study. Am J Respir Crit Care Med 1999;159:502–7.

[33] Kezirian EJ, Litwack S, Ancoli-Israel S, et al. Sleep disordered breathing and daytime sleepiness in older women: a prospective study with objective measures of sleep [abstract]. Sleep 2005;28:A196.

[34] Martin J, Stepnowsky C, Ancoli-Israel S. Sleep apnea in the elderly. In: McNicholas WT, Phillipson EA, editors. Breathing disorders during sleep. London: WB Saunders; 2002. p. 278–87.

[35] Hoch CC, Dew MA, Reynolds CF III, et al. Longitudinal changes in diary- and laboratory-based sleep measures in healthy "old old" and "young old" subjects: a three-year follow-up. Sleep 1997;20:192–202.

[36] Young T, Peppard PE, Gottlieb DJ. Epidemiology of obstructive sleep apnea: a population health perspective. Am J Respir Crit Care Med 2002;165:1217–39.

[37] Kim J, In K, You S, et al. Prevalence of sleep-disordered breathing in middle-aged Korean men and women. Am J Respir Crit Care Med 2004;170:1108–13.

[38] Young T, Shahar E, Nieto FJ, et al. Predictors of sleep-disordered breathing in community-dwelling adults: the Sleep Heart Health Study. Arch Intern Med 2002;162:893–900.

[39] Ancoli-Israel S, Parker L, Sinaee R, et al. Sleep fragmentation in patients from a nursing home. J Gerontol 1989;44:M18–21.

[40] Hoch CC, Reynolds CF. Cognitive function and sleep disordered breathing in dementia: the Pittsburgh experience. In: Kuna ST, Suratt PM, Remmers JE, editors. Sleep and respiration in aging adults. New York: Elsevier; 1991. p. 245–50.

[41] Taylor W, Phillipson EA, Moldofsky H. Cognitive function and sleep disordered breathing

in normal elderly and patients with Alzheimer's disease. In: Kuna ST, Suratt PM, Remmers JE, editors. Sleep and respiration in aging adults. New York: Elsevier; 1991. p. 251–8.

[42] Erkinjuntti T, Partinen M, Sulkava R, et al. Sleep apnea in multiinfarct dementia and Alzheimer's disease. Sleep 1987;10:419–25.

[43] Peppard PE, Young T, Palta M, et al. Longitudinal study of moderate weight change and sleep-disordered breathing. JAMA 2000; 284:3015–21.

[44] Redline S, Schluchter MD, Larkin EK, et al. Predictors of longitudinal change in sleep-disordered breathing in a nonclinic population. Sleep 2003;26:703–9.

[45] Tishler PV, Larkin EK, Schluchter MD, et al. Incidence of sleep-disordered breathing in an urban adult population: the relative importance of risk factors in the development of sleep-disordered breathing. JAMA 2003; 289:2230–7.

[46] Newman AB, Foster G, Givelber R, et al. Progression and regression of sleep-disordered breathing with changes in weight: the Sleep Heart Health Study. Arch Intern Med 2005; 165:2408–13.

[47] Phillips B, Ancoli-Israel S. Sleep disorders in the elderly. Sleep Med 2001;2:99–114.

[48] Kripke DF, Ancoli-Israel S, Klauber MR, et al. Prevalence of sleep-disordered breathing in ages 40–64 years: a population-based survey. Sleep 1997;20:65–76.

[49] Vgontzas AN, Papanicolaou DA, Bixler EO, et al. Sleep apnea and daytime sleepiness and fatigue: relation to visceral obesity, insulin resistance, and hypercytokinemia. J Clin Endocrinol Metab 2000;85:1151–8.

[50] Vanitallie TB. Frailty in the elderly: contributions of sarcopenia and visceral protein depletion. Metabolism 2003;52(Suppl 2):22–6.

[51] Fried LP, Tangen CM, Walston J, et al. Frailty in older adults: evidence for a phenotype. J Gerontol A Biol Sci Med Sci 2001;56:M146–56.

[52] Dempsey JA, Skatrud JB, Jacques AJ, et al. Anatomic determinants of sleep-disordered breathing across the spectrum of clinical and nonclinical male subjects. Chest 2002; 122:840–51.

[53] Redline S, Kump K, Tishler PV, et al. Gender differences in sleep disordered breathing in a community-based sample. Am J Respir Crit Care Med 1994;149(3 Pt 1):722–6.

[54] Redline S, Tishler PV, Hans MG, et al. Racial differences in sleep-disordered breathing in African-Americans and Caucasians. Am J Respir Crit Care Med 1997;155:186–92.

[55] Young T, Finn L, Austin D, et al. Menopausal status and sleep-disordered breathing in the Wisconsin Sleep Cohort Study. Am J Respir Crit Care Med 2003;167:1181–5.

[56] Shahar E, Redline S, Young T, et al. Hormone replacement therapy and sleep-disordered breathing. Am J Respir Crit Care Med 2003; 167:1186–92.

[57] Bixler EO, Vgontzas AN, Lin HM, et al. Prevalence of sleep-disordered breathing in women: effects of gender. Am J Respir Crit Care Med 2001;163(3 Pt 1):608–13.

[58] Newman AB, Nieto FJ, Guidry U, et al. Relation of sleep-disordered breathing to cardiovascular disease risk factors: the Sleep Heart Health Study. Am J Epidemiol 2001;154:50–9.

[59] Foley DJ, Monjan AA, Masaki KH, et al. Associations of symptoms of sleep apnea with cardiovascular disease, cognitive impairment, and mortality among older Japanese American men. J Am Geriatr Soc 1999;47:524–8.

[60] Lavie P, Silverberg D, Oksenberg A, et al. Obstructive sleep apnea and hypertension: from correlative to causative relationship. J Clin Hypertens (Greenwich) 2001;3:296–301.

[61] Lavie P, Herer P, Hoffstein V. Obstructive sleep apnoea syndrome as a risk factor for hypertension: population study. BMJ 2000;320: 479–82.

[62] Giles TL, Lasserson TJ, Smith BJ, et al. Continuous positive airways pressure for obstructive sleep apnoea in adults. Cochrane Database Syst Rev 2006;1:CD001106.

[63] Haas DC, Foster GL, Nieto FJ, et al. Age-dependent associations between sleep-disordered breathing and hypertension: importance of discriminating between systolic/diastolic hypertension and isolated systolic hypertension in the Sleep Heart Health Study. Circulation 2005; 111:614–21.

[64] Stoohs RA, Gingold J, Cohrs S, et al. Sleep-disordered breathing and systemic hypertension in the older male. J Am Geriatr Soc 1996; 44:1295–300.

[65] Berry DT, Phillips BA, Cook YR, et al. Sleep-disordered breathing in healthy aged persons: one-year follow-up of daytime sequelae. Sleep 1989;12:211–5.

[66] Javaheri S, Parker TJ, Liming JD, et al. Sleep apnea in 81 ambulatory male patients with stable heart failure: types and their prevalences, consequences, and presentations. Circulation 1998; 97:2154–9.

[67] Chan J, Sanderson J, Chan W, et al. Prevalence of sleep-disordered breathing in diastolic heart failure. Chest 1997;111:1488–93.

[68] Ryan CM, Bradley TD. Pathogenesis of obstructive sleep apnea. J Appl Physiol 2005; 99:2440–50.

[69] Verrier RL. Cardiovascular disorders and sleep. In: Lee-Chiong TL, Sateia MJ, Carskadon MA, editors. Sleep medicine. Philadelphia: Hanley & Belfus; 2002. p. 447–53.

[70] Jennum P, Schultz-Larsen K, Davidsen M, et al. Snoring and risk of stroke and ischaemic heart disease in a 70 year old population: a 6-year follow-up study. Int J Epidemiol 1994;23: 1159–64.

[71] Yaggi H, Mohsenin V. Obstructive sleep apnoea and stroke. Lancet Neurol 2004;3:333–42.

[72] Levy P, Pepin JL, Malauzat D, et al. Is sleep apnea syndrome in the elderly a specific entity? Sleep 1996;19(3 Suppl):S29–38.

[73] Bassetti CL, Milanova M, Gugger M. Sleep-disordered breathing and acute ischemic stroke: diagnosis, risk factors, treatment, evolution, and long-term clinical outcome. Stroke 2006; 37(4):967–72.

[74] Martinez-Garcia MA, Galiano-Blancart R, Roman-Sanchez P, et al. Continuous positive airway pressure treatment in sleep apnea prevents new vascular events after ischemic stroke. Chest 2005;128:2123–9.

[75] Mehra R, Benjamin EJ, Shahar E, et al. Association of nocturnal arrhythmias with sleep-disordered breathing: the Sleep Heart Health Study. Am J Respir Crit Care Med 2006;173(8): 910–6.

[76] Nieto FJ, Herrington DM, Redline S, et al. Sleep apnea and markers of vascular endothelial function in a large community sample of older adults. Am J Respir Crit Care Med 2004; 169:354–60.

[77] Faulx MD, Larkin EK, Hoit BD, et al. Sex influences endothelial function in sleep-disordered breathing. Sleep 2004;27:1113–20.

[78] Naylor E, Penev PD, Orbeta L, et al. Daily social and physical activity increases slow-wave sleep and daytime neuropsychological performance in the elderly. Sleep 2000;23:87–95.

[79] Millman RP, Carlisle CC, McGarvey ST, et al. Body fat distribution and sleep apnea severity in women. Chest 1995;107:362–6.

[80] Derderian SS, Rajagopal KR. Obesity, gender and sleep. Chest 1988;93:900–1.

[81] Lakka HM, Laaksonen DE, Lakka TA, et al. The metabolic syndrome and total and cardiovascular disease mortality in middle-aged men. JAMA 2002;288:2709–16.

[82] Brown LK. A waist is a terrible thing to mind: central obesity, the metabolic syndrome, and sleep apnea hypopnea syndrome. Chest 2002; 122:774–8.

[83] Smith GS, Reynolds CF III, Houck PR, et al. Glucose metabolic response to total sleep deprivation, recovery sleep, and acute antidepressant treatment as functional neuroanatomic correlates of treatment outcome in geriatric depression. Am J Geriatr Psychiatry 2002; 10:561–7.

[84] de la Eva RC, Baur LA, Donaghue KC, et al. Metabolic correlates with obstructive sleep apnea in obese subjects. J Pediatr 2002;140: 654–9.

[85] Grunstein RR, Stenlof K, Hedner J, et al. Impact of obstructive sleep apnea and sleepiness on metabolic and cardiovascular risk factors in the Swedish Obese Subjects (SOS) Study. Int J Obes Relat Metab Disord 1995;19: 410–8.

[86] Spiegel K, Leproult R, Van Cauter E. Impact of sleep debt on metabolic and endocrine function. Lancet 1999;354:1435–9.

[87] Mullington JM, Hinze-Selch D, Pollmacher T. Mediators of inflammation and their interaction with sleep: relevance for chronic fatigue syndrome and related conditions. Ann N Y Acad Sci 2001;933:201–10.

[88] Shamsuzzaman AS, Winnicki M, Lanfranchi P, et al. Elevated C-reactive protein in patients with obstructive sleep apnea. Circulation 2002; 105:2462–4.

[89] Brunner EJ, Hemingway H, Walker BR, et al. Adrenocortical, autonomic, and inflammatory causes of the metabolic syndrome: nested case-control study. Circulation 2002;106:2659–65.

[90] Vgontzas AN, Papanicolaou DA, Bixler EO, et al. Elevation of plasma cytokines in disorders of excessive daytime sleepiness: role of sleep disturbance and obesity. J Clin Endocrinol Metab 1997;82:1313–6.

[91] Vgontzas A, Papanicolaou D, Bixler E, et al. Circadian interleukin-6 secretion and quantity and depth of sleep. J Clin Endocrinol Metab 1999; 84:2603–7.

[92] Saarelainen S, Lehtimaki T, Kallonen E, et al. No relation between apolipoprotein E alleles and obstructive sleep apnea. Clin Genet 1998; 53:147–8.

[93] Reichmuth KJ, Austin D, Skatrud JB, et al. Association of sleep apnea and type II diabetes: a population-based study. Am J Respir Crit Care Med 2005;172:1590–5.

[94] Al-Delaimy WK, Manson JE, Willett WC, et al. Snoring as a risk factor for type II diabetes mellitus: a prospective study. Am J Epidemiol 2002; 155:387–93.

[95] Babu AR, Herdegen J, Fogelfeld L, et al. Type 2 diabetes, glycemic control, and continuous positive airway pressure in obstructive sleep apnea. Arch Intern Med 2005;165:447–52.

[96] Harsch IA, Schahin SP, Bruckner K, et al. The effect of continuous positive airway pressure treatment on insulin sensitivity in patients with obstructive sleep apnoea syndrome and type 2 diabetes. Respiration 2004;71:252–9.

[97] Ayas NT, White DP, Al-Delaimy WK, et al. A prospective study of self-reported sleep duration and incident diabetes in women. Diabetes Care 2003;26:380–4.

[98] Aloia MS, Arnedt JT, Davis JD, et al. Neuropsychological sequelae of obstructive sleep apnea-hypopnea syndrome: a critical review. J Int Neuropsychol Soc 2004;10:772–85.

[99] Foley DJ, Masaki K, White L, et al. Sleep-disordered breathing and cognitive impairment in elderly Japanese-American men. Sleep 2003; 26:596–9.

[100] Bedard MA, Montplaisir J, Richer F, et al. Nocturnal hypoxemia as a determinant of vigilance impairment in sleep apnea syndrome. Chest 1991;100:367–70.

[101] Findley LJ, Barth JT, Powers DC, et al. Cognitive impairment in patients with obstructive sleep apnea and associated hypoxemia. Chest 1986; 90:686–90.

[102] Lojander J, Kajaste S, Maasilta P, et al. Cognitive function and treatment of obstructive sleep apnea syndrome. J Sleep Res 1999;8:71–6.

[103] Cohen-Zion M, Stepnowsky C, Marler M, et al. Changes in cognitive function associated with sleep disordered breathing in older people. J Am Geriatr Soc 2001;49:1622–7.

[104] Kim HC, Young T, Matthews CG, et al. Sleep-disordered breathing and neuropsychological deficits: a population-based study. Am J Respir Crit Care Med 1997;156:1813–9.

[105] Bliwise DL. Sleep in normal aging and dementia. Sleep 1993;16:40–81.

[106] Bliwise DL. Cognivier function and sleep disordered breathing in aging adults. In: Kuna ST, Remmers JE, Suratt PM, editors. Sleep and respiration in aging adults. New York: Elsevier; 1991. p. 237–44.

[107] Ancoli-Israel S. Epidemiology of sleep disorders. Philadelphia: WB Saunders; 1989.

[108] Ancoli-Israel S, Klauber MR, Gillin JC, et al. Sleep in non-institutionalized Alzheimer's disease patients. Aging (Milano) 1994;6:451–8.

[109] Gehrman PR, Martin JL, Shochat T, et al. Sleep-disordered breathing and agitation in institutionalized adults with Alzheimer disease. Am J Geriatr Psychiatry 2003;11:426–33.

[110] Prinz PN, Vitaliano PP, Vitiello MV, et al. Sleep, EEG and mental function changes in senile dementia of the Alzheimer's type. Neurobiol Aging 1982;3:361–70.

[111] Arnulf I, Konofal E, Merino-Andreu M, et al. Parkinson's disease and sleepiness: an integral part of PD. Neurology 2002;58:1019–24.

[112] Maria B, Sophia S, Michalis M, et al. Sleep breathing disorders in patients with idiopathic Parkinson's disease. Respir Med 2003; 97:1151–7.

[113] Emre M. Dementia associated with Parkinson's disease. Lancet Neurol 2003;2:229–37.

[114] Schapira AH. Excessive daytime sleepiness in Parkinson's disease. Neurology 2004;63(Suppl 3): S24–7.

[115] Lavie P, Herer P, Peled R, et al. Mortality in sleep apnea patients: a multivariate analysis of risk factors. Sleep 1995;18:149–57.

[116] He J, Kryger MH, Zorick FJ, et al. Mortality and apnea index in obstructive sleep apnea: experience in 385 male patients. Chest 1988; 94:9–14.

[117] Gonzalez-Rothi RJ, Foresman GE, Block AJ. Do patients with sleep apnea die in their sleep? Chest 1988;94:531–8.

[118] Bliwise DL, Bliwise NG, Partinen M, et al. Sleep apnea and mortality in an aged cohort. Am J Public Health 1988;78:544–7.

[119] Hoch CC, Reynolds CF III, Houck PR, et al. Predicting mortality in mixed depression and dementia using EEG sleep variables. J Neuropsychiatry Clin Neurosci 1989;1:366–71.

[120] Mant A, King M, Saunders NA, et al. Four-year follow-up of mortality and sleep-related respiratory disturbance in non-demented seniors. Sleep 1995;18:433–8.

[121] Ancoli-Israel S, DuHamel ER, Stepnowsky C, et al. The relationship between congestive heart failure, sleep apnea, and mortality in older men. Chest 2003;124:1400–5.

[122] Newman AB, Spiekerman CF, Enright P, et al. Daytime sleepiness predicts mortality and cardiovascular disease in older adults: the Cardiovascular Health Study Research Group. J Am Geriatr Soc 2000;48:115–23.

[123] Cohen MC, Rohtla KM, Lavery CE, et al. Meta-analysis of the morning excess of acute myocardial infarction and sudden cardiac death. Am J Cardiol 1997;79:1512–6.

[124] Gami AS, Howard DE, Olson EJ, et al. Day-night pattern of sudden death in obstructive sleep apnea. N Engl J Med 2005;352:1206–14.

[125] Nevitt MC, Cummings SR, Kidd S, et al. Risk factors for recurrent nonsyncopal falls: a prospective study. JAMA 1989;261:2663–8.

[126] Nevitt MC, Cummings SR, Hudes ES. Risk factors for injurious falls: a prospective study. J Gerontol 1991;46:M164–70.

[127] O'Loughlin JL, Robitaille Y, Boivin JF, et al. Incidence of and risk factors for falls and injurious falls among the community-dwelling elderly. Am J Epidemiol 1993;137:342–54.

[128] Stone KL, Blackwell T, Ensrud KE, et al. Sleep disordered breathing increases the risk of falls in older men [abstract]. Sleep, in press.

[129] Stone KL, Ewing SK, Lui L, et al. Self-reported sleep and nap habits and risk of falls and fractures in older women: the Study of Osteoporotic Fractures. J Am Geriatr Soc, in press.

[130] Wauquier A, van Sweden B, Lagaay AM, et al. Ambulatory monitoring of sleep-wakefulness patterns in healthy elderly males and females (greater than 88 years): the "Senieur" protocol. J Am Geriatr Soc 1992;40:109–14.

[131] Barbe F, Mayoralas LR, Duran J, et al. Treatment with continuous positive airway pressure is not effective in patients with sleep apnea but no daytime sleepiness. a randomized, controlled trial. Ann Intern Med 2001;134:1015–23.

[132] Grunstein R. Continuous positive airway pressure treatment for obstructive sleep apnea–hypopnea syndrome. In: Kryger MH, Roth T, Dement WC, editors. Principles and practice of sleep medicine. Philadelphia: Elsevier; 2005. p. 1066–80.

[133] Bradley TD, Logan AG, Kimoff RJ, et al. Continuous positive airway pressure for central sleep apnea and heart failure. N Engl J Med 2005; 353:2025–33.

[134] Guilleminault C, Lin CM, Goncalves MA, et al. A prospective study of nocturia and the quality of life of elderly patients with obstructive sleep

apnea or sleep onset insomnia. J Psychosom Res 2004;56:511–5.

[135] Aloia MS, Ilniczky N, Di Dio P, et al. Neuropsychological changes and treatment compliance in older adults with sleep apnea. J Psychosom Res 2003;54:71–6.

[136] Ayalon L, Ancoli-Israel S, Stepnowsky C, et al. Adherence to continuous positive airway pressure treatment in patients with Alzheimer's disease and obstructive sleep apnea. Am J Geriatr Psychiatry 2006;14:176–80.

[137] Chong MS, Ayalon L, Marler M, et al. Continuous positive airway pressure improves subjective daytime sleepiness in mild-moderate Alzheimer's disease patients with sleep disordered breathing. J Am Geriatr Soc 2006;54(5): 777–81.

[138] Ferguson KA, Lowe AA. Oral appliances for sleep disordered breathing. In: Kryger MH, Roth T, Dement WC, editors. Principles and practice of sleep medicine. Philadelphia: Elsevier; 2005. p. 1098–108.

[139] Sher AE, Schechtman KB, Piccirillo JF. The efficacy of surgical modifications of the upper airway in adults with obstructive sleep apnea syndrome. Sleep 1996;19:156–77.

[140] Fletcher EC, Munafo DA. Role of nocturnal oxygen therapy in obstructive sleep apnea: when should it be used? Chest 1990;98: 1497–504.

[141] Bixler EO, Vgontzas AN, Ten Have T, et al. Effects of age on sleep apnea in men: I. Prevalence and severity. Am J Respir Crit Care Med 1998; 157:144–8.

[142] Ancoli-Israel S, Gehrman P, Kripke DF, et al. Long-term follow-up of sleep disordered breathing in older adults. Sleep Med 2001; 2:511–6.

SLEEP
MEDICINE
CLINICS

Sleep Med Clin 1 (2006) 263–271

ELSEVIER
SAUNDERS

Periodic Leg Movements in Sleep and Restless Legs Syndrome: Considerations in Geriatrics

Donald L. Bliwise, PhD

- Periodic leg movements in sleep: prevalence and associated factors
- Technical considerations in the recording of periodic leg movements in sleep as a function of age
- Restless legs syndrome: prevalence and associated factors
- Restless legs syndrome in dementia
- Treatment considerations
- Summary
- References

Both periodic leg movements in sleep (PLMS) and restless legs syndrome (RLS) are common conditions in elderly populations. This article reviews relevant knowledge regarding their prevalence and associated conditions, discusses technical considerations related to the polysomnographic characterization of PLMS in relation to age, evaluates possible manifestations of these conditions in dementia, and offers some brief perspectives on treatment considerations. Although PLMS does not approach 100% sensitivity and 100% specificity as a marker of RLS (specificity lags because many patients without RLS still demonstrate PLMS), both conditions show a high prevalence in the older adult. PLMS and RLS are defined from different data sources (polysomnographic criteria for PLMS, clinical criteria for RLS), although their considerable overlap has led many researchers [1] to argue that PLMS represents the single best objective marker of a condition (ie, RLS) that may be complex and variegated, and may have somewhat unique characterization in geriatrics [2].

Periodic leg movements in sleep: prevalence and associated factors

PLMS are stereotypic, repetitive, nonepileptiform movements of the lower limbs typically occurring during non–rapid eye movement sleep but occasionally occurring in rapid eye movement sleep and in some situations discernible in the waking state. PLMS typically consist of dorsiflexion of the anterior tibialis muscle, although movements may involve the hip or be confined to the great toe (extensor hallucis longus). PLMS represent a physiologic finding made with polysomnography or ankle-mounted actigraphy. The best single-night estimate of PLMS prevalence is about 45% in an unselected geriatric population derived from the San Diego [3]. In a population of similar demographics, over 85% of elderly subjects showed a mean PLMS Index (PLMS per hour of sleep) in excess of 5 [4] across 5 nights of recordings. Somewhat lower estimates of PLMS prevalence (29%) have also been reported [5]. Longitudinal data on

This work was supported by the following grants: AG-020269, AG-025688, NS-35345, NS-050595, AT-00611, and a grant from the Alzheimer's Association
Program in Sleep, Aging and Chronobiology, Department of Neurology, Emory University Medical School, Wesley Woods Geriatric Hospital, 1841 Clifton Road, Atlanta, GA 30329, USA
E-mail address: dbliwis@emory.edu

1556-407X/06/$ – see front matter © 2006 Elsevier Inc. All rights reserved.
doi:10.1016/j.jsmc.2006.04.005

whether PLMS increase with aging are scarce and/or disagree, with some studies showing increases [6] and other studies showing no change [7] over time.

A substantial number of studies have examined symptomatic correlates of PLMS in middle-aged and aged populations and have shown decidedly mixed results. Complaints of poor altered sleep architecture were not apparent in conjunction with PLMS in the early studies of Bixler and coworkers [5] and Kales and coworkers [8] and Mosko and colleagues [9]. Ancoli-Israel and coworkers [3] noted that the myoclonus index (based solely on recorded movements without reference to electroencephalogram) was related to a history of kicking at night and some history of respiratory symptoms, but many symptoms that might be expected to be correlated with disrupted sleep (eg, lower total sleep time, prolonged sleep onset latency) were not. The strongest single correlate of PLMS in that study was the report of the estimated number of awakenings on the night of recording. Another study in the elderly noted relationships between PLMS and sleep latency problems but not nocturnal awakenings [10]. Youngstedt and coworkers [11] examined PLMS polysomnographically without reference to arousal and noted relationships with lower total sleep times and wake after sleep onset. By contrast, across a broader age range of subjects, Mendelson [12] evaluated leg movements accompanied by electroencephalogram arousals and was unable to find relationships between PLMS and symptoms. Montplaisir and coworkers [13] noted no differences in PLMS among controls, individuals with insomnia, and individuals with hypersomnia. Karadeniz and coworkers [14] found no modifications in macrosleep or microsleep architecture associated with the presence of PLMS in 40- to 64-year-old patients with insomnia. Hornyak and Trenkwalder [15] reported no association between PLMS and sleep quality in non-RLS insomniac patients. More recently, Carrier and coworkers [16] reported that the presence of PLMS was unrelated to polysomnographic measurements of sleep quality in a group of 70 normal subjects between the ages of 40 and 60, although in male subjects a significant (but very small size) effect was noted for lower sleep quality in association with PLMS Index (number of movements per sleep hour) greater than 10.

The absence of associations between subjectively or objectively disturbed sleep and PLMS in many of these studies stands in contrast to early published case series of patients from sleep disorder clinics where the diagnosis of the condition seemed to be clearly related to disturbed sleep [17,18]. These were highly selected, clinic-based populations, however, and also included a substantial portion of patients with frank RLS, which is less ambiguously related to poor sleep (poor sleep is a feature associated with diagnosis) [2]. The meaning of such studies for the clinical correlates of PLMS in the general population remains doubtful. Of note is a recent epidemiologic study suggesting that the clinical conditions of RLS and reported leg jerking may be relatively tightly coupled [19], but because PLMS in that study were defined atypically (ie, by self-report and not electrophysiologically), it is difficult to draw inferences from these data. Some have claimed that when PLMS are defined symptomatically by the concurrent presence of sleep complaints (ie, periodic leg movement disorder [PLMD]), specific polysomnographic features (eg, higher number of PLMS with arousal) may distinguish this group of patients from those with RLS [20].

Technical considerations in the recording of periodic leg movements in sleep as a function of age

A possible reason that many of the aforementioned studies may have failed to find unequivocal relationships between PLMS and symptoms is the large night-to-night variability that exists in the nightly measurement of PLMS, particularly in the aged [4,21–23]. Extensive variability in the measurement of PLMS is expected to introduce error into the detection of any relationships between such metrics and symptoms. Potentially, the variability could also underlay the inconsistencies across those few longitudinal studies to date. Factors influencing the variability in PLMS between nights remain ill-defined. Some have speculated that, in the patient with RLS, extreme variability in sleep length or quality may impact on the variability [1], such that if an individual sleeps very little on a given night their PLMS Index is low by necessity. Some data support that the variability of the PLMS index is higher in RLS than in other sleep-disorder patients [24], but higher mean levels make this conclusion equivocal on a purely statistical basis. Other studies of internight variability of PLMS in RLS suggest considerably less variability [25]. Considerable night-to-night variability also occurs in PLMS in elderly individuals who do not have apparent RLS, as has been noted in several studies [4,21–23].

Several other potential age-associated aspects related to characterization of the movements have been examined. Within bouts of PLMS, both duration of movements [26] and intermovement interval [9] were unrelated to age. Nicholas and coworkers [26], however, noted the intermovement interval for waking periodic leg movements decreased with age. An analysis of time of night effects noted similarly that older subjects, who had an earlier time-of-night predominance in their PLMS, also had shorter intermovement intervals [27]. Finally, given the known disruption of sleep continuity with aging, it is hardly surprising that several studies have reported that, consistent with greater fragmentation of sleep with aging, the number of PLMS with arousals or awakening increases with age [12,17,28]. Heightened reactivity to movements cannot be assumed to crossover into the autonomic domain, however, because Gosselin and coworkers [29] reported that older subjects had reduced magnitude of heart rate variability accompanying PLMS relative to younger subjects.

Restless legs syndrome: prevalence and associated factors

RLS is a clinical syndrome, now consensually agreed on to be defined by four cardinal features: (1) the urge to move legs often accompanied by unpleasant leg sensations, (2) the urge to move or unpleasant sensations begin or worsen during periods of inactivity, (3) the urge to move or unpleasant sensations are relieved by movement, (4) the urge to move or unpleasant sensations are worse in the evening or at night [2]. Supportive features include positive family history; treatment responsiveness; and a finding of PLMS (measured electrophysiologically).

Many [30–35] but not all [19,36–41] epidemiologic studies have suggested that the prevalence of RLS increases with age. Interpretation of age effects in population-based work is complicated by the fact that the upper age limit varies among studies and various studies use different definitions of RLS. The wide range of prevalence figures is depicted in Fig. 1. Because of the age range of peak prevalence (from 50–59 to as high as 80 and above) reported in these studies, it remains unclear whether RLS shows true age dependence (ie, the likelihood of its prevalence increases nearly linearly with chronologic age), or whether the age effect is better characterized as age-related (ie, encompassing a distinct chronologic window of vulnerability) [42]. Additionally, because these studies encompass diverse populations from the United States [32,33,38,40], the United Kingdom [33,34,40], French and non-French speaking Canadian provinces [31], Germany [33,37,39,40], Scandinavian countries [19,30], France [35,40], Italy [33,36,41], and Spain [33,40], age differences in peak prevalence could represent the partial influence of varying genetic predispositions for RLS, consistent with several gene loci that have been implicated with the condition [43,44].

Many conditions have been associated with RLS in these epidemiologic studies. Perhaps because many of the RLS definitions used encompass

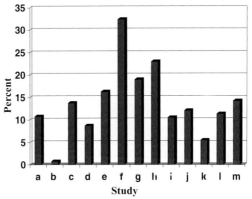

Fig. 1. Prevalence of restless legs syndrome across various studies. Prevalence figures reflect oldest age groups with peak prevalence with data averaged for men and women when available. Studies (and references) are as follows: a [36], b [34], c [37], d [33], e [39], f [38], g [32], h [31], i [30], j [41], k [40], l [35], and m [19].

elements of disturbed sleep, only a limited number of prevalence studies have presented data on relationships between RLS and independently ascertained insomnia questions. Not surprisingly, RLS was associated with complaints of poor sleep in those studies [19,30,34,40]. More commonly, medical or psychiatric conditions have been studied in association with RLS including hypertension and cardiovascular disease [30,33,39], diabetes or possible neuropathy [32,33,39], depressive symptomatology [30,34,37] or poor mental health [32,33], musculoskeletal disease [33], treated hyperthyroidism [39], renal disease [34], habitual lack of exercise [32], and smoking [33,39]. Not every study reports data on all the aforementioned conditions, and particular medication classes have also been associated with RLS (or PLMS) (see section below on Treatment Considerations). At least some of these conditions (eg, cardiovascular disease, depressive symptoms, diabetes, sedentary lifestyle) are expected to occur in higher frequency in elderly populations; however, there is only limited evidence that age prevalence per se is caused primarily by any one of these factors. Such a contention requires that observed age prevalence no longer occurred subsequent to multivariate adjustment for any particular associated factor. To date, no study has shown this.

Altered iron metabolism represents a condition associated with RLS deserving special note in the context of aged populations. Following the report of O'Keeffe and coworkers [45] that elderly RLS patients were likely to demonstrate low serum ferritin levels, several important lines of evidence have pursued this work. Although frank anemia and lower serum iron may not always be apparent in association with RLS, neuroimaging and cerebrospinal fluid studies have suggested that total brain iron concentrations are reduced in RLS, which is consistent with an alteration in blood-brain transport [46,47]. Because anemia is a common problem in elderly populations, it is possible that such derangements in some aspect of iron metabolism underlie the high prevalence of RLS in the aged. Few studies have tested this hypothesis in elderly populations. O'Keeffe [48] published a small additional case series suggesting that serum ferritin levels <50 ng/mL were significantly more likely in elderly patients with recent-onset RLS, but other population-based studies show a more complex picture. Although RLS was not accompanied by low levels of serum ferritin or by higher levels of soluble transferrin receptor in one population-based study, it seemed that mid-range levels (cf. highest ranges) of serum iron and transferrin saturation may have exerted protective effects [49]. Neither anemia (defined by hemoglobin levels less than 2 SDs below gender-expected values) nor ferritin values were significant factors in RLS in another study of a German population across a broader age range (20–79) [39]. By contrast, in a northern Italian elderly population (South Tyrol), lower serum iron and higher soluble transferrin receptor levels (often seen in early stage anemia) were related to RLS [41]. Finally, recent data have suggested that cerebrospinal fluid ferritin in older, late-onset RLS patients was unrelated to onset of symptoms and that elderly patients had higher levels of cerebrospinal fluid ferritin than younger patients [50]. These data cast doubt on whether iron deficiency may be a relevant risk factor for RLS presenting in the aged population, unless the condition also had early onset.

Restless legs syndrome in dementia

The recent National Institutes of Health (NIH) Diagnosis and Workshop Conference regarding definitions of RLS [2] acknowledged that different definitions of the syndrome might be relevant in geriatrics and children. Although dementia patients may be too verbally compromised to express their condition in language, several essential features, such as rubbing or kneading legs, excessive motor activity in lower limbs (including fidgeting and pacing), and worsening of leg discomfort during rest or activity and its diminishment with activity, are suggestive of the condition, as is the temporally specific occurrence of leg discomfort or motor activity in the late afternoon or early evening. Although not explicitly described in the NIH Conference Report, wandering (cf. pacing), a widely acknowledged clinical management issue in dementia patients [51], may

represent an unrecognized RLS phenotype of particular note and importance in geriatric care. For example, typical treatments for wandering may involve medications that exert dopaminergic blockage, which might otherwise be expected to worsen, rather than improve, the wandering behaviors (see section below on Treatment Considerations).

Wandering has long been recognized as one of the most difficult and intractable components of dementia in general [52] and Alzheimer's disease (AD) specifically [53]. Patients may place themselves at grave risk wandering outside their homes, and their recovery often involves police and other emergency service personnel [54]. Several studies have noted that nocturnal wandering was the most distressing of all sleep-related behaviors of AD patients [53,55]. Wandering represents a particular conundrum for clinical researchers attempting to understand the mechanisms underlying these peculiar behaviors. Some descriptive research has focused on tracking the specific vectors of the ambulation [56], whereas others have focused on wandering as escape-like behavior [57]. Perhaps the most thorough neurobiologic perspective on wandering to date has been the work of Kavcic and Duffy [58] and Tetewsky and Duffy [59] who have suggested that wandering may be a function of a modified processing system in which aberrant visual attention systems undermine spatial orientation or, as so aptly stated by Duffy: "Alzheimer's patients do not get lost because they have forgotten where they are going, rather, they get lost because they cannot keep track of where they have been" [52a]. Also of mechanistic interest are the positron emission tomography studies of Meguro and colleagues [60] and Tanaka and coworkers [61], who showed that wandering AD patients (relative to those who do not wander) demonstrated lower dopamine uptake in caudate and putamen; those decreases also correlated with decreased cerebral glucose use in frontal and temporal, but not parietal, regions. Comparable findings have been reported more recently by Rolland and coworkers [62]. These results in wandering AD patients bear resemblance to some neuroimaging findings in RLS patients, who showed reduced dopamine terminal storage [63,64]. These parallels assume a major role for nigrostriatal dysfunction in RLS, however, which may be open to question (see later).

Within the context of the NIH Workshop statement [2], there is now increasing recognition that at least some cases of wandering could represent unrecognized RLS, and the tendency for wandering to occur in the early evening hours [65] is consistent with RLS in dementia. A patient with a long-standing personal history suggestive of RLS or other (perhaps younger) family members with known RLS also serves as partial corroboration for RLS in the dementia patient. Of note in this regard is that wanderers were more likely to have lifelong patterns of walking or strolling when stressed, at least as recalled retrospectively by family members [56]. Factors associated with RLS in the general population (anemia, diabetes, musculoskeletal disease, or neuropathy), when present in a dementia patient who wanders, also might be suggestive of RLS. Curiously, as a group, AD patients were reported by their caregivers to be no more likely to have RLS symptoms or leg twitches than elderly controls [66], implying that only a subset of patients show such symptomatology. RLS patients have been reported recently to have deficits in cognitive tasks implicated in prefrontal cortex localization, which have been interpreted as the effects of sleep loss [67]. These data can be viewed as broadly compatible with the presence of RLS in dementia.

A discussion of the phenotypic presentation of RLS in neurodegenerative disease (such as AD) invariably raises the issue of RLS in parkinsonism, which can often but not invariably be accompanied by dementia (eg, Lewy body dementia). Although RLS and parkinsonism are both characterized as dopamine-deficient conditions, one could expect the prevalence of the former to be considerably higher in the latter. Some data suggest that PLMS prevalence is higher in Parkinson's disease (PD) than in control populations [68]; however, evidence to date linking PD and RLS has been negative [34,36,49,69], mixed [70,71], or in one study, positive [72]. Low serum ferritin has been shown to be a relevant mediating variable for older-onset RLS in PD [70]; however, as described above, there is some evidence of decreased salience of reduced iron stores as relevant for later-onset RLS [50]. The relative independence of RLS and PD may reflect the relative contribution of putative postsynaptic and/or diencephalospinal dysfunction in RLS [73]. Abnormalities of flexor reflex and the sensory abnormalities accompanying RLS are compatible with dysfunction of dopaminergic efferents and afferents within the dorsal horn that are rarely, if ever, seen in PD [73]. Comparisons of single-photon emission CT of the dopamine transporter in age-matched RLS and PD patients showed better preserved binding in the RLS patients [74]. Finally, a small neuropathologic case series of RLS patients did not demonstrate Lewy bodies or α-synuclein deposits (exceedingly common in PD), again reiterating the relative independence of the two conditions [75].

Treatment considerations

Empirical evidence for treatment options for RLS and symptomatic PLMS (ie, PLMD) have been summarized in a practice parameters publication from the American Academy of Sleep Medicine [76] and an accompanying review of empirical evidence as of 2002 [77]. These publications clearly indicate the efficacy of levodopa and the dopamine agonists pergolide, pramipexole, and ropinirole as effective for RLS and PLMD. Other dopamine agonists, and amantadine and selegiline, were viewed as possibly effective. With the exception of ropinirole (which has a Food and Drug Administration–approved indication for use in RLS), usage of all of these other medications constitutes off-label use. Since the publication of the American Academy of Sleep Medicine guidelines, a number of phase III, multisite, randomized clinical trials of some of these medications (eg, ropinirole) have been published that confirm the original report [78,79]. Some data also suggest use of dopamine agonists having longer half-lives, such as cabergoline [80], and, under development in transdermal formulation, rotigotine [81] and lisuride [82]. In practice, oral pramipexole and ropinirole probably see the most widespread current usage. The two can be distinguished by primarily hepatic (ropinirole) versus renal (pramipexole) excretion and by half-life (6 hours for ropinirole; 8–12 hours for pramipexole). Iron supplementation may also be useful in selected cases, but, as suggested above, this may be less relevant for the aged population.

In the wandering dementia patient with a history of RLS or a medical condition associated with RLS, an empirical trial of a low-dose dopaminergic agonist (0.25–0.5 mg ropinirole; 0.125–0.25 mg pramipexole) may represent an avenue of treatment; however, because of possible dopamine-induced psychosis, judicious usage, and careful dose escalation is advised. An initial approach should examine potential exacerbating medications already in use before adding new ones. In nondemented populations, some evidence suggests that selective serotonin-reuptake inhibitors [33,83] and antidepressants, such as venlafaxine [83] and mirtazapine [84,85], can be associated with PLMD or RLS, although one recent study presented data to the contrary [86].

Case reports with atypical antipsychotics (olanzapine, quetiapine, risperidone) having at least partial blockade at specific dopaminergic receptors (eg, olanzapine at D1-D4, quetiapine at D1-D2, risperidone at D2) have been reported both to aggravate RLS or PLMS [87–89], but also treat nocturnal wandering in one case series in AD patients [90]. Neuroleptic use was significant [34] or borderline significant [37] in predicting RLS in population-based studies. At least in theory, for the dementia patient with long-standing RLS whose evening wandering and agitation represents a continuation or exacerbation of their premorbid condition, such medication is expected only to aggravate, rather than improve, the behavior. In a secondary analysis of a double-blind, placebo-controlled trial of risperidone in dementia patients, baseline wandering predicted higher rates of falls at 2 mg/day but was protective at 1 mg, although it was unclear whether any of the wandering patients may have represented unrecognized RLS [91]. In normal adults, quetiapine (25 mg and 100 mg) was shown to improve polysomnographically defined sleep architecture in a double-blind, placebo-controlled trial, although the number of PLMS was increased under the higher dose [92]. Taken together, these results suggest that usage of atypical antipsychotics to treat wandering (an off-label indication) should be entertained cautiously with careful ascertainment of premorbid predisposition for RLS or PLMS.

Summary

PLMS and RLS are exceedingly common in ambulatory, noninstitutionalized, noncognitively impaired elderly populations and may occur in demented patients, where they may be manifested by signs of late afternoon and evening wandering. Risk factors operating for these conditions in geriatrics include many of the same factors acknowledged to be of importance in middle-aged patients (eg, diabetes, neuropathy or radiculopathy, renal insufficiency, cardiovascular disease) but occurring with relatively high prevalence in the elderly and particularly salient in this age group. Altered iron metabolism may also be a risk if the RLS is long-standing. It must never be assumed that PLMS, in the absence of frank RLS symptomatology, represents a cause of poor sleep or daytime sleepiness in old age. Ample evidence demonstrates that many geriatric patients present with PLMS who have no symptomatic correlate. In such cases, intervention is premature and unnecessary. There are no natural history data that suggest that the presence of asymptomatic PLMS is a harbinger for any later pathology, and overlap between RLS and parkinsonism remains in doubt. Nonetheless, symptomatic RLS is a major problem for many geriatric patients and deserves full recognition as a highly treatable condition. Particularly in the dementia population with nocturnal wandering (as a potential sign of RLS) implementation of new treatment should be carefully entertained, and cessation of potentially aggravating medications always should be considered initially.

References

[1] Allen RP. The resurrection of periodic limb movements (PLM): leg activity monitoring and the restless legs syndrome (RLS). Sleep Med 2005;6:385–7.

[2] Allen RP, Picchietti D, Hening WA, et al. Restless legs syndrome: diagnostic criteria, special considerations, and epidemiology: a report from the restless legs syndrome diagnosis and epidemiology workshop at the National Institutes of Health. Sleep Med 2003;4:101–19.

[3] Ancoli-Israel S, Kripke DF, Klauber MR, et al. Periodic limb movements in sleep in community-dwelling elderly. Sleep 1991;14:496–500.

[4] Youngstedt SD, Kripke DF, Klauber MR, et al. Periodic leg movements during sleep and sleep disturbances in elders. J Gerontol A Biol Sci Med Sci 1998;53:M391–4.

[5] Bixler EO, Kales A, Vela-Bueno A, et al. Nocturnal myoclonus and nocturnal myoclonic activity in the normal population. Res Commun Chem Pathol Pharmacol 1982;36:129–40.

[6] Coleman R, Bliwise D, Sajben N, et al. Epidemiology of periodic leg movements during sleep. In: Guilleminault C, Lugaresi E, editors. Sleep/wake disorders: natural history, epidemiology, and long-term evolution. New York: Raven Press; 1983. p. 217–29.

[7] Gehrman P, Stepnowsky C, Cohen-Zion M, et al. Long-term follow-up of periodic limb movements in sleep in older adults. Sleep 2002;25:340–3.

[8] Kales A, Bixler EO, Soldatos CR, et al. Biopsychobehavioral correlates of insomnia, part 1: Role of sleep apnea and nocturnal myoclonus. Psychosomatics 1982;23:589–600.

[9] Mosko SS, Dickel MJ, Paul T, et al. Sleep apnea and sleep-related periodic leg movements in community resident seniors. J Am Geriatr Soc 1988;36:502–8.

[10] Bliwise D, Petta D, Seidel W, et al. Periodic leg movements during sleep in the elderly. Arch Gerontol Geriatr 1985;4:273–81.

[11] Youngstedt SD, Kripke DF, Elliott JA, et al. Circadian abnormalities in older adults. J Pineal Res 2001;31:264–72.

[12] Mendelson WB. Are periodic leg movements associated with clinical sleep disturbance? Sleep 1996;19:219–23.

[13] Montplaisir J, Michaud M, Denesle R, et al. Periodic leg movements are not more prevalent in insomnia or hypersomnia but are specifically associated with sleep disorders involving a dopaminergic impairment. Sleep Med 2000;1:163–7.

[14] Karadeniz D, Ondze B, Besset A, et al. Are periodic leg movements during sleep (PLMS) responsible for sleep disruption in insomnia patients? Eur J Neurol 2000;7:331–6.

[15] Hornyak M, Trenkwalder C. Restless legs syndrome and periodic limb movement disorder in the elderly. J Psychosom Res 2004;56:543–8.

[16] Carrier J, Frenette S, Montplaisir J, et al. Effects of periodic leg movements during sleep in middle-aged subjects without sleep complaints. Mov Disord 2005;20:1127–32.

[17] Coleman RM, Miles LE, Guilleminault CC, et al. Sleep-wake disorders in the elderly: polysomnographic analysis. J Am Geriatr Soc 1981; 29:289–96.

[18] Roehrs T, Zorick F, Sicklesteel J, et al. Age-related sleep-wake disorders at a sleep disorder center. J Am Geriatr Soc 1983;31:364–70.

[19] Bjorvatn B, Leissner L, Ulfberg J, et al. Prevalence, severity and risk factors of restless legs syndrome in the general adult population in two Scandinavian countries. Sleep Med 2005;6: 307–12.

[20] Eisenschr I, Ehrenberg BI, Noachtar S. Different sleep characteristics in restless legs syndrome and periodic limb movement disorder. Sleep Med 2003;4:147–52.

[21] Bliwise DL, Carskadon MA, Dement WC. Nightly variation of periodic leg movements in sleep in middle aged and elderly individuals. Arch Gerontol Geriatr 1988;7:273–9.

[22] Mosko SS, Dickel MJ, Ashurst J. Night-to-night variability in sleep apnea and sleep-related periodic leg movements in the elderly. Sleep 1988; 11:340–8.

[23] Edinger JD, McCall WV, Marsh GR, et al. Periodic limb movement variability in older DIMS patients across consecutive nights of home monitoring. Sleep 1992;15:156–61.

[24] Hornyak M, Kopasz M, Feige B, et al. Variability of periodic leg movements in various sleep disorders: implications for clinical and pathophysiologic studies. Sleep 2005;28:331–5.

[25] Sforza E, Haba-Rubio J. Night-to-night variability in periodic leg movements in patients with restless legs syndrome. Sleep Med 2005;6: 259–67.

[26] Nicolas A, Michaud M, Lavigne G, et al. The influence of sex, age and sleep/wake state on characteristics of periodic leg movements in restless legs syndrome patients. Clin Neurophysiol 1999;110:1168–74.

[27] Culpepper WJ, Badia P, Shaffer JI. Time-of-night patterns in PLMS activity. Sleep 1992;15:306–11.

[28] Chabli A, Michaud M, Montplaisir J. Periodic arm movements in patients with the restless legs syndrome. Eur Neurol 2000;44:133–8.

[29] Gosselin N, Lanfranchi P, Michaud M, et al. Age and gender effects on heart rate activation associated with periodic leg movements in patients with restless legs syndrome. Clin Neurophysiol 2003;114:2188–95.

[30] Ulfberg J, Nystrom B, Carter N, et al. Prevalence of restless legs syndrome among men aged 18 to 64 years: an association with somatic disease and neuropsychiatric symptoms. Mov Disord 2001; 16:1159–63.

[31] Lavigne GJ, Montplaisir JY. Restless legs syndrome and sleep bruxism: prevalence and association among Canadians. Sleep 1994;17:739–43.

[32] Phillips B, Young T, Finn L, et al. Epidemiology of restless legs symptoms in adults. Arch Intern Med 2000;160:2137–41.

[33] Ohayon MM, Roth T. Prevalence of restless legs syndrome and periodic limb movement disorder in the general population. J Psychosom Res 2002;53:547–54.

[34] Van De Vijver DA, Walley T, Petri H. Epidemiology of restless legs syndrome as diagnosed in UK primary care. Sleep Med 2004;5:435–40.

[35] Tison F, Crochard A, Leger D, et al. Epidemiology of restless legs syndrome in French adults: a nationwide survey: the INSTANT Study. Neurology 2005;65:239–46.

[36] Wenning GK, Kiechl S, Seppi K, et al. Prevalence of movement disorders in men and women aged 50–89 years (Bruneck Study cohort): a population-based study. Lancet Neurol 2005;4:815–20.

[37] Rothdach AJ, Trenkwalder C, Haberstock J, et al. Prevalence and risk factors of RLS in an elderly population: the MEMO study. Memory and Morbidity in Augsburg Elderly. Neurology 2000; 54:1064–8.

[38] Nichols DA, Allen RP, Grauke JH, et al. Restless legs syndrome symptoms in primary care: a prevalence study. Arch Intern Med 2003;163:2323–9.

[39] Berger K, Luedemann J, Trenkwalder C, et al. Sex and the risk of restless legs syndrome in the general population. Arch Intern Med 2004; 164:196–202.

[40] Allen RP, Walters AS, Montplaisir J, et al. Restless legs syndrome prevalence and impact: REST general population study. Arch Intern Med 2005; 165:1286–92.

[41] Hogl B, Kiechl S, Willeit J, et al. Restless legs syndrome: a community-based study of prevalence, severity, and risk factors. Neurology 2005;64:1920–4.

[42] Brody JA, Schneider EL. Diseases and disorders of aging: an hypothesis. J Chronic Dis 1986; 39:871–6.

[43] Ferini-Strambi L, Bonati MT, Oldani A, et al. Genetics in restless legs syndrome. Sleep Med 2004; 5:301–4.

[44] Bonati MT, Ferini-Strambi L, Aridon P, et al. Autosomal dominant restless legs syndrome maps on chromosome 14q. Brain 2003;126:1485–92.

[45] O'Keeffe ST, Gavin K, Lavan JN. Iron status and restless legs syndrome in the elderly. Age Ageing 1994;23:200–3.

[46] Earley CJ, Connor JR, Beard JL, et al. Abnormalities in CSF concentrations of ferritin and transferrin in restless legs syndrome. Neurology 2000,54:1698–700.

[47] Allen RP, Barker PB, Wehrl F, et al. MRI measurement of brain iron in patients with restless legs syndrome. Neurology 2001;56:263–5.

[48] O'Keeffe ST. Secondary causes of restless legs syndrome in older people. Age Ageing 2005; 34:349–52.

[49] Berger K, von Eckardstein A, Trenkwalder C, et al. Iron metabolism and the risk of restless legs syndrome in an elderly general population: the MEMO-Study. J Neurol 2002;249:1195–9.

[50] Earley CJ, Connor JR, Beard JL, et al. Ferritin levels in the cerebrospinal fluid and restless legs

syndrome: effects of different clinical pheno-
types. Sleep 2005;28:1069–75.

[51] Algase DL. Wandering in dementia. Annu Rev
Nurs Res 1999;17:185–217.

[52] Silverstein NM, Flaherty G, Tobin TS. Dementia
and wandering behavior: concern for the lost elder. New York: Springer Publishing Company;
2002.

[52a] Duffy CJ. Introduction. In: Silverstein NM,
Flaherty G, Tobin TS. Dementia and wandering behavior: concern for the lost elder. New
York: Springer Publishing Company; 2002.
p. xi.

[53] Logsdon RG, Teri L, McCurry SM, et al. Wandering: a significant problem among community-
residing individuals with Alzheimer's disease.
J Gerontol B Psychol Sci Soc Sci 1998;53:294–9.

[54] Rowe MA, Glover JC. Antecedents, descriptions
and consequences of wandering in cognitive-
ly-impaired adults and the Safe Return (SR) program. Am J Alzheimers Dis Other Demen 2001;
16:344–52.

[55] Tractenberg RE, Singer CM, Cummings JL, et al.
The Sleep Disorders Inventory: an instrument
for studies of sleep disturbance in persons with
Alzheimer's disease. J Sleep Res 2003;12:331–7.

[56] Snyder LH, Rupprecht P, Pyrek J, et al. Wandering. Gerontologist 1978;18:272–80.

[57] Nasman B, Bucht G, Eriksson S, et al. Behaviou-
ral symptoms in the institutionalized elderly: relationship to dementia. Inter J Geriatr Psych
1993;8:843–9.

[58] Kavcic V, Duffy CJ. Attentional dynamics and
visual perception: mechanisms of spatial disorientation in Alzheimer's disease. Brain 2003;
126(Pt 5):1173–81.

[59] Tetewsky SJ, Duffy CJ. Visual loss and getting lost
in Alzheimer's disease. Neurology 1999;52:
958–65.

[60] Meguro K, Yamaguchi S, Itoh M, et al. Striatal
dopamine metabolism correlated with fronto-
temporal glucose utilization in Alzheimer's disease: a double-tracer PET study. Neurology
1997;49:941–5.

[61] Tanaka Y, Meguro K, Yamaguchi S, et al. Decreased striatal D2 receptor density associated
with severe behavioral abnormality in Alzheimer's
disease. Ann Nucl Med 2003;17:567–73.

[62] Rolland Y, Payoux P, Lauwers-Cances V, et al.
SPECT study of wandering behavior in Alzheimer's disease. Int J Geriatr Psychiatry 2005;
20:816–20.

[63] Turjanski N, Lees AJ, Brooks DJ. Striatal dopaminergic function in restless legs syndrome:
18F-dopa and 11C-raclopride PET studies. Neurology 1999;52:932–7.

[64] Garcia-Borreguero D, Odin P, Serrano C. Restless
legs syndrome and PD: a review of the evidence
for a possible association. Neurology 2003;
61(Suppl 3):S49–55.

[65] Martino-Saltzman D, Blasch BB, Morris RD,
et al. Travel behavior of nursing home residents

perceived as wanderers and nonwanderers. Gerontologist 1991;31:666–72.

[66] Tractenberg RE, Singer CM, Kaye JA. Characteriz-
ing sleep problems in persons with Alzheimer's
disease and normal elderly. J Sleep Res 2006;
15:97–103.

[67] Pearson VE, Allen RP, Dean T, et al. Cognitive
deficits associated with restless legs syndrome
(RLS). Sleep Med 2006;7:25–30.

[68] Wetter TC, Collado-Seidel V, Pollmacher T, et al.
Sleep and periodic leg movement patterns in
drug-free patients with Parkinson's disease and
multiple system atrophy. Sleep 2000;23:361–7.

[69] Tan EK, Lum SY, Wong MC. Restless legs syndrome in Parkinson's disease. J Neurol Sci
2002;196:33–6.

[70] Ondo WG, Vuong KD, Jankovic J. Exploring the
relationship between Parkinson disease and restless legs syndrome. Arch Neurol 2002;59:421–4.

[71] Nomura T, Inoue Y, Miyake M, et al. Prevalence
and clinical characteristics of restless legs syndrome in Japanese patients with Parkinson's disease. Mov Disord 2006;21(3):380–4.

[72] Krishnan PR, Bhatia M, Behari M. Restless legs
syndrome in Parkinson's disease: a case-con-
trolled study. Mov Disord 2003;18:181–5.

[73] Rye DB. Parkinson's disease and RLS: the dopaminergic bridge. Sleep Med 2004;5:317–28.

[74] Linke R, Eisensehr I, Wetter TC, et al. Presynaptic
dopaminergic function in patients with restless
legs syndrome: are there common features with
early Parkinson's disease? Mov Disord 2004;
19:1158–62.

[75] Pittock SJ, Parrett T, Adler CH, et al. Neuropathology of primary restless leg syndrome: absence of specific tau- and alpha-synuclein
pathology. Mov Disord 2004;19:695–9.

[76] Littner MR, Kushida C, Anderson WM, et al.
Practice parameters for the dopaminergic treatment of restless legs syndrome and periodic limb
movement disorder. Sleep 2004;27:557–9.

[77] Hening WA, Allen RP, Earley CJ, et al. An update
on the dopaminergic treatment of restless legs
syndrome and periodic limb movement disorder. Sleep 2004;27:560–83.

[78] Walters AS, Ondo WG, Dreykluft T, et al. Ropinirole is effective in the treatment of restless legs
syndrome. TREAT RLS 2: a 12-week, double-
blind, randomized, parallel-group, placebo-controlled study. Mov Disord 2004;19:1414–23.

[79] Bogan RK, Fry JM, Schmidt MH, et al. Ropinirole
in the treatment of patients with restless legs syndrome: a US-based randomized, double-blind,
placebo-controlled clinical trial. Mayo Clin Proc
2006;81:17–27.

[80] Zucconi M, Oldani A, Castronovo C, et al. Cabergoline is an effective single-drug treatment
for restless legs syndrome: clinical and actigraphic evaluation. Sleep 2003;26:815–8.

[81] Stiasny-Kolster K, Kohnen R, Schollmayer E,
et al. Patch application of the dopamine agonist
rotigotine to patients with moderate to advanced

stages of restless legs syndrome: a double-blind, placebo-controlled pilot study. Mov Disord 2004;19:1432–8.

[82] Benes H. Transdermal lisuride: short-term efficacy and tolerability study in patients with severe restless legs syndrome. Sleep Med 2006; 7:31–5.

[83] Yang C, White DP, Winkelman JW. Antidepressants and periodic leg movements of sleep. Biol Psychiatry 2005;58:510–4.

[84] Agargun MY, Kara H, Ozbek H, et al. Restless legs syndrome induced by mirtazapine. J Clin Psychiatry 2002;63:1179.

[85] Bahk WM, Pae CU, Chae JH, et al. Mirtazapine may have the propensity for developing a restless legs syndrome? A case report. Psychiatry Clin Neurosci 2002;56:209–10.

[86] Brown LK, Dedrick DL, Doggett JW, et al. Antidepressant medication use and restless legs syndrome in patients presenting with insomnia. Sleep Med 2005;6:443–50.

[87] Pinninti NR, Mago R, Townsend J, et al. Periodic restless legs syndrome associated with quetiapine use: a case report. J Clin Psychopharmacol 2005;25:617–8.

[88] Kraus T, Schuld A, Pollmacher T. Periodic leg movements in sleep and restless legs syndrome probably caused by olanzapine. J Clin Psychopharmacol 1999;19:478–9.

[89] Wetter TC, Brunner J, Bronisch T. Restless legs syndrome probably induced by risperidone treatment. Pharmacopsychiatry 2002;35:109–11.

[90] Meguro K, Meguro M, Tanaka Y, et al. Risperidone is effective for wandering and disturbed sleep/wake patterns in Alzheimer's disease. J Geriatr Psychiatry Neurol 2004;17:61–7.

[91] Katz IR, Rupnow M, Kozma C, et al. Risperidone and falls in ambulatory nursing home residents with dementia and psychosis or agitation: secondary analysis of a double-blind, placebo-controlled trial. Am J Geriatr Psychiatry 2004; 12:499–508.

[92] Cohrs S, Rodenbeck A, Guan Z, et al. Sleep-promoting properties of quetiapine in healthy subjects. Psychopharmacology (Berl) 2004; 174:421–9.

SLEEP
MEDICINE
CLINICS

Sleep Med Clin 1 (2006) 273–292

Sleep and Neurologic Problems in the Elderly

Alon Y. Avidan, MD, MPH

The geriatric patient population is growing very fast around the world. The rates of dementia are similarly on the rise. In the year 2000, 34 million Americans were older than 65 years. By the year 2025, this number is expected to double to 62 million [1]. This anticipated increase is expected to have significant medical, economic, and psychosocial consequences. Older adults are often dissatisfied with the quality of their sleep [2]. Almost half of seniors over age 65 who live at home are not happy with their sleep and nearly two thirds of those residing in nursing home facilities suffer from sleep disorders [3]. Sleep disorders increase with age, and clinicians who care for older patients need to become familiar with

the age-related sleep changes and recognize the sleep disorders that are likely to impact this patient population.

Sleep disturbances in elderly patients may be caused by primary sleep disorders, such as sleep apnea, periodic leg movements, and restless leg syndrome, or may arise secondary to medical problems, psychiatric conditions, polypharmacy, or psychosocial factors [4]. Conversely, when sleep disorders become chronic, they may exacerbate coexisting medical and psychiatric illnesses. Chronic sleep disorders are often associated with excessive daytime sleepiness and may result in disturbed cognition, impaired intellect, confusion, and psychomotor retardation, which may be misinterpreted as

Sleep Disorders Center UCLA, Department of Neurology, 710 Westwood Blvd., Room 4238 Reed Bldg., Los Angeles, CA 90095, USA
E-mail address: avidan@mednet.ucla.edu

1556-407X/06/$ – see front matter © 2006 Elsevier Inc. All rights reserved.
sleep.theclinics.com

doi:10.1016/j.jsmc.2006.04.010

dementia. Sleep disturbances may also increase the risk of injury, compromise the quality of life, and create social and economic burdens for caregivers.

Sleep disturbances in patients with neurodegenerative diseases

Dementia refers to a syndrome that is characterized by progressive deterioration of cognitive functions [5]. Patients also exhibit neuropsychiatric symptoms, such as apathy, agitation, and depression. With increasing loss of function, a patient with dementia is gradually robbed of his or her independence, eventually necessitating placement in a nursing home [5]. Dementia affects about 6% of individuals over 65 years of age and has a strong age-dependent prevalence [5]. Alzheimer's disease (AD) is by far the most important and common cause of dementia, accounting for approximately 70% of all cases of dementia [2]. This is followed by dementia with Lewy bodies, which is currently considered the second most common irreversible cause of dementia, accounting for approximately 20% to 25% of cases.

Patients with dementia can have a variety of underlying sleep disturbances consisting of insomnia, hypersomnia, circadian rhythm disturbances, excessive motor activity at night, nocturnal agitation, and wandering and abnormal nocturnal behaviors [6]. Increased irritability, impaired motor and cognitive skills, depression, and fatigue are also common [7]. Many of these symptoms have multiple underlying causes and pathophysiologies. Patients with dementia are at risk for additional sleep disturbances, such as obstructive sleep apnea (OSA) and periodic limb movement disorder of sleep, which occur at higher incidence with aging. Many of these sleep disruptions can cause considerable caregiver burden and may put the patient at increased risk for institutionalization within nursing home facilities [8,9].

Sleep disturbances in dementia may be caused by direct and indirect mechanisms [6,7]. Direct mechanisms are related to specific lesions in neuroanatomic pathways involved in sleep physiology and neurochemistry. Structural alteration of the sleep-wake generating neurons located in the suprachiasmatic nucleus (SCN) is one example of the direct mechanism, whereas insufficient light exposure and excessive noise at the patient's living quarter are examples of the indirect (external) mechanisms disturbing sleep (Fig. 1).

Alzheimer's disease

Memory disturbance is the most common initial sign in AD and consists of short-term memory loss

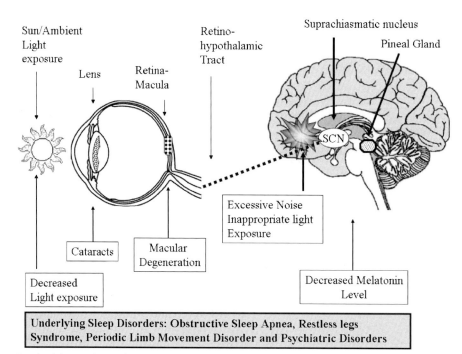

Fig. 1. Pathophysiology of circadian rhythm disturbances in patients with dementia. Potential environmental and intrinsic factors. SCN, suprachiasmatic nucleus.

and difficulties incorporating new information into memory. As the disease progresses, patient present with severe memory impairment, causing difficulties in correctly identifying family members, friends, and place of residence [10]. AD is characterized by classic pathologic changes including senile plaques, neurofibrillary tangles, and loss of subcortical cells, including particularly the cholinergic cells of the nucleus basalis complex and progressive degeneration of the cortical and subcortical cerebral structures [11,12].

In AD, degeneration of the neurons of the SCN may be responsible for circadian rhythm abnormalities, sundown syndrome, and other sleep-wake schedule disturbances (Fig. 2) [6,7]. The severity of circadian rhythm disturbances was correlated with the severity of dementia [13,14]. Sleep recordings in patients with dementia show increased diffuse slow wave activity, decreased sleep efficiency, and reversal of their circadian rhythmicity, which, after incontinence, is the second most common cause for institutionalization [15].

Degeneration of the cholinergic neurons in the nucleus basalis of Meynert, the pedunculopontine tegmental and laterodorsal tegmental nuclei, and noradrenergic neurons of the brainstem may be responsible for decreased rapid eye movement (REM) sleep in AD patients (see Fig. 2) [6,7]. Degeneration

of the brainstem respiratory neurons and the supramedullary respiratory pathways may cause sleep-disordered breathing (SDB) and other respiratory dysrhythmias in sleep in AD (see Fig. 2) [6,7].

Indirect mechanisms include medication-related side effects; underlying psychiatric diagnosis, such as mood disorders; increasing incidence of periodic limb movements in elderly AD patients; and age-related alterations in sleep (see Fig. 1). Other indirect mechanisms include general medical diseases affecting the cardiovascular and respiratory systems and environmental factors, such as insufficient or dim light and excessive environmental noise in nursing homes or other long-term care institutions (see Fig. 1).

Sleep architecture in Alzheimer's disease

Patients with AD have significant sleep architecture abnormalities. The hallmarks include reduction in sleep efficiency, increase in non-REM stage 1 sleep, increase in arousal and awakening frequency, decrease in total sleep time, and reduction in sleep spindles and K complexes. A profound disruption in sleep-wake rhythmicity occurs primarily early in the onset of the disease. Sleep fragmentation subsequently leads to increased daytime sleepiness, nocturnal insomnia, nocturnal wandering, increase in cognitive decline, increase in the number of

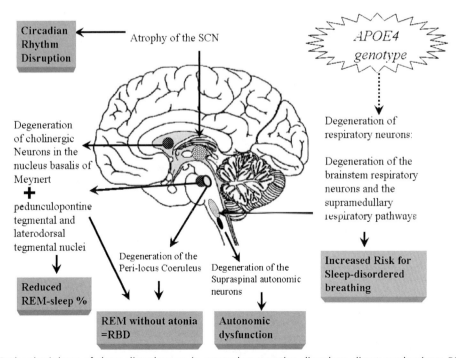

Fig. 2. Pathophysiology of sleep disturbances in neurodegenerative disorders: direct mechanisms. RBD, REM sleep behavior disorder; REM, rapid eye movement; SCN, suprachiasmatic nucleus. Broken arrow demonstrates a hypothetical relationship.

daytime naps, increase in time in bed and time spent awake in bed, increase in the frequency of nocturnal wandering, disorientation, and confusion [6,16–21].

Later on, as the disease progresses, patients with AD present with a more dramatic reduction of REM sleep, increased REM sleep latency, and a marked alteration of the circadian rhythm resulting in hypersomnolence [7]. Sleep and cognitive dysfunction are positively correlated in AD. Patients with AD are also susceptible to "sundowning," which is described as the nocturnal exacerbation of disruptive behavior or agitation in older people [22]. It is frequently encountered in dementia and remains a frequent cause of institutionalization in patients with AD.

The medications often used for patients with AD also effect sleep. Current pharmacotherapy for cognitive loss in AD involves the use of cholinesterase inhibitors, which may increase REM sleep and may also induce insomnia and vivid dreams [23].

Circadian rhythm disturbances in Alzheimer's disease

The symptoms of insomnia and hypersomnia can reflect a primary circadian dysrhythmia. Patients with AD tend to sleep more during the day and be active more during the night. This increased motor activity at night is the major contributing factor to significant caregiver distress.

Direct mechanisms thought to contribute to circadian dysrhythmia in patients with AD and other dementing conditions are related to degenerative changes that take place in the SCN of the hypothalamus and are caused by decreased melatonin production in the pineal gland (see Figs. 1 and 2) [24–27]. Indirect mechanisms include medications prescribed for these patients that cause nocturnal confusion or sundowning. Patients with AD are commonly affected by the irregular sleep-wake rhythm, which is characterized by a lack of discernable sleep-wake circadian rhythm. Instead of having a major sleep period, sleep is fragmented into three or more periods during the 24-hour day with the longest sleep period occurring between 2:00 and 6:00 AM. Patients with irregular sleep-wake rhythm may present with insomnia, hypersomnia, or needing frequent naps throughout the day. The disorder also affects the sleep quality of the caregiver.

Important factors that may contribute to irregular sleep-wake rhythm may include weak external entraining stimuli, such as reduced exposure to environmental light and diminished daytime activity. The diagnosis of irregular sleep-wake rhythm is made by reviewing the patient's sleep log or actigraphy confirming the lack of periodic circadian rhythmicity. A history of isolation or reclusion can often aid in diagnosis. The differential diagnosis of irregular sleep-wake rhythm includes other sleep or psychiatric disorders that can cause fragmented sleep, poor sleep hygiene, or voluntary maintenance of irregular sleep schedules.

Sleep disordered breathing in Alzheimer's disease

Sleep-related breathing disorders, such as OSA, are very common in AD compared with nondemented elderly and with younger adults [28,29]. One study demonstrated that the severity of AD is proportional to the severity of the OSA [30,31]. Furthermore, anecdotal reports of dementia-like symptoms associated with OSA have led to the speculation that there may be a causal relationship between SDB and AD [32].

In AD, sleep apnea could be a consequence of cell loss in the brainstem respiratory center. Conversely, neuronal degradation in AD could be hastened by nightly insults of intermittent cerebral hypoxemia related to the underlying sleep apnea. One of the key genotypic markers for AD is the apolipoprotein E epsilon 4 (APOE4) allele. A recent discovery that SDB is associated with the APOE4 allele in the general population has sparked an interest in this topic, because OSA is characterized by multiple genetic vulnerabilities [33,34]. In individuals under age 65, the APOE4 allele was more significantly associated with increased risk of OSA [35]. Other studies did not replicate the result, however, in part because of different genetic populations and different age-cohorts [36,37]. In a recent study of 1775 participants age 40 to 100 years with an OSA prevalence rate of 19%, after adjustment for age, sex, and body mass index, the presence of any APOE4 allele was associated with increased odds of having OSA [38].

Treatment of sleep disturbances in Alzheimer's disease

SDB is related to agitation in AD, and treatment of the underlying SDB may decrease agitation, easing the burden of caregiving and prolonging the time that patients are able to remain at home [39]. Neuropsychologic analyses have revealed that in patients with OSA, cognitive flexibility, attention, processing speed, and memory all improve with continuous positive airway pressure (CPAP) therapy [4,40–43]. Compliance with CPAP was also associated with greater improvements in attention, psychomotor speed, executive functioning, and nonverbal delayed recall [40].

Recent studies showed that melatonin, an indoleamine secreted by the pineal gland, may play an important role in aging and AD as an antioxidant and neuroprotector. Melatonin levels diminish with aging and patients with AD have a more profound reduction in this hormone [44]. Data from clinical trials indicate that melatonin supplementation improves sleep and slows down the progression of cognitive impairment in AD [44]. Other data show that melatonin protects neuronal cells by antioxidant and anti–amyloid-mediated activity properties, arrests the formation of amyloid fibrils, attenuates Alzheimer-like tau hyperphosphorylation, and protects cholinergic neurons but may not be an effective sleep agent [45–50]. A misleading labeling of the hormone melatonin as a food supplement and the lack of quality control over melatonin preparations on the market unfortunately continue to be a serious concern and heath care providers should use caution when prescribing it to elderly patients with dementia [51]. To date, there have been no randomized clinical trials of sedative-hypnotic medications specifically targeted at AD patients with sleep problems [23].

Treatment for circadian rhythm disturbances in Alzheimer's disease

Treatments for circadian rhythm sleep disorders including the irregular sleep-wake type are aimed at consolidating the sleep-wake cycle. Most of the studies have examined the effect of melatonin or the effect of increased bright light exposure in patients living in nursing homes. In one study, combination therapy of vitamin B_{12}, bright light, chronotherapy, and hypnotics produced a 45% success rate in one cohort of patients suffering from AD [52]. A recent multicenter, randomized, double-blind, placebo-controlled clinical trial using actigraphically derived measures of sleep demonstrated no beneficial effects of melatonin, 2.5 or 10 mg, on sleep disturbance, however, in a well-characterized, large AD population (N = 157) [23,46].

Light therapy has been shown to be effective in the management of circadian rhythm disturbances in patients with dementia; however, the optimal timing, duration, and intensity of light have not yet been determined [53,54]. A more practical approach to the management of irregular sleep-wake rhythm is to begin with behavioral and environmental strategies. In addition to increased bright light exposure, structured social and physical activities and avoidance of naps during the day have been shown to improve sleep [55–58]. During the sleep period, the environment should be conducive to sleep and consist of minimal noise, a darkened room, and a comfortable room temperature. The use of hypnotic or sedating psychoactive medications should be used with caution in elderly patients with dementia. Time exposure to bright light in the morning may be helpful in some patients. Evening bright light pulses ameliorated sleep-wake cycle disturbances in some patients with

AD [54]. Ancoli-Israel and coworkers [59] examined the effect of light on sleep and circadian activity rhythms in nursing home patients with probable or possible AD. The results of her study showed that both morning and evening bright light resulted in more consolidated sleep at night, as measured with wrist actigraphy. The authors suggested that nursing homes increase ambient light in activity rooms where patients spend most of their days [59]. The authors hypothesized that whereas the SCN of patients with severe AD is more likely to be degenerated, and the circadian activity rhythms deteriorate as AD progresses, it is still possible that patients with more intact SCNs (ie, patients with mild-to-moderate AD) might benefit from light treatment even more than those with severe AD [60]. Fig. 1 provides a summary of the therapy of circadian sleep rhythm disruption in dementia. Because most of the light treatment studies of sleep in dementia have taken place in the institutionalized setting, more studies of AD patients living at home are needed.

Data evaluating the use of antipsychotic agents and benzodiazepines have demonstrated improvements in sleep or nocturnal behavior but lacked real-time behavioral observations as relevant outcomes [61]. Such agents as the antipsychotics often have adverse effects, such as sedation, confusion, orthostatic hypotension, and parkinsonism, which are often clinically significant in elderly patients with dementia [61]. The high-potency antipsychotics are associated with an increased risk of producing extrapyramidal side effects, whereas the low-potency agents have more sedating, anticholinergic, and orthostatic hypotensive properties [61] and extrapyramidal side effects.

Parkinson's disease

Parkinson's disease (PD), the most common movement disorder, affects approximately 500,000 people in the United States [62]. The neuropathologic hallmark of PD is the finding of Lewy bodies in the brainstem nuclei and depigmentation of the substantia nigra. PD is a clinical diagnosis based on the signs of resting tremor, bradykinesia, cogwheel rigidity, and loss of postural reflexes [63]. Bradykinesia, or slowness of voluntary movements, may cause disturbances in common, yet simple motor tasks, such as dressing or turning in bed. Falls can become quite common as the disease progresses. Among the behavioral and cognitive troubles experienced in PD, depression and dementia affect approximately one third of patients [64,65]. Sleep disorders are encountered in most PD patients, adversely affecting their quality of life [66]. Pathologic daytime sleepiness and fatigue are common in patients with PD and are two of the most disabling features [67]. Sleep problems in PD patients also correlate with increased severity of disease.

The frequency of sleep complaints in patients with PD is estimated to be between 60% and 90%, and a variety of other mechanisms, which are either disease-related or secondary mechanisms, may come into play including prescribed therapy for PD using dopaminergic treatment [68]. Patients with PD may experience a number of sleep disorders including insomnia; parasomnia; and daytime somnolence (including excessive daytime sleepiness and sleep attacks) [7]. Excessive nocturia can disturb sleep, particularly in those with severe PD, and may be related to the natural evolution of dysautonomia in PD [69].

Patients with PD often have difficulties or total inability to turn over during the night and get out of bed. This is most likely secondary to bradykinesia. Leg cramps and leg jerks are also very common and dystonic spasms of the limbs, face, and back. One community-based survey evaluating 245 patients with PD demonstrated that nearly two thirds of patients reported sleep disorders, significantly more than among patients with diabetes (46%) and healthy control subjects (33%) [70]. About a third of the patients with PD rated their overall nighttime problem as moderate to severe [70]. The most commonly reported sleep disorders included frequent awakening (sleep fragmentation) and early awakening [70]. The study found a strong correlation between depression and sleep disorders in patients with PD, which underlines the importance of identifying and treating both conditions in these patients [70].

The underlying biologic basis of sleep disruption in PD is possibly related to the alteration of dopaminergic, noradrenergic, serotonergic, and cholinergic neurons in the brainstem [68]. Typical sleep abnormalities include fragmented sleep with increased number of arousals and awakenings, and PD-specific motor phenomena, such as nocturnal immobility, rest tremor, eye-blinking, dyskinesias, and other phenomena, such as periodic limb movements in sleep, restless legs syndrome, fragmentary myoclonus, and respiratory dysfunction in sleep [68]. Sleep maintenance problems and difficulties with sleep initiation are the earliest and most frequent sleep disorders observed in these patients [68]. Close to 90% of these patients often have sleep maintenance insomnia associated with frequent awakenings [6,71]. Sleep fragmentation and spontaneous daytime dozing occurred much more frequently in PD patients than in controls [72]. Sleep fragmentation in PD may be caused by an increased skeletal muscle activity, disturbed breathing, and REM to non-REM variations of the dopaminergic receptor sensitivity [68].

These complaints manifest on polysomnographic recordings as reduction of sleep efficiency; increased wake after sleep onset; increased sleep fragmentation; reduction of slow wave sleep and REM sleep; disruption of non-REM to REM cyclicity; loss of muscle atonia; and increased electromyography activity, which is the basis for REM behavior disorder (RBD) [66,68,73,74].

Motor abnormalities in PD during sleep include the parkinsonism tremor and REM-onset blepherospasm, which disappears during REM sleep. Patients have rapid blinking at sleep onset and REM intrusion into non-REM sleep. RBD is very common in patients with PD [6,73] and may also precede the onset of PD [75]. Patients with PD who have posture reflex abnormalities and autonomic impairment are at an increased risk for sleep-related breathing disorder in the form of central sleep apnea, OSA, and alveolar hypoventilation syndrome [76]. PD may lead to a restrictive pulmonary disease. Patients with PD are also found to have circadian rhythm abnormalities and depression [77]. Circadian rhythm disturbances in PD may be related to mesocorticolimbic dopaminergic abnormalities and mesostriatal system abnormalities [68]. Abnormalities of dopaminergic neurons in the ventral tegmentum area often lead to EEG desynchronization and abnormal sleep-wake schedule disorder [78]. Additional attempts to explain the sleep-wake disruption in PD have been linked to reduction in serotonergic neurons of the dorsal raphe, noradrenergic neurons of the locus coeruleus. and cholinergic neurons of the pedunculopontine nucleus [68].

Patients with PD who are already on medications may have additional sleep difficulties. Low-dose dopaminergic agonists are often sedating. High-dose dopaminergic agonists, however, may lead to increased hallucinations, nightmares, and increased arousals. Levodopa is often associated with increased sleep latency but an increased sleep continuity [79,80]. In patients with PD who developed motor fluctuations (on-off phenomenon, wearing-off) during the day, other common sleep-related motor complaints including nocturnal akinesia, dystonia, and painful cramps are observed [68]. Chronic release formulation of levodopa-carbidopa has been demonstrated to improve nocturnal akinesia and increase sleep efficiency of patients with PD with underlying sleep-related motor disturbances [68].

Treatment of sleep disorders in patients with PD deserves special consideration. Patients with PD who suffer from insomnia are often treated by improving sleep hygiene abnormalities.

Pharmacologic treatment with small-dose dopaminergic preparation (ie, levodopa-carbidopa 25/100) and small doses of sedating tricyclic antidepressants may be tried. Problems with bradykinesia and nocturia are often improved by providing patients with a portable bedside commode. For patients with restless leg syndrome symptoms, an evening and nocturnal dose of dopaminergic agonist, such as carbidopa-levodopa, or a dopamine (D_3) agonist, is useful [81]. Patients with OSA are often improved with CPAP. Patients who are diagnosed with OSA in addition to autonomic dysfunction can be treated effectively with CPAP. A definitive treatment (with tracheostomy) is indicated, however, and is often mandatory because of the increased risk of fatal cardiac arrhythmias.

Rapid eye movement sleep behavior disorder

RBD is characterized by pathologic augmentation of skeletal muscle tone during REM sleep (Fig. 3). Patients present with unusual, complex, and intense motor activity during a dream sequence. The range of motor activities can vary from a simple limb movement to very complex quasipurposeful movements suggestive of dream content enactment [6]. The potential for self injury and bed partner injury is high, especially during severe episodes [82]. Current speculations suggest that the pontine tegmentum is the locus of muscle tone inhibitor system, which normally causes muscle atonia during REM sleep (Fig. 4) [81]. The peril-locus coeruleus of the rostral tegmentum of the pons produces activation of the medullary inhibitory zone by tegmentoreticular tract. RBD is characterized by a loss of atonia during REM sleep, which facilitates the motor behaviors during dreaming [83–85]. Fig. 4 summarizes the possible neuroanatomic explanation for RBD.

RBD is a common sleep disorder seen in PD [86,87]. Recent findings from various studies suggest a high percentage of patients with PD without sleep complaints may have subclinical or clinical RBD, and RBD can be the heralding manifestation of parkinsonism by many years in older male patients [68,87–93]. In addition to its high prevalence

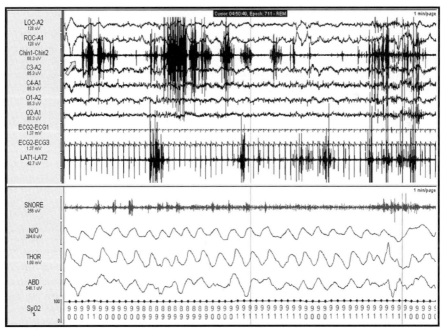

Fig. 3. Polysomnographic example of REM sleep behavior disorder. A 60-second epoch from a diagnostic polysomnogram of an 80-year-old man with Parkinson's disease who was referred to the sleep disorders clinic for evaluation of recurrent violent nighttime awakenings. Illustrated in this figure is a typical spell that this patient was experiencing during the night. He was noted to yell, jump from bed, and have complex body movements. The figure shows abnormal augmentation REM-muscle atonia in the left anterior tibialis muscle and chin electromyography channel. The patient was diagnosed with REM sleep behavior disorder and was treated successfully with 0.25 mg of clonazepam. Channels are as follows: electro-oculogram (left: LOC-A2; right: ROC-A1); chin electromyogram; electroencephalogram (left central, right central, left occipital, right occipital); two ECG channels; limb electromyogram (LAT); snore channel; nasal-oral airflow; respiratory effort (thoracic, abdominal); and oxygen saturation (Sao2).

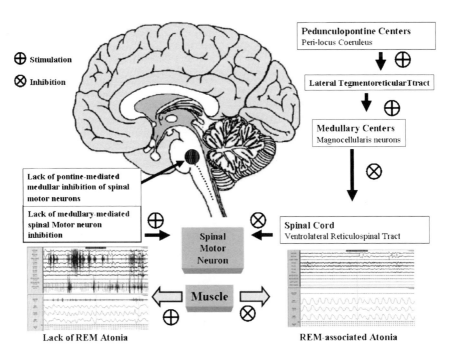

Fig. 4. Pathophysiology of REM sleep behavior disorder. Muscle atonia during REM sleep results from pontine-mediated perilocus ceruleus inhibition of motor activity. This pontine activity exerts an excitatory influence on medullary centers (magnocellularis neurons) by the lateral tegmentoreticular tract (- - - - - -). These neuronal groups hyperpolarize the spinal motor neuron postsynaptic membranes by the ventrolateral reticulospinal tract. In REM sleep behavior disorder (RBD), the brainstem mechanisms generating muscle is disrupted. The pathophysiology of RBD in humans is based on the cat model. In the cat model, bilateral pontine lesions result in a persistent absence of REM atonia associated with prominent motor activity during REM sleep, similar to that observed in RBD in humans. The pathophysiology of the idiopathic form of RBD in humans is still not very well understood but may be related to reduction of striatal presynaptic dopamine transporters. REM, rapid eye movement. (*Modified from* Avidan AY. Sleep disorders in the elderly. Primary Care Clinics in Office Practice 2005;32:536–87.)

in patients with PD, RBD is a common sleep disturbance in other neurodegenerative disorders, such as multiple system atrophy (MSA) and dementia with Lewy bodies [93–95].

Most cases occur with advancing age; approximately 60% are idiopathic, whereas the remaining 40% may have an underlying neuropathology. RBD typically manifests itself in the sixth or seventh decade of life. This disorder has a particular predilection to occur in a number of synucleinopathies and other neurodegenerative disorders in addition to PD, such as Lewy body dementia, olivopontocerebellar degeneration, Shy-Drager syndrome, and MSA [83,94,96–99].

Secondary causes of RBD include diseases that disrupt brainstem centers involved in REM-generated muscle atonia, such as multiple sclerosis, cerebral vascular accidents, and brainstem neoplasm. Twenty-five percent of patients may have a prodrome of subclinical behavioral release during sleep. The acute onset of RBD is related to drugs,

such as tricyclic antidepressants, monamine oxidase inhibitors, selective serotonin reuptake inhibitors, and acute withdrawal of alcohol and barbiturates. In extreme cases, excessive caffeine intake has been implicated in RBD [97,98,83,100].

In many cases, the diagnosis is suspected clinically based on the patient's and the bed partner's reports of recurrent dream-enacting behaviors. The diagnosis is confirmed by polysomnography using multiple-limb electromyography leads with simultaneous continuous video monitoring demonstrating evidence of increased electromyographic bursts of chin electromyography or limb electrodes during REM sleep. Clinically, the diagnosis of RBD based on the International Classification of Sleep Disorders Revised, has some intrinsic limitations based on the patient report and terminologic ambiguity, whereas diagnosis based on polysomnography has a better reliability [101,102]. The sleep study may also capture the actual spells during which the abnormal activity is demonstrated (limb jerk, complex, vigorous, violent behaviors). If there is evidence of an abnormal neurologic examination, a full neurologic work-up including a brain MRI may also be needed [81,98].

The differential diagnosis of RBD includes sleep-walking, nocturnal seizures, posttraumatic stress disorder, sleep terrors, nocturnal panic disorders, delirium, sleep-related gastroesophageal reflux, periodic limb movement disorder of sleep, psychogenic dissociative state, and confusional arousals with sleep apnea. Distinguishing RBD from nocturnal seizures may sometimes be difficult. Unlike nocturnal seizures, however, the typical RBD spell is usually not stereotyped and is often variable [82,98,83,103]. Additional laboratory studies may be needed especially if the clinical history remains vague or ambiguous. When the possibility of nocturnal seizures cannot be reliably excluded additional sleep testing may be warranted.

Rapid eye movement sleep behavior disorder treatment

Environmental safety is crucial in every patient with likely RBD. This may include making the sleeping environment safe by removing sharp objects and padding the bed area. Suggested pharmacotherapy for RBD includes clonazepam (0.25 to 1 mg orally at bedtime), which is effective in 90% of cases [98]. There is little evidence of tolerance or abuse with this form of treatment. Caution should be exercised when using it in patients with chronic respiratory diseases or impaired renal function, and it is contraindicated in patients with documented hypersensitivity, severe liver disease, or acute narrow-angle glaucoma. Abrupt discontinuation of clonazepam can precipitate withdrawal symptoms [98]. Other agents that can be helpful include imipramine (25 mg orally QHS); carbamazepine (100 mg, orally three times a day); and levodopa, in cases where RBD is associated with PD. Recent studies have also demonstrated improvement with melatonin, which is believed to exert its therapeutic effect by restoring REM sleep atonia. One study reported that melatonin was effective in 87% of patients taking 3 to 9 mg at bedtime [104], whereas a later study reported resolution in those taking 6 to 12 mg of melatonin at bedtime [105]. Tacrine, donepezil, and serzone, drugs used in AD and other dementing disorders, may exacerbate RBD. Some antidepressants may potentially increase total REM sleep, which may worsen RBD.

Diffuse Lewy body dementia

Diffuse Lewy body disease is a neurodegenerative disorder characterized by parkinsonism, dementia, fluctuations in mental status, and hallucinations. RBD is now recognized as a feature of diffuse Lewy body disease [106,107]. Nightmares without atonia may be an early symptom of diffuse Lewy body disease and is very often the initial manifestation of diffuse Lewy body disease [96,108].

Multiple-system atrophy

MSA is characterized clinically by any combination of autonomic, extrapyramidal, or cerebellar signs and symptoms. Patients with MSA experience degeneration of the pontine tegmentum, nucleus tractus solitarius, nucleus ambiguous, hypoglossal nucleus, reticular formation of the brainstem, and at times the cervical and thoracic spinal cord. The diffuse neurodegenerative process that encompasses these key structures involved in the regulation of the sleep-wake transition and respiratory function in MSA may account for the most frequent sleep disturbances in MSA, SDB, and RBD [109,110].

Patients with MSA are commonly affected with RBD, which represents the most common clinical sleep manifestation and polysomnographic finding in patients with MSA. In a large study involving MSA patients, RBD was diagnosed by polysomnographic monitoring in 90%, dream-enacting behaviors were reported in 69%, and RBD preceded the clinical presentation of MSA in 44% patients [94]. Because RBD can frequently herald the appearance of other MSA symptoms by years, expanded polysomnographic montage consisting of multiple limbs and video monitoring is recommended in patients with MSA when these spells are suspected [81,94]. Increasing evidence points to the role of basal ganglia dysfunction in the underlying pathophysiology of RBD in MSA. A recent study from the author's center has revealed that decreased nigrostriatal dopaminergic projections may contribute to RBD in MSA [111].

Patients with MSA frequently manifest a variety of sleep-related respiratory disturbances, some which are life-threatening. Above all, a common and serious complication is upper-airway OSA associated with stridor, which is caused by vocal cord abductor paralysis and may lead to sudden death during sleep [112]. For this reason, nocturnal stridor in MSA has been considered a poor prognostic feature [113]. For the early diagnosis of vocal cord abductor paralysis, it is critical to perform laryngoscopy during sleep, because vocal cord abductor paralysis does not appear during wakefulness in the early stage of MSA [114]. Polysomnography study should be obtained to assess the severity of respiratory disturbances and tracheostomy is the most reliable treatment for respiratory disturbances caused by vocal cord abductor paralysis. Although CPAP may be a useful treatment for some patients, absolute compliance is mandatory. Tracheostomy is probably the only effective measure for emergency treatment of severe respiratory dysfunction and hypoxia in patients with marked laryngeal stridor, as can be seen in laryngeal abductor paralysis in patients with MSA [113,114].

Olivopontocerebellar degeneration

Patients with olivopontocerebellar atrophy (OPCA) present with parkinsonism, atrophy of the pontine nuclei and cerebellar cortex, and degeneration of the olivopontocerebellar region. The sleep problems encountered in this condition include central, obstructive, and mixed sleep apnea, probably caused by bulbar muscle weakness [7]. Patients may also have nocturnal stridor and RBD [115,116]. Patients, unaware of their nocturnal sleep disturbance, complained only of the resulting daytime tiredness and sleepiness [116]. Nocturnal polyuria has also been reported in OPCA, possibly related to a disturbance in the circadian rhythm for arginine vasopressin secretion caused by degeneration of SCN and marked increase in the secretion of atrial natriuretic peptide caused by abnormal diurnal variation in blood pressure [117].

Shy-Drager syndrome

Progressive autonomic failure and progressive somatic neurologic manifestations characterize patients with Shy-Drager syndrome. Neuropathologic findings include striatonigral degeneration, OPCA, and autonomic neuronal degeneration [6]. The neuropathologic hallmarks of this disease include argyrophilic oligodendroglionic cytoplasmic inclusions in the cortical motor, premotor, supplementary motor association regions, extrapyramidal, corticocerebellar, brainstem, reticular formation, and the supraspinal autonomic system.

Patients with Shy-Drager syndrome most commonly present with sleep-related respiratory dysregulation with frequent arousals and hypoxemia [118]. Apneas encountered in this syndrome include obstructive, mixed, and central apneas. Cheyne-Stokes respiratory dysfunction, apneustic breathing, and inspiratory gasping are commonly seen. The hypersomnia seen in these patients is probably secondary to the dramatic sleep disruption. Patients may be at risk of dying from sudden cardiac death related to the underlying sleep-related breathing disorder. RBD disorder and insomnia are also common in this disease.

The mechanism of sleep disruption in this condition is probably caused by pathology in the brainstem structures regulating sleep-wake transition. Patients with Shy-Drager syndrome are at increased risk for developing brainstem ischemia secondary to nocturnal hypotensive episodes, which may subsequently potentiate the tendency to develop RBD

[119]. Sleep studies in patients with Shy-Drager syndrome demonstrate reduced slow wave sleep, reduced REM sleep, reduced total sleep time, increased sleep latency, increase in the frequency of awakenings, absence of atonia in REM sleep, and an increase in respiratory dysrhythmias [6,7].

Progressive supranuclear palsy

Patients with progressive supranuclear palsy often present with dementia, axial rigidity, dystonia, gait disturbances, and supranuclear eye movement abnormalities leading to impairment of vertical eye gaze. Other features include pseudobulbar paresis, axial rigidity, gait disturbances, and subcortical dementia. Neuropathologic hallmarks of progressive supranuclear palsy include neuronal loss and gliosis in brainstem nuclei and the locus coeruleus. Sleep disturbance is universal in progressive supranuclear palsy [7,120]. Insomnia is probably the most severe sleep problem noted by decreased total sleep time and significant sleep disruption without a specific clinical complaint [7]. Insomnia in progressive supranuclear palsy is worse than insomnia in PD or AD and may be caused by degenerative changes in brain structures responsible for sleep maintenance and marked nigrostriatal dopamine deficiency [121,122]. Other sleep disturbances may be related to the well-documented immobility in bed and difficulty with transfers, depression, dysphagia, and frequent nocturia seen in progressive supranuclear palsy. RBD and SDB are not common features in progressive supranuclear palsy [7,120].

The polysomnographic features of progressive supranuclear palsy are unique. When one evaluates the eye leads of the recording, it is interesting to note the absence of vertical eye movement during REM sleep. Horizontal eye movements are present but are slower and reduced in amplitude. During REM sleep, polysomnography may show increased phasic twitching and increased fast activity with alpha intrusion. The minority of patients with progressive supranuclear palsy may have periodic leg movements of sleep and OSA. Sleep architecture profile consists of increased sleep latency, increased arousal and awakening frequency, decreased stage 2 non-REM, reduced REM sleep, and reduced REM latency [6,7].

Epilepsy

Consideration of epilepsy and epileptic-like spells in the elderly is important, because these are frequent problems in elderly patients referred to epilepsy centers. A recent study from the Cleveland Clinic Foundation looked at the frequency of non-epileptic seizures in elderly patients referred for epilepsy monitoring, and found that 43% had a diagnosis other than epilepsy, including transient ischemic attacks, syncope, movement disorders, and sleep disorders [123]. Although most of the patients did not have any evidence for epilepsy, more than two thirds of these patients had been placed on anticonvulsive drugs [123].

Sleep and epilepsy have a reciprocal relationship. Sleep can affect the frequency and distribution of epileptiform discharges, whereas epileptic discharges can change sleep regulation and induce sleep disruption. Patients with epilepsy complain of symptoms, such as hypersomnia, insomnia, and even greater breakthrough seizures attributed to sleep disruptions. Sleep disturbances in epilepsy patients probably indicate the presence of an underlying sleep disorder rather than the effect of epilepsy or medication on sleep. Physicians must be able to identify and differentiate between potential underlying sleep disorders and sleep dysfunction related to epilepsy and direct therapy to improve the patient's symptoms [124].

Sleep deprivation was noted to increase interictal discharges in patients with generalized epilepsy [125]. The sleep state can promote interictal activity in as many as a third of patients with epilepsy and up to 90% of patients with sleep state–dependent epilepsy [124,126]. Up to one third of patients with medically refractory epilepsy had evidence of OSA and treatment of the underlying sleep apnea with CPAP can improve seizure frequency [127–129].

Nocturnal seizures and certain types of parasomnia can have similar clinical semiologies and can become a diagnostic dilemma. Common sleep disorders and manifestations, such as cataplexy, sleep attacks in the setting of narcolepsy, night terrors, and RBD, may be confused with epilepsy [130]. Some epilepsy syndromes, such as benign rolandic and nocturnal frontal lobe epilepsies, occur predominantly or exclusively during sleep.

Antiepileptic drugs also affect sleep architecture [131]. Phenytoin increases the amount of non-REM sleep, decreases sleep efficiency, and reduces sleep latency [132]. Carbamazepine increases the number of sleep-stage shifts and decreases REM sleep [133]. Benzodiazepines decrease sleep latency and reduce slow wave sleep [131,134]. Gabapentin has been shown to improve sleep efficiency and slow wave sleep, and increase REM sleep [135,136]. In clinical practice, understanding the unique effects of these antiepileptic drugs may offer the clinician an opportunity to improve sleep and wakefulness; medications that improve sleep disorders may require tailored dosing schedules to maximize their benefit [124].

Multiple sclerosis

Multiple sclerosis is the most common nontraumatic cause of neurologic disability in young adults [137]. With improved therapy, many patients survive to older age. Sleep disturbances in multiple sclerosis are common but poorly recognized and almost half of all patients demonstrate sleep disturbances caused by leg spasms, pain, immobility, nocturia, or medication [138]. Common sleep disorders in patients with multiple sclerosis include insomnia, restless legs syndrome, narcolepsy, and RBD. Sleep disruption in multiple sclerosis may result in hypersomnolence, increased fatigue, and a lowered pain threshold. An increased clinical awareness of sleep-related problems is warranted in this patient population because they are extremely common and have the potential negatively to impact overall health and quality of life [139].

Sleep and stroke

Stroke is the most common neurologic disease and the leading cause of adult disability in Western countries [140]. The number of patients affected by stroke increases as a function of aging [140]. Sleep and stoke interact in a number of complex ways. Probably the most important of these interactions is the fact that patients with sleep apnea or nocturnal hypoxemia often present with cardiac arrhythmias, intellectual decline, and increased risk of stroke. Habitual snoring affects 4% to 24% of the adult population with a maximum prevalence around the age of 50 to 60, and is strongly associated with OSA [141]. Habitual snoring may have adverse effects on long-term stroke outcome. Snoring was found adversely to affect prognosis in stroke survivors [142]. Hypersomnolence and prolonged sleep, which can be symptoms of SDB, may also represent independent risk factors for stroke [143,144]. SDB is common among stroke patients as defined by an apnea-hypopnea index ≥ 10 per hour [145–147].

Treatment of SDB has been recently shown to improve subjective well-being and mood in stroke patients with SDB [148,149]. Based on blood pressure–lowering effects of CPAP, treatment of SDB may lead to a stroke risk reduction of about 20% [150].Currently, it remains to be establishes if SDB represents an independent risk factor for stroke. The relationship may be a genetically determined one because of the increased vascular risk associated with SDB.

Central sleep apnea and sometimes Cheyne-Stokes breathing may be a latent phenomena after the stroke, and may predominate in as many as 30% to 40% of patients [151,152]. Subsequent to the stroke, patients may present with the coexistence of both OSA during REM sleep, and Cheyne-Stokes breathing during light NREM sleep [151,153,154]. Central hypoventilation syndrome and failure of automatic breathing (Ondine's curse) are more typically associated with brainstem strokes and are less common presentations [154].

Bilateral lacunar ischemic infarcts in the tegmentum of the pons, periventricular white matter damage can present as REM sleep without atonia, which leads to RBD [155,156]. Patients with Binswanger's disease or subcortical leukoencephalopathy are at an increased risk for developing RBD primarily because white matter ischemia in the vicinity of the supratentorial system is often involved in modulating REM related atonia. Brain MRI studies in patients with RBD with underlying strokes show ischemic lesions in the pontine tegmentum, which is the locus of muscle tone inhibitor system. Stroke can impair the regulation of sleep-wake and breathing control mechanisms. Secondary consequences from the stroke, such as immobilization, pain, hypoxia, and depression, can also impact sleep.

Amyotrophic lateral sclerosis

Amyotrophic lateral sclerosis is a neurodegenerative disease of middle age and elderly patients. The incidence of the disease increases with age, with a peak occurrence between 55 and 75 years of age. Pathology shows degeneration of the lateral corticospinal tracts, loss of motor neurons and astrogliosis in the brain and brainstem, and neuronal inclusions. This produces both upper and lower motor neuron deficits [157]. Amyotrophic lateral sclerosis has a relentless progression with no impairment of the mental function, or sensorium. Respiratory failure in this disorder occurs late in the course of the disease and may also be the presenting feature of this disease. It is not uncommon for physicians to encounter patients with breathing difficulties, bulbar weakness, and stridor in the emergency room only later to diagnose amyotrophic lateral sclerosis. The major sleep complaint of these patients includes excessive daytime sleepiness likely caused by sleep-related respiratory disturbances and insomnia [158–161].

The mechanism of respiratory disturbance in this disorder may be a result of the weakness of the upper airways caused by bulbar weakness; diaphragmatic weakness (caused by a phrenic nerve lesion); and intercostal muscle weakness (caused by the degeneration of intercostal nerve nuclei). Degeneration of the central respiratory neurons accounts for both central sleep apnea and OSA. Polysomnographic findings include apneas in the form of central, obstructive, and mixed events; increased awakenings; sleep fragmentation; and reduced nocturnal oxygen saturation [158,159,162–164].

Noninvasive positive pressure upper airway ventilation provides a long-lasting benefit on symptoms and quality of life indicators for amyotrophic lateral sclerosis patients and should be offered to all patients with symptoms of SDB or inspiratory muscle dysfunction [165]. Positive pressure therapy can also prolong tracheostomy-free survival [166].

Spinal cord diseases

Patients with spinal cord injury often present with sleep disturbances related to respiratory dysfunction, particularly when the lesion occurs in the upper cervical spinal cord within the vicinity of the phrenic nerve nuclei [167]. Patients with spinal cord injury have a greater difficulty in falling asleep, describe more frequent awakenings, are more likely to be prescribed sleeping pills, sleep more hours, take more frequent and longer naps, and are more likely to snore than compared with controls [168]. In particular, spasms, pain, paresthesia, and voiding difficulties have a higher association with sleep problems [168].

The incidence of SDB in spinal cord injury is high in patients with tetraplegia, especially when the patient is elderly, has an increased large neck circumference, has a long duration of the disease, and is on cardiac medications [169]. The increased use of cardiac medication in tetraplegics with SDB may implicate a link between SDB and cardiovascular morbidity, one of the leading causes of death in tetraplegia. OSA seems to be more common in older patients with spinal cord injury than in the general population and is related to ventilatory dysfunction secondary to spinal cord [170].

Neurologic conditions likely to damage and disrupt the phrenic and intercostal motor neurons in the spinal cord include poliomyelitis; amyotrophic lateral sclerosis; spinal cord tumors; spinal trauma; spinal surgery (eg, cervical cordotomy or anterior spinal surgery); and nonspecific or demyelinating myelitis [167]. Patients with syringobulbia present with severe abnormalities in respiratory rhythm generation during sleep [171]. The respiratory disturbances are not caused by muscle weakness and they are not correlated with the size of the cavity [171]. Phrenic nerve damage may cause diaphragmatic paralysis and whereas unilateral paralysis is asymptomatic, bilateral paralysis presents with orthopnea manifesting as difficulty on inspiration out of proportion to the cardiopulmonary status and may be life-threatening [167].

Postpolio syndrome

Postpolio syndrome describes the new, late manifestations that occur in patients three to four decades after the occurrence of acute poliomyelitis [172]. Postpolio syndrome is more common at the present time because of the large epidemics of poliomyelitis in the 1940s and 1950s. Neurologic manifestations of postpolio syndrome consist of neurologic, musculoskeletal, and systemic symptoms and signs. The most prominent neurologic manifestation is a new progressive weakness, at times accompanied by atrophy referred to as "post-polio progressive muscular atrophy" when affecting the extremities. A new weakness can also affect respiratory and bulbar muscles, however, which can be more serious causing dysphagia, dysphonia, and respiratory failure [173,174]. Respiratory failure in postpolio syndrome may be treated with CPAP, Bilevel positive airway pressure (BiPAP), or tracheotomy and permanent ventilation if necessary [175]. Other sleep disturbances include random myoclonus, periodic movements in sleep with muscle contractions, ballistic movements of the legs, and restless legs syndrome [176]. Poliovirus-induced damage to the spinal cord and brain may be implicated as a possible cause of these abnormal movements in sleep [176]. It is suggested that polysomnography be performed on postpolio syndrome patients with excessive daytime sleepiness and respiratory complaints [177].

Huntington's disease

Huntington's disease is a hereditary progressive, neurodegenerative condition characterized by significant motor dysfunction (typically appearing as involuntary and spasmodic movements); cognitive impairment; and psychiatric difficulties. It is caused by an expanded CAG repeat in the gene encoding huntingtin, a protein of unknown function. Sleep disturbances are common in Huntington's disease and consist of disturbed sleep pattern with increased sleep-onset latency, reduced sleep efficiency, increased arousals and sleep fragmentation, decreased slow wave sleep, frequent nocturnal awakenings, increased density of sleep spindles, increased time spent awake, and reduced sleep efficiency [178–180]. Patients who have Huntington's disease have also shown higher-density sleep spindles, in contrast with findings in other neurodegenerative dementia populations [179]. These abnormalities correlated in part with duration of illness, severity of clinical symptoms, and degree of atrophy of the caudate nucleus [180].

Based on actigraphy data, patients with Huntington's disease demonstrate significant activity and spend more time making high acceleration movements compared with age-matched controls [181]. No increase in sleep-related breathing disorders has been demonstrated in Huntington's disease, also in contrast with findings in other neurodegenerative dementias [182]. Circadian-rhythm sleep disturbances, however, are an important pathologic feature of Huntington's disease, and may arise from a disruption of the expression of the circadian clock genes mPer2 and mBmal1 in the SCN, the principal circadian pacemaker in the brain [183].

Myotonic dystrophy

Myotonic dystrophy or dystrophia myotonica (DM) is a multisystem disorder with myotonia, muscle weakness, cataracts, endocrine dysfunction, and intellectual impairment. This disorder is caused by a CTG triplet expansion of the DMPK gene on 19q13. Sleep abnormalities in patients with DM include hypersomnia, sharing with narcolepsy a short sleep latency and the presence of sleep-onset REM periods during the Multiple Sleep Latency Test [184]. Hypersomnia is found in almost a third of patients with DM and the severity of daytime sleepiness correlated with the severity of muscular impairment [185]. Corpus callosum atrophy might occur in DM patients, and the size of the corpus callosum anterior area might be associated with the hypersomnia [186]. Patients with DM report a longer sleep period, a less restorative sleep, difficulties with sleep initiation, and hypersomnia comparable with those found in idiopathic hypersomnia [185]. In DM, hypersomnia may be aggravated by alveolar hypoventilation and SDB, but is not entirely reversed by satisfactory application of positive pressure airway ventilation, suggesting that hypersomnia is partially related to an intrinsic hypersomnia caused by central nervous system alteration [165].

A dysfunction of the hypothalamic hypocretin system has recently been found in patients with DM and may mediate the underlying hypersomnia [184]. Modafinil, a wake-promoting agent, was recently found to reduce hypersomnolence and improves mood, quality-of-life measures of energy, and health change in patients with DM [187,188].

Patients with DM are found have increased risk of OSA, central sleep apnea, and excessive daytime sleepiness [163,165,189]. These patients are also thought to have a centrally mediated impairment in breathing probably related to brainstem respiratory center disorder rather than respiratory muscle weakness [190,191]. Non-OSAs and alveolar hypoventilation may be related to an underlying central neurologic pathology in DM, muscle weakness and myotonia may underlie development of obstructive SDB [165].

Neuropathologic findings include severe neuronal loss and gliosis in the midbrain and pontine raphe (particularly in dorsal raphe nucleus), superior central nucleus, and medullary reticular formation [192]. Alveolar hypoventilation and the hypersomnia in DM may be attributed to these morphologic abnormalities, and seems to be central in nature [192].

Diagnostic approaches to sleep disturbances in neurologic disorders

Clinical assessment

The first and most important step in the work-up of sleep disturbances of patients with neurologic disturbances is a detailed inventory of sleep complaints. The history should consist of present and past sleep history; family history; medication and substance use (eg, caffeine, nicotine, and alcohol); and information about underlying medical or psychiatric pathologies. The history should also be specifically directed at possible respiratory disturbances during sleep. It is important to perform a physical examination for the diagnosis of the primary condition or associated medical conditions, including neurologic disorders, which may be responsible for the sleep disturbances.

Laboratory assessment

Laboratory investigations should be undertaken to diagnose the nature of the sleep disturbance and the primary neurologic disorder. Overnight polysomnography and the Multiple Sleep Latency Test are the two most important laboratory tests for the diagnosis of sleep disturbances. Sometimes, pulmonary-function tests are needed to address the question of sleep-related respiratory disturbances, specifically in the setting of underling motor neuron disease or neuromuscular disorder and underlying respiratory pathologies.

Sleep tests

Polysomnography

Polysomnography should be performed in patients suspected of sleep-related respiratory disorders [4,41,193,194]. Unfortunately, the diagnosis and treatment of sleep disturbances may be problematic in neurodegenerative diseases with severe functional impairment given difficulties in ascertaining the clinical history from the patient. All-night polysomnography is critical in the assessment of the severity of the SDB and in documenting the consequences on the sleep architecture. Sleep itself may adversely affect breathing and the primary neurologic disorder; conversely, primary neurologic disorders may adversely affect sleep. In addition to the typical montage obtained in patients without neurodegenerative disorders, in suspected cases of upper airway resistance syndrome, which can sometimes be encountered in extrapyramidal disorders, measurement of the esophageal pressure manometry is important and can be accomplished by inserting an esophageal pressure monitor [195]. Comprehensive electroencephalogram monitoring

is also helpful in the context of neurodegenerative disorders further to characterize sleep architectural disturbances and when focal or diffuse cerebral lesions and epileptiform activities are suspected [196,197]. As detailed in the previous sections, more specific polysomnography montages (including multiple limb electrodes and electroencephalogram) may be helpful in the evaluation of potential parasomnia and nocturnal seizures.

Multiple Sleep Latency Test

When patients with neurodegenerative diseases present with pathologic sleepiness, the Multiple Sleep Latency Test can be helpful in documenting the extent of sleepiness. A mean sleep latency of less than 5 minutes is consistent with pathologic excessive sleepiness. Abnormalities of REM-sleep regulatory mechanisms and circadian rhythm sleep disturbances may also lead to REM abnormalities during the Multiple Sleep Latency Test.

Additional laboratory tests

Multichannel, continuous video polysomnographic monitoring may be helpful when abnormal motor activities are encountered in patients with MSA, OPCA, PD, and AD. Actigraphy, a recently developed technique that uses a motion detector to record activities during sleep and waking, may be useful in the diagnosis of circadian rhythm sleep disorders in patients with neurodegenerative diseases. Neuroimaging is of particular help when patients present with a variety of complaints with unusual features, such as dream enactment behavior (in a young woman); severe hypersomnia (following head trauma); and apneic episodes (following a brainstem stroke).

Summary

Sleep changes dramatically with old age and even more dramatically with dementia. When encountering daytime sleepiness in an older patient with dementia or neurodegenerative disorders, it is crucial first to review the patient's medical history, psychiatric history, medications, underlying medical illnesses, and sleep-wake schedule pattern. The prevalence of SDB, periodic limb movements, restless legs syndrome, and RBD increases with age and may lead to excessive daytime sleepiness or insomnia. Many sleep disorders are potentially reversible. A carefully thought out clinical decision-making process can greatly benefit the patient and family. Sleep problems of the elderly contribute heavily to the decision to institutionalize an elder and to the social and economic cost of institutional care and seem to do this largely by interfering with the sleep of caregivers. The nature, prevalence, and treatability of the sleeping problems of both elders and their caregivers need further study [15].

References

[1] Census USBot. Population projects program [Internet Source]. Available at: www.census.gov. Accessed February 10, 2004.

[2] Janssens JPPS, Hilleret H, Michel J-P. Sleep disordered breathing in the elderly. Aging Clin Exp Res 2000;12:417–29.

[3] Burger CSJ. Sleep-disordered breathing and aging. New York: Marcel Dekker; 1993.

[4] Avidan AY. Sleep in the geriatric patient population. Semin Neurol 2005;25:52–63.

[5] van der Flier WM, Scheltens P. Epidemiology and risk factors of dementia. J Neurol Neurosurg Psychiatry 2005;76(Suppl 5):v2–7.

[6] Chokroverty S. Sleep and degenerative neurologic disorders. Neurol Clin 1996;14:807–26.

[7] Bhatt MH, Podder N, Chokroverty S. Sleep and neurodegenerative diseases. Semin Neurol 2005;25:39–51.

[8] Little JT, Satlin A, Sunderland T, et al. Sundown syndrome in severely demented patients with probable Alzheimer's disease. J Geriatr Psychiatry Neurol 1995;8:103–6.

[9] Pollak CP, Perlick D, Linsner JP, et al. Sleep problems in the community elderly as predictors of death and nursing home placement. J Community Health 1990;15:123–35.

[10] Storandt M, Kaskie B, Von Dras DD. Temporal memory for remote events in healthy aging and dementia. Psychol Aging 1998;13:4–7.

[11] Wisniewski HM, Wegiel J. The neuropathology of Alzheimer's disease. Neuroimaging Clin N Am 1995;5:45–57.

[12] Blass JP. Alzheimer's disease. Dis Mon 1985;31:1–69.

[13] Ancoli-Israel S, Klauber MR, Jones DW, et al. Variations in circadian rhythms of activity, sleep, and light exposure related to dementia in nursing-home patients. Sleep 1997;20:18–23.

[14] Ancoli-Israel S, Klauber MR, Gillin JC, et al. Sleep in non-institutionalized Alzheimer's disease patients. Aging (Milano) 1994;6:451–8.

[15] Pollak CP, Perlick D. Sleep problems and institutionalization of the elderly. J Geriatr Psychiatry Neurol 1991;4:204–10.

[16] Bliwise DL, Tinklenberg J, Yesavage JA, et al. REM latency in Alzheimer's disease. Biol Psychiatry 1989;25:320–8.

[17] Vitiello MV, Prinz PN, Williams DE, et al. Sleep disturbances in patients with mild-stage Alzheimer's disease. J Gerontol 1990;45:M131–8.

[18] Vitiello MV, Prinz PN. Alzheimer's disease: sleep and sleep/wake patterns. Clin Geriatr Med 1989;5:289–99.

[19] Vitiello MV, Poceta JS, Prinz PN. Sleep in Alzheimer's disease and other dementing disorders. Can J Psychol 1991;45:221–39.

[20] Vitiello MV, Borson S. Sleep disturbances in patients with Alzheimer's disease: epidemiology, pathophysiology and treatment. CNS Drugs 2001;15:777–96.

[21] Vitiello MV, Bliwise DL, Prinz PN. Sleep in Alzheimer's disease and the sundown syndrome. Neurology 1992;42(Suppl 6):83–93. [discussion: 84–93].

[22] Taylor JL, Friedman L, Sheikh J, et al. Assessment and management of "sundowning" phenomena. Semin Clin Neuropsychiatry 1997;2:113–22.

[23] Bliwise DL. Sleep disorders in Alzheimer's disease and other dementias. Clin Cornerstone 2004;6(Suppl 1A):S16–28.

[24] Stopa EG, Volicer L, Kuo-Leblanc V, et al. Pathologic evaluation of the human suprachiasmatic nucleus in severe dementia. J Neuropathol Exp Neurol 1999;58:29–39.

[25] Czeisler C, Dumont M, Duffy JF. Association of sleep-wake habits in older people with changes in output of circadian pacemaker. Lancet 1992;340:933–6.

[26] Swaab DF, Fisser B, Kamphorst W, et al. The human suprachiasmatic nucleus; neuropeptide changes in senium and Alzheimer's disease. Basic Appl Histochem 1988;32:43–54.

[27] Swaab DF, Fliers E, Partiman TS. The suprachiasmatic nucleus of the human brain in relation to sex, age and senile dementia. Brain Res 1985;342:37–44.

[28] Hoch CC, Reynolds CF, Kupfer DJ, et al. Sleep disordered breathing in normal and pathological aging. J Clin Psychiatry 1986;47:499–503.

[29] Erkinjuntti TPM, Partinen M, Sulkava R, et al. Sleep apnea in multiinfarct dementia and Alzheimer's disease. Sleep 1987;10:419–25.

[30] Janssens JP, Pautex S, Hilleret H, et al. Sleep disordered breathing in the elderly. Aging (Milano) 2000;12:417–29.

[31] Ancoli-Israel S, Klauber MR, Butters N, et al. Dementia in institutionalized elderly: relation to sleep apnea. J Am Geriatr Soc 1991;39:258–63.

[32] Schletens PVF, Van Keimpema A, Lindebloom J, et al. Sleep apnea syndrome presenting with cognitive impairment. Neurology 1991;41:155–6.

[33] Bliwise DL. Sleep apnea, APOE4 and Alzheimer's disease 20 years and counting? J Psychosom Res 2002;53:539–46.

[34] Kadotani H, Kadotani T, Young T, et al. Association between apolipoprotein E epsilon4 and sleep-disordered breathing in adults. JAMA 2001;285:2888–90.

[35] Punjabi NM, Shahar E, Redline S, et al. Sleep-disordered breathing, glucose intolerance, and insulin resistance: the Sleep Heart Health Study. Am J Epidemiol 2004;160:521–30.

[36] Foley DJ, Masaki K, White L, et al. Relationship between apolipoprotein E epsilon4 and sleep-disordered breathing at different ages. JAMA 2001;286:1447–8.

[37] Saarelainen S, Lehtimaki T, Kallonen E, et al. No relation between apolipoprotein E alleles and obstructive sleep apnea. Clin Genet 1998; 53:147–8.

[38] Gottlieb DJ, DeStefano AL, Foley DJ, et al. APOE epsilon4 is associated with obstructive sleep apnea/hypopnea: the Sleep Heart Health Study. Neurology 2004;63:664–8.

[39] Gehrman PR, Martin JL, Shochat T, et al. Sleep-disordered breathing and agitation in institutionalized adults with Alzheimer disease. Am J Geriatr Psychiatry 2003;11:426–33.

[40] Aloia MSIN, Di Dio P, Perlis ML, et al. Neuropsychological changes and treatment compliance in older adults with sleep apnea. J Psychosom Res 2003;54:71–6.

[41] Avidan AY. Sleep disorders in the older patient. Prim Care 2005;32:563–86.

[42] Mazza M, Della Marca G, De Risio S, et al. Sleep disorders in the elderly. Clin Ther 2004; 155:391–4.

[43] Cohen-Zion M, Stepnowsky C, Marler, et al. Changes in cognitive function associated with sleep disordered breathing in older people. J Am Geriatr Soc 2001;49:1622–7.

[44] Wu YH, Swaab DF. The human pineal gland and melatonin in aging and Alzheimer's disease. J Pineal Res 2005;38:145–52.

[45] Frank B, Gupta S. A review of antioxidants and Alzheimer's disease. Ann Clin Psychiatry 2005; 17:269–86.

[46] Singer C, Tractenberg RE, Kaye J, et al. A multicenter, placebo-controlled trial of melatonin for sleep disturbance in Alzheimer's disease. Sleep 2003;26:893–901.

[47] Skene DJ, Swaab DF. Melatonin rhythmicity: effect of age and Alzheimer's disease. Exp Gerontol 2003;38:199–206.

[48] Srinivasan V, Pandi-Perumal SR, Maestroni GJ, et al. Role of melatonin in neurodegenerative diseases. Neurotox Res 2005;7:293–318.

[49] Wang JZ, Wang ZF. Role of melatonin in Alzheimer-like neurodegeneration. Acta Pharmacol Sin 2006;27:41–9.

[50] Olakowska E, Marcol W, Kotulska K, et al. The role of melatonin in the neurodegenerative diseases. Bratisl Lek Listy 2005;106:171–4.

[51] Zhdanova IV, Tucci V. Melatonin, circadian rhythms, and sleep. Curr Treat Options Neurol 2003;5:225–9.

[52] Asayama K, Yamadera H, Ito T, et al. Double blind study of melatonin effects on the sleep-wake rhythm, cognitive and non-cognitive functions in Alzheimer type dementia. J Nippon Med Sch 2003;70:334–41.

[53] Lyketsos CG, Lindell Veiel L, Baker A, et al. A randomized, controlled trial of bright light therapy for agitated behaviors in dementia patients residing in long-term care. Int J Geriatr Psychiatry 1999;14:520–5.

[54] Satlin A, Volicer L, Ross V, et al. Bright light treatment of behavioral and sleep disturbances in patients with Alzheimer's disease. Am J Psychiatry 1992;149:1028–32.

[55] Alessi CA, Martin JL, Webber AP, et al. Randomized, controlled trial of a nonpharmacological intervention to improve abnormal sleep/wake patterns in nursing home residents. J Am Geriatr Soc 2005;53:803–10.

[56] Alessi CA, Schnelle JF, MacRae PG, et al. Does physical activity improve sleep in impaired nursing home residents? J Am Geriatr Soc 1995;43:1098–102.

[57] Alessi CA, Yoon EJ, Schnelle JF, et al. A randomized trial of a combined physical activity and environmental intervention in nursing home residents: do sleep and agitation improve? J Am Geriatr Soc 1999;47:784–91.

[58] Schnelle JF, Cruise PA, Alessi CA, et al. Sleep hygiene in physically dependent nursing home residents: behavioral and environmental intervention implications. Sleep 1998;21:515–23.

[59] Ancoli-Israel S, Gehrman P, Martin JL, et al. Increased light exposure consolidates sleep and strengthens circadian rhythms in severe Alzheimer's disease patients. Behav Sleep Med 2003;1:22–36.

[60] Ancoli-Israel S, Martin JL, Gehrman P, et al. Effect of light on agitation in institutionalized patients with severe Alzheimer disease. Am J Geriatr Psychiatry 2003;11:194–203.

[61] McGaffigan S, Bliwise DL. The treatment of sundowning: a selective review of pharmacological and nonpharmacological studies. Drugs Aging 1997;10:10–7.

[62] Tanner CM, Aston DA. Epidemiology of Parkinson's disease and akinetic syndromes. Curr Opin Neurol 2000;13:427–30.

[63] Sethi KD. Clinical aspects of Parkinson disease. Curr Opin Neurol 2002;15:457–60.

[64] McDonald WM, Richard IH, DeLong MR. Prevalence, etiology, and treatment of depression in Parkinson's disease. Biol Psychiatry 2003; 54:363–75.

[65] Elmer L. Cognitive issues in Parkinson's disease. Neurol Clin 2004;22(3 Suppl):S91–106.

[66] Partinen M. Sleep disorder related to Parkinson's disease. J Neurol 1997;244(Suppl 1):S3–6.

[67] Fabbrini G, Barbanti P, Aurilia C, et al. Excessive daytime sleepiness in de novo and treated Parkinson's disease. Mov Disord 2002;17:1026–30.

[68] Stocchi F, Barbato L, Nordera G, et al. Sleep disorders in Parkinson's disease. J Neurol 1998; 245(Suppl 1):S15–8.

[69] Young A, Home M, Churchward T, et al. Comparison of sleep disturbance in mild versus severe Parkinson's disease. Sleep 2002;25:573–7.

[70] Tandberg E, Larsen JP, Karlsen K. A community-based study of sleep disorders in patients with Parkinson's disease. Mov Disord 1998; 13:895–9.

[71] Frucht S, Greene P, Fahn S. Sleep episodes in Parkinson's disease: a wake-up call. Mov Disord 2000;15:601–3.

[72] Factor SA, McAlarney T, Sanchez-Ramos JR, et al. Sleep disorders and sleep effect in Parkinson's disease. Mov Disord 1990;5:280–5.

[73] Comella CL. Sleep disturbances in Parkinson's disease. Curr Neurol Neurosci Rep 2003;3:173–80.

[74] Schenck CH, Mahowald MW. REM parasomnias. Neurol Clin 1996;14:697–720.

[75] Tan A, Salgado M, Fahn S. Rapid eye movement sleep behavior disorder preceding Parkinson's disease with therapeutic response to levodopa. Mov Disord 1996;11:214–6.

[76] Apps MC, Sheaff PC, Ingram DA, et al. Respiration and sleep in Parkinson's disease. J Neurol Neurosurg Psychiatry 1985;48:1240–5.

[77] Trenkwalder C. Sleep dysfunction in Parkinson's disease. Clin Neurosci 1998;5:107–14.

[78] Eisensehr I, Linke R, Noachtar S, et al. Reduced striatal dopamine transporters in idiopathic rapid eye movement sleep behavior disorder: comparison with Parkinson's disease and controls. Brain 2000;123:1155–60.

[79] Askenasy JJ, Yahr MD. Reversal of sleep disturbance in Parkinson's disease by antiparkinsonian therapy: a preliminary study. Neurology 1985;35:527–32.

[80] Pappert EJ, Goetz CG, Niederman FG, et al. Hallucinations, sleep fragmentation, and altered dream phenomena in Parkinson's disease. Mov Disord 1999;14:117–21.

[81] Schenck CH, Bundlie SR, Patterson AL, et al. Rapid eye movement sleep behavior disorder: a treatable parasomnia affecting older adults. JAMA 1987;257:1786–9.

[82] Aldrich MS. Sleep Medicine, vol 53. New York: Oxford University Press; 1999.

[83] Schenck CH, Mahowald MW. REM sleep parasomnias. Neurol Clin 1996;14:697–720.

[84] Morrison AR. The pathophysiology of REM-sleep behavior disorder. Sleep 1998;21:446–9.

[85] Parkes JD. The parasomnias. Lancet 1986; 2:1021–5.

[86] Lowe AD. Sleep in Parkinson's disease. J Psychosom Res 1998;44:613–7.

[87] Gagnon JF, Bedard MA, Fantini ML, et al. REM sleep behavior disorder and REM sleep without atonia in Parkinson's disease. Neurology 2002; 59:585–9.

[88] Wetter TC, Trenkwalder C, Gershanik O, et al. Polysomnographic measures in Parkinson's disease: a comparison between patients with and without REM sleep disturbances. Wien Klin Wochenschr 2001;113:249–53.

[89] Poryazova RG, Zachariev ZI. REM sleep behavior disorder in patients with Parkinson's disease. Folia Med (Plovdiv) 2005;47:5–10.

[90] Larsen JP, Tandberg E. Sleep disorders in patients with Parkinson's disease: epidemiology and management. CNS Drugs 2001;15:267–75.

[91] Boeve BF, Silber MH, Ferman TJ, et al. Association of REM sleep behavior disorder and neurodegenerative disease may reflect an underlying synucleinopathy. Mov Disord 2001;16:622–30.

[92] Boeve BF, Silber MH, Ferman TJ. REM sleep behavior disorder in Parkinson's disease and dementia with Lewy bodies. J Geriatr Psychiatry Neurol 2004;17:146–57.

[93] Abad VC, Guilleminault C. Review of rapid eye movement behavior sleep disorders. Curr Neurol Neurosci Rep 2004;4:157–63.

[94] Plazzi G, Corsini R, Provini F, et al. REM sleep behavior disorders in multiple system atrophy. Neurology 1997;48:1094–7.

[95] Iranzo A, Santamaria J, Rye DB, et al. Characteristics of idiopathic REM sleep behavior disorder and that associated with MSA and PD. Neurology 2005;65:247–52.

[96] Boeve BF, Silber MH, Ferman T. REM sleep behavior disorder and degenerative dementia: an association likely reflecting Lewy body disease. Neurology 1998;51:363–70.

[97] Ferini-Strambi L, Zucconi M. REM sleep behavior disorder. Clin Neurophysiol 2000;111(Suppl 2): S136–40.

[98] Mahowald MW, Schenck CH. REM sleep behavior disorder. Philadelphia: WB Saunders; 1994.

[99] Schenck CH, Bundlie SR, Mahowald MW. Delayed emergence of a parkinsonian disorder in 38% of 29 older men initially diagnosed with idiopathic rapid eye movement sleep behavior disorder. Neurology 1996;46:388–93.

[100] Stolz SE, Aldrich MS. REM sleep behavior disorder associated with caffeine abuse. Sleep Res 1991;20:341.

[101] Bologna, Genera, Parma, and Pisa Universities group for the study of REM Sleep Behaviour Disorders in Parkinson's Disease. Interobserver reliability of ICSD-R criteria for REM sleep behaviour disorder. J Sleep Res 2003;12(3): 255–7.

[102] Consens FB, Chervin RD, Koeppe RA, et al. Validation of a polysomnographic score for REM sleep behavior disorder. Sleep 2005;28:993–7.

[103] Kowey PR, Mainchak RA, Rials SJ. Things that go bang in the night. N Engl J Med 1992;327:1884.

[104] Takeuchi N, Uchimura N, Hashizume Y, et al. Melatonin therapy for REM sleep behavior disorder. Psychiatry Clin Neurosci 2001;55:267–9.

[105] Boeve B. Melatonin for treatment of REM sleep behavior disorder: response in 8 patients. Sleep 2001;24:A35.

[106] Zesiewicz TA, Baker MJ, Dunne PB, et al. Diffuse Lewy body disease. Curr Treat Options Neurol 2001;3:507–18.

[107] Turner RS, Chervin RD, Frey KA, et al. Probable diffuse Lewy body disease presenting as REM sleep behavior disorder. Neurology 1997; 49:523.

[108] de Brito-Marques PR, de Mello RV, Montenegro L. Nightmares without atonia as an early symptom of diffuse Lewy bodies disease. Arq Neuropsiquiatr 2003;61:936–41.

[109] Ghorayeb I, Bioulac B, Tison F. Sleep disorders in multiple system atrophy. J Neural Transm 2005;112:1669–75.

[110] Chokroverty S, Sharp JT, Barron KD. Periodic respiration in erect posture in Shy-Drager syndrome. J Neurol Neurosurg Psychiatry 1978; 41:980–6.

[111] Gilman S, Koeppe RA, Chervin RD, et al. REM sleep behavior disorder is related to striatal monoaminergic deficit in MSA. Neurology 2003;61:29–34.

[112] Munschauer FE, Mador J, Ahuja A, et al. Selective paralysis of voluntary but not limbically influenced automatic respiration. Arch Neurol 1991;48:1190–2.

[113] Olson EJ, Boeve BF, Silber MH. Rapid eye movement sleep behaviour disorder: demographic, clinical and laboratory findings in 93 cases. Brain 2000;123(Pt 2):331–9.

[114] Sakakibara R, Odaka T, Uchiyama T, et al. Colonic transit time and rectoanal videomanometry in Parkinson's disease. J Neurol Neurosurg Psychiatry 2003;74:268–72.

[115] Hughes RJ, Sack RL, Lewy AJ. The role of melatonin and circadian phase in age-related sleep-maintenance insomnia: assessment in a clinical trial of melatonin replacement. Sleep 1998; 21:52–68.

[116] Salva MA, Guilleminault C. Olivopontocerebellar degeneration, abnormal sleep, and REM sleep without atonia. Neurology 1986;36:576–7.

[117] Miyamoto T, Miyamoto M, Yokota N, et al. A case of nocturnal polyuria in olivopontocerebellar atrophy. Psychiatry Clin Neurosci 1999; 53:279–81.

[118] Briskin JG, Lehrman KL. Shy-Drager syndrome and sleep apnea. New York: Liss; 1978.

[119] Pauletto G, Belgrado E, Marinig R, et al. Sleep disorders and extrapyramidal diseases: an historical review. Sleep Med 2004;5:163–7.

[120] Gross RA, Spehlmann R, Daniels JC. Sleep disturbances in progressive supranuclear palsy. Electroencephalogr Clin Neurophysiol 1978; 45:16–25.

[121] Kish SJ, Chang LJ, Mirchandani L, et al. Progressive supranuclear palsy: relationship between extrapyramidal disturbances, dementia, and brain neurotransmitter markers. Ann Neurol 1985;18:530–6.

[122] Aldrich MS, Foster NL, White RF, et al. Sleep abnormalities in progressive supranuclear palsy. Ann Neurol 1989;25:577–81.

[123] Kellinghaus C, Loddenkemper T, Dinner DS, et al. Non-epileptic seizures of the elderly. J Neurol 2004;251:704–9.

[124] Vaughn BV, D'Cruz OF. Sleep and epilepsy. Semin Neurol 2004;24:301–13.

[125] Degen R, Degen HE. Sleep and sleep deprivation in epileptology. Epilepsy Res Suppl 1991; 2:235–60.

[126] Dinner DS. Effect of sleep on epilepsy. J Clin Neurophysiol 2002;19:504–13.

[127] Malow BA, Bowes RJ, Lin X. Predictors of sleepiness in epilepsy patients. Sleep 1997; 20:1105–10.

[128] Vaughn BV, D'Cruz OF, Beach R, et al. Improvement of epileptic seizure control with treatment of obstructive sleep apnoea. Seizure 1996;5:73–8.

[129] Devinsky O, Ehrenberg B, Barthlen GM, et al. Epilepsy and sleep apnea syndrome. Neurology 1994;44:2060–4.

[130] Bazil CW. Nocturnal seizures. Semin Neurol 2004;24:293–300.

[131] Sammaritano M, Sherwin A. Effect of anticonvulsants on sleep. Neurology 2000;54 (Suppl 1):S16–24.

[132] Wolf P, Roder-Wanner UU, Brede M. Influence of therapeutic phenobarbital and phenytoin medication on the polygraphic sleep of patients with epilepsy. Epilepsia 1984;25:467–75.

[133] Gigli GL, Placidi F, Diomedi M, et al. Nocturnal sleep and daytime somnolence in untreated patients with temporal lobe epilepsy: changes after treatment with controlled-release carbamazepine. Epilepsia 1997;38:696–701.

[134] Copinschi G, Van Onderbergen A, L'Hermite-Baleriaux M, et al. Effects of the short-acting benzodiazepine triazolam, taken at bedtime, on circadian and sleep-related hormonal profiles in normal men. Sleep 1990; 13:232–44.

[135] Placidi F, Diomedi M, Scalise A, et al. Effect of anticonvulsants on nocturnal sleep in epilepsy. Neurology 2000;54(Suppl 1):S25–32.

[136] Foldvary-Schaefer N, De Leon Sanchez I, Karafa M, et al. Gabapentin increases slow-wave sleep in normal adults. Epilepsia 2002; 43:1493–7.

[137] Johnson RT. Current therapy in neurologic disease. St. Louis: BC Decker; 1985.

[138] Tachibana N, Howard RS, Hirsch NP, et al. Sleep problems in multiple sclerosis. Eur Neurol 1994;34:320–3.

[139] Fleming WE, Pollak CP. Sleep disorders in multiple sclerosis. Semin Neurol 2005;25:64–8.

[140] Carolei A, Sacco S, De Santis F, et al. Epidemiology of stroke. Clin Exp Hypertens 2002; 24:479–83.

[141] Bassetti CL, Milanova M, Gugger M. Sleep-disordered breathing and acute ischemic stroke: diagnosis, risk factors, treatment, evolution, and long-term clinical outcome. Stroke 2006; 37(4):967–72.

[142] Spriggs DA, French JM, Murdy JM, et al. Snoring increases the risk of stroke and adversely affects prognosis. Q J Med 1992;303:555–62.

[143] Qreshi AI, Giles WH, Croft JB, et al. Habitual sleep patterns and risk for stroke and coronary disease: a 10-year follow-up from NHANES I. Neurology 1997;48:904–10.

[144] Davies DP, Rodgers H, Walshaw D, et al. Snoring, daytime sleepiness and stroke: a case-control study of first-ever stroke. J Sleep Res 2003; 12:313–8.

[145] Bassetti C, Aldrich M, Chervin R, et al. Sleep apnea in the acute phase of TIA and Stroke. Neurology 1996;47:1167–73.

[146] Dyken ME, Somers VK, Yamada T, et al. Investigating the relationship between stroke and obstructive sleep apnea. Stroke 1996;27:401–7.

[147] Good DC, Henkle JQ, Gelber D, et al. Sleep-disordered breathing and poor functional outcome after stroke. Stroke 1996;27:252–9.

[148] Sandberg O, Franklin KA, Bucht G, et al. Nasal continuous positive airway pressure in stroke patients with sleep apnoea: a randomized treatment study. Eur Respir J 2001;18:619–22.

[149] Wessendorf TE, Wang YM, Thilmann AF, et al. Treatment of obstructive sleep apnoea with nasal continuous positive airway pressure. Eur Respir J 2001;18:623–9.

[150] Pepperell JCT, Ramdassingh-Dow S, Crosthwaite N, et al. Ambulatory blood pressure after therapeutic and subtherapeutic nasal continuous positive airway pressure for obstructive sleep apnoea: a randomized parallel trial. Lancet 2001;359:204–10.

[151] Parra O, Arboix A, Bechich S, et al. Time course of sleep-related breathing disorders in first-ever stroke or transient ischemic attack. Am J Respir Crit Care Med 2000;161:375–80.

[152] Iranzo A, Santamaria J, Berenguer J, et al. Prevalence and clinical importance of sleep apnea in the first night after cerebral infarction. Neurology 2002;58:911–6.

[153] Power WR, Mosko SS, Sassin JF. Sleep-stage dependent Cheyne-Stokes respiration after cerebral infarct: a case study. Neurology 1982;32:763–6.

[154] Bassetti C, Aldrich MS, Quint D. Sleep-disordered breathing in patients with acute supraand infratentorial stroke. Stroke 1997;28:1765–72.

[155] Bahro M, Katzmann KJ, Guckel F, et al. REM sleep parasomnia. Nervenarzt 1994;65:568–71.

[156] Schenck CH, Mahowald MW. Injurious sleep behavior disorders (parasomnias) affecting patients on intensive care units. Intensive Care Med 1991;17:219–24.

[157] Gordon PH, Mitsumoto H, Hays AP. Amyotrophic lateral sclerosis. Sci Aging Knowl Environ 2003;2003:dn2.

[158] Ferguson KA, Strong MJ, Ahmad D, et al. Sleep-disordered breathing in amyotrophic lateral sclerosis. Chest 1996;110:664–9.

[159] Ferguson KA, Strong MJ, Ahmad D, et al. Sleep and breathing in amyotrophic lateral sclerosis. Sleep 1995;18:514.

[160] Arnulf I, Similowski T, Salachas F, et al. Sleep disorders and diaphragmatic function in patients with amyotrophic lateral sclerosis. Am J Respir Crit Care Med 2000;161(3 Pt 1):849–56.

[161] Arnulf I, Derenne JP. Respiratory disorders during sleep in degenerative diseases of the brain stem. Rev Neurol (Paris) 2001;157(11 Pt 2):S148–51.

[162] Minz M, Autret A, Laffont F, et al. A study on sleep in amyotrophic lateral sclerosis. Biomedicine 1979;30:40–6.

[163] Culebras A. Sleep and neuromuscular disorders. Neurol Clin 1996;14:791–805.

[164] Aboussouan LS, Lewis RA. Sleep, respiration and ALS. J Neurol Sci 1999;164:1–2.

[165] Culebras A. Sleep disorders and neuromuscular disease. Semin Neurol 2005;25:33–8.

[166] Butz M, Wollinsky KH, Wiedemuth-Catrinescu U, et al. Longitudinal effects of noninvasive positive-pressure ventilation in patients with amyotrophic lateral sclerosis. Am J Phys Med Rehabil 2003;82:597–604.

[167] Culebras A. Sleep and neuromuscular disorders. Neurol Clin 2005;23(4):ix, 1209–23.

[168] Biering-Sorensen F, Biering-Sorensen M. Sleep disturbances in the spinal cord injured: an epidemiological questionnaire investigation, including a normal population. Spinal Cord 2001;39:505–13.

[169] Stockhammer E, Tobon A, Michel F, et al. Characteristics of sleep apnea syndrome in tetraplegic patients. Spinal Cord 2002;40:286–94.

[170] Short DJ, Stradling JR, Williams SJ. Prevalence of sleep apnoea in patients over 40 years of age with spinal cord lesions. J Neurol Neurosurg Psychiatry 1992;55:1032–6.

[171] Nogues M, Gene R, Benarroch E, et al. Respiratory disturbances during sleep in syringomyelia and syringobulbia. Neurology 1999;52:1777–83.

[172] Jubelt B. Post-polio syndrome. Curr Treat Options Neurol 2004;6:87–93.

[173] Dalakas MC, Sever JL, Madden DL, et al. Late postpoliomyelitis muscular atrophy: clinical, virologic, and immunologic studies. Rev Infect Dis 1984;6(Suppl 2):S562–7.

[174] Jubelt B, Cashman NR. Neurological manifestations of the post-polio syndrome. Crit Rev Neurobiol 1987;3:199–220.

[175] Bach JR. Management of post-polio respiratory sequelae. Ann N Y Acad Sci 1995;753:96–102.

[176] Bruno RL. Abnormal movements in sleep as a post-polio sequelae. Am J Phys Med Rehabil 1998;77:339–43.

[177] Steljes DG, Kryger MH, Kirk BW, et al. Sleep in postpolio syndrome. Chest 1990;98:133–40.

[178] Hansotia P, Wall R, Berendes J. Sleep disturbances and severity of Huntington's disease. Neurology 1985;35:1672–4.

[179] Emser W, Brenner M, Stober T, et al. Changes in nocturnal sleep in Huntington's and Parkinson's disease. J Neurol 1988;235:177–9.

[180] Wiegand M, Moller AA, Lauer CJ, et al. Nocturnal sleep in Huntington's disease. J Neurol 1991;238:203–8.

[181] Hurelbrink CB, Lewis SJ, Barker RA. The use of the Actiwatch-Neurologica system to objectively assess the involuntary movements and sleep-wake activity in patients with mild-moderate Huntington's disease. J Neurol 2005;252:642–7.

[182] Bollen EL, Den Heijer JC, Ponsioen C, et al. Respiration during sleep in Huntington's chorea. J Neurol Sci 1988;84:63–8.

[183] Morton AJ, Wood NI, Hastings MH, et al. Disintegration of the sleep-wake cycle and circadian timing in Huntington's disease. J Neurosci 2005;25:157–63.

[184] Martinez-Rodriguez JE, Lin L, Iranzo A, et al. Decreased hypocretin-1 (Orexin-A) levels in the cerebrospinal fluid of patients with myotonic dystrophy and excessive daytime sleepiness. Sleep 2003;26:287–90.

[185] Laberge L, Begin P, Montplaisir J, et al. Sleep complaints in patients with myotonic dystrophy. J Sleep Res 2004;13:95–100.

[186] Giubilei F, Iannilli M, Vitale A, et al. Sleep patterns in acute ischemic stroke. Acta Neurol Scand 1992;86:567–71.

[187] Damian MS, Gerlach A, Schmidt F, et al. Modafinil for excessive daytime sleepiness in myotonic dystrophy. Neurology 2001;56:794–6.

[188] MacDonald JR, Hill JD, Tarnopolsky MA. Modafinil reduces excessive somnolence and enhances mood in patients with myotonic dystrophy. Neurology 2002;59:1876–80.

[189] Sivak ED, Shefner JM, Sexton J. Neuromuscular disease and hypoventilation. Curr Opin Pulm Med 1999;5:355–62.

[190] Takasugi T, Ishihara T, Kawamura J, et al. Respiratory failure: respiratory disorder during sleep in patients with myotonic dystrophy. Rinsho Shinkeigaku 1995;35:1486–8.

[191] Ververs CC, Van der Meche FG, Verbraak AF, et al. Breathing pattern awake and asleep in myotonic dystrophy. Respiration (Herrlisheim) 1996;63:1–7.

[192] Ono S, Kurisaki H, Sakuma A, et al. Myotonic dystrophy with alveolar hypoventilation and hypersomnia: a clinicopathological study. J Neurol Sci 1995;128:225–31.

[193] Ancoli-Israel S. Sleep problems in older adults: putting myths to bed. Geriatrics 1997;52: 20–30.

[194] Phillips BA-IS. Sleep disorders in the elderly. Sleep Med 2001;2:99–114.

[195] Guilleminault C, Stoohs R, Clerk A, et al. From obstructive sleep apnea syndrome to upper airway resistance syndrome: consistency of daytime sleepiness. Sleep 1992;15(6 Suppl): S13–6.

[196] Loewenstein RJ, Weingartner H, Gillin JC, et al. Disturbances of sleep and cognitive functioning in patients with dementia. Neurobiol Aging 1982;3:371–7.

[197] Montplaisir J, Petit D, Gauthier S, et al. Sleep disturbances and EEG slowing in Alzheimer's disease. Sleep Res Online 1998;1:147–51.

SLEEP
MEDICINE
CLINICS

Sleep Med Clin 1 (2006) 293–298

Sleep Disturbances in Nursing Home Patients

Lavinia Fiorentino, MS, Sonia Ancoli-Israel, PhD*

- Methods used to study sleep in nursing home patients
- Sleep disruption in nursing home patients
- Environmental influences on sleep
- Consequences of disturbed sleep in nursing homes
- Treatment of sleep disturbances in the nursing home

- *Pharmacologic treatments*
- *Behavioral treatments*
- Sleep disordered breathing
- Interventions to reduce daytime sleeping in the nursing home
- Summary
- References

Although sleep complaints are common in all older adults, elderly people living in institutionalized settings are more susceptible to sleep disturbances for a variety of reasons and their sleep disturbances tend to be more severe when compared with nondemented elderly [1]. Nursing home patients often suffer from dementia, and it has been reported that sleep disturbances in demented patients are a contributing cause to institutionalization and represent a significant source of physical and psychologic distress for the patients' caregivers [2–4].

Factors associated with older age, including age-related sleep architecture changes (eg, more light sleep, less deep sleep), changes in the internal biologic clock (ie, propensity toward an advanced sleep phase), increased medical burden (eg, dementia, depression, chronic illness), medications used to treat possible illnesses, disrupted daily routines because of lack of a work schedule, low levels of exercise, and low exposure to daily sunlight all contribute to the deregulation of the sleep-wake cycle in this population. In addition, older people who live in institutionalized settings have even greater risk of developing sleep disturbance than community-dwelling older adults because of such factors as social isolation, low levels of activity, common sleeping rooms, and extended time spent in bed.

Some environmental factors in nursing homes also contribute to the reduction in the quality of sleep. Noise and light exposure occur intermittently throughout the night and are known to contribute to the sleep disruption. Institutionalized patients spend a significant amount of the 24-hour day in bed, leading to rapid cycling between sleep and wake during this time and poor bed-sleep stimulus control. Sleep hygiene education and changes in the sleep environment of nursing home patients (eg, darker and quiet rooms at night) may greatly improve the sleep quality in this population [5,6].

Supported by NIA 08415, NCI CA112035, CBCRP 11IB-0034, CBCRP 11GB0049, NIH grant # M01 RR00827, and NIA AG15301
Department of Psychiatry, University of California San Diego, 9500 Gilman Drive #0603, La Jolla, CA 92093, USA
* Corresponding author.
E-mail address: sancoliisrael@ucsd.edu (S. Ancoli-Israel).

1556-407X/06/$ – see front matter © 2006 Elsevier Inc. All rights reserved.
sleep.theclinics.com

doi:10.1016/j.jsmc.2006.04.002

Methods used to study sleep in nursing home patients

Behavioral observation and actigraphy are good ways to study sleep in nursing home patients because they are nonintrusive and feasible. Polysomnography is often too cumbersome and invasive for this population especially if used to record daytime and nighttime sleep. Sleep diaries and questionnaires are often excessively complicated, particularly given that dementia is prevalent in nursing home patients.

Sleep disruption in nursing home patients

It has been reported that most institutionalized older adults have one or more sleep-related complaints [7]. The sleep of patients living in nursing homes who have severe dementia has been shown to be severely disturbed and fragmented. A study by Ancoli-Israel and coworkers [8,9] showed that in nursing home patients, there is often not a single hour in a 24-hour period that is spent fully awake or fully asleep. In this study, the 200 nursing home patients sampled slept on average for only 40 minutes per hour during the night and half of the patients woke up at least twice per hour between midnight and 6:00 AM. There were no differences found in sleep fragmentation based on age, ambulation status, sleep-disordered breathing, or use of sedatives [9]. Schnelle and coworkers [10] also found that nighttime sleep percentage in nursing home patients was low (ie, 66%), and that the average duration of a nighttime sleep episode was only 20 minutes. In addition to nighttime sleep disruption, nursing home patients spend a lot of time asleep during the day. A summary of daytime behavioral observations in 230 nursing home patients from eight different institutions found that patients were asleep during 24% of the observations, and that during 36% of the observations the patients were in bed. The typical pattern consisted of returning back into bed by 2:00 to 3:00 PM and remaining in bed for the rest of the day [11]. Recently, Martin and coworkers [12] reported that 69% of 492 observed nursing home patients slept during the daytime and 60% of these had disturbed nighttime sleep. These patients also had high levels of sleep-wake cycle disturbance, which was associated with modifiable sleep hygiene factors (eg, time in bed). In addition, residents spent one third of the day in their rooms, typically in bed, seldom went outdoors, or were exposed to bright light; more time in bed and less social activity were significant predictors of daytime sleepiness. Importantly, sleep disturbance and daytime sleeping were rarely documented in medical records.

Entering the nursing home can itself result in disrupted sleep. In a study of 102 residents in three nursing homes, napping, number of awakenings at night, problems falling asleep, and sleeping pill use all increased when compared with preinstitutionalization [13]. These sleep disturbances are often precipitated and perpetuated by the poor sleep hygiene practiced in nursing home patients, including having an irregular sleep schedule, spending too much time in bed, not being exposed to sufficient bright light during the day, or sleeping in an environment that is not conducive to a good night's sleep [14].

Environmental influences on sleep

It has long been known that bright light exposure is one of the strongest cues for a good sleep-wake cycle. In the nursing home, patients are exposed to very little bright light. In a series of studies by Ancoli-Israel and colleagues [15,16], the median amount of daily light exposure in patients with dementia living in a nursing home was only 1 minute for very bright light (more than 2500 lux) and 10.5 minutes for moderate bright light (more than 1000 lux). Four percent of the patients were never exposed to any bright light. In addition, those patients exposed to higher average illumination levels during the day had more consolidated sleep at night, even when level of dementia was included in the model [15].

Noise is also a major problem in the nursing home. Schnelle and coworkers [10,17] measured noise levels at night and found that there were 32 episodes of loud noise (≥ 60 dB) per night. Noise levels increased until midnight, then decreased from 1:00 to 4:00 AM. The source of noise was most often related to nursing staff speaking loudly or staff creating other noise with squeaking medication carts or pill crushing. A minority of the time the noise was caused by the participants or their roommates [17]. The authors also measured light levels at night and found that there was an average of five light changes (ie, light being turned on and off) per night. In this study, 50% of awakenings of ≥ 4 minutes in duration were associated with either noise or light [10,17].

Consequences of disturbed sleep in nursing homes

Not sleeping at night results in daytime consequences and potential health consequences. In a study of 272 nursing home residents by Manabe and coworkers [18], data suggested that insomnia at night and particularly sleep onset delay resulted in a 1.5 to 1.8 increased risk of shorter survival at

2-year follow-up, even after adjustment for age, gender, and activities of daily living.

In a population where falls are common, there is always the fear of whether poor sleep or the treatments for poor sleep (ie, a sedating drug) will result in an increased number of falls. In one recent study, hypnotics were identified as a leading cause of falls in older adults [19]. In a second recent study, data suggested that when possible confounding variables were controlled, it was the insomnia and not the use of hypnotics that was associated with falls in nursing home patients [20]. Because these results were based on the minimal data set, randomized controlled clinical trials are needed to answer the question of the relationship between hypnotics, insomnia, and falls.

Treatment of sleep disturbances in the nursing home

Pharmacologic treatments

The treatment of sleep problems in elderly people with dementia is particularly challenging. In an older study, when compared with independent and service home living adults, institutionalized older adults had increased usage of prescribed hypnotics [21]. The pharmaceuticals used to manage the dementia (eg, sedative hypnotics and antipsychotics) may exacerbate the sleep problems [22] however, and there is some evidence that hypnotics may not be aiding the sleep of institutionalized elderly. A second older study conducted in a nursing home showed no relationship between increased or decreased use of hypnotics and degree of sleep complaints [7]. These studies were conducted before Food and Drug Administration approval of many of the newer, shorter-acting benzodiazepine receptor and melatonin receptor agonists.

Often sedating antidepressants, antipsychotics, and anticonvulsants are used off-label to help nursing home residents sleep at night. A recent National Institutes of Health panel on the state-of-the-science of insomnia concluded, however, that all of these agents have potentially significant adverse effects, raising concerns about the risk-benefit ratio, and their use in the treatment of chronic insomnia cannot be recommended [23].

Behavioral treatments

Given the environmental problems that contribute to sleep disturbances in this population, many studies have examined whether manipulating the environment results in improved sleep. Behavioral treatments, such as bright light therapy [24,25], increased physical activity, and restriction of time in bed [25–27], have been suggested as promising tools to consolidate sleep in this population.

Increased bright light exposure in the morning or evening has been shown to consolidate nighttime sleep and make circadian rhythms more robust in nursing home patients [24,25,28]. Other behavioral treatments have also been studied. Naylor and coworkers [29] examined the effect of an enforced schedule of structured social and physical activity (9:00–10:30 AM, 7:00–8:30 PM, daily for 2 weeks) in 23 residents in a continued care retirement facility. The results showed an increase in slow wave sleep and an improvement in memory-oriented tasks.

Alessi and colleagues [30], in a series of studies, examined the effect of increasing physical activity, increasing light exposure, and decreasing noise. In the first study of 65 residents, increasing physical activity during the day had no effect on sleep [30]. In a second study, 267 incontinent patients in eight nursing homes were assigned to either a delayed intervention or a behavioral intervention to decrease noise and individualize nighttime incontinence care. The results showed a decrease in nighttime noise and light and decreased awakenings associated with noise and light, but no other significant effects on sleep [31]. The third study was a multidimensional, nonpharmacologic intervention to change lifestyle and environmental factors and resulted in decreased time in bed and increased bright light exposure during the day among participants; a modest decrease in duration of awakenings at night (by wrist actigraphy); and a decrease in observed daytime sleep [27].

Alessi and coworkers [32] also examined a treatment that consisted of keeping patients out of bed during the daytime, exposure to sunlight for 30 minutes daily, increased physical activity, and structured bedtime routine that resulted in a slight decrease in duration of nighttime awakenings and a decrease in daytime sleeping. A second recent nursing home study, however, using a nonpharmacologic intervention to improve sleep that also included physical activity, attempts to keep patients out of bed during the day, and evening bright light found no significant improvement in any sleep variables [33].

A study that looked at the effects of individualized social activity on sleep in nursing home patients with dementia found that patients with an initial sleep efficiency <50% slept less during the day, had a lower day/night sleep ratio, fell asleep faster, and spent less time awake at night compared with the control group [34]. This study is particularly interesting because it sheds light on the possible relationships between little social contact and isolation and quality of sleep in nursing home patients.

Overall, the results of these interventional studies suggest that physical activity and light need to be increased during the day, whereas light and noise levels need to be decreased at night. In addition to studies that manipulated the environment, one study of acupressure was shown to decrease nocturnal awakenings and wake time after sleep onset compared with the sham-acupressure group and with a control group [35].

Sleep disordered breathing

Sleep-disordered breathing is a condition in which people stop breathing while asleep as a function of their upper-airways being obstructed or collapsed. It is characterized by hypopneas (partial respiration) or apneas (complete cessation of respiration) during sleep. The prevalence of sleep-disordered breathing is higher in older adults (45%–62% in those over 60 years old) compared with younger and middle-aged adults (4%–9% in those 30–60 years old) [36,37], and even higher in demented nursing home patients [38,39].

In one of the first studies of sleep apnea and dementia in the nursing home, Ancoli-Israel and coworkers [38] found that most patients had sleep apnea. In addition, those with severe dementia had significantly more severe sleep apnea and those with severe sleep apnea had significantly more severe dementia. A second study from the same laboratory confirmed that 90% of the patients had more than five respiratory disturbances per hour of sleep (mean RDI = 32; SD = 26.1); 63% had greater than 15 (mean = 40.6; SD = 26.7); and 50% had more than 20 events per hour of sleep (mean = 46.9; SD = 26.6) [39]. A more recent study of 109 nursing home patients with daytime sleepiness found that 40% of the patients had abnormal oxygen desaturation indices (>5), which were correlated with loud breathing [40]. This study found no correlation between other symptoms of sleep-disordered breathing, such as loud snoring and discontinuous thoracic movements, and oxygen desaturation indices.

Assessment and treatment of sleep-disordered breathing in the nursing home population is important because respiratory events lead to repeated arousals from sleep and reductions in blood oxygen levels over the course of the night, which results in nighttime hypoxemia. This in turn may cause excessive daytime sleepiness and affect levels of alertness, time spent sleeping, and the overall functioning. Sleep-disordered breathing and excessive daytime sleepiness may lower the quality of life of nursing home patients by causing reduced vigilance, and cognitive deficits, including decreased concentration, slowed response time, and memory and attention difficulties. Nursing home patients are at risk of developing these symptoms as a reflection of age, but also concomitantly with neurologic diseases, such as Alzheimer's or Parkinson's disease. It is particularly important to recognize and treat sleep-disordered breathing in a timely manner to avoid further exacerbation of the cognitive deficits. Furthermore, sleep-disordered breathing is a risk factor for other health problems, particularly hypertension and cardiac and pulmonary problems [41,42], which may lead to increased risk of mortality [43–45].

Interventions to reduce daytime sleeping in the nursing home

Although many studies have attempted to improve nighttime sleep in the nursing home setting and studies suggest that increasing exposure to bright light can have some modest beneficial effects on nighttime sleep and circadian rhythms [24,25,46], less work has focused on interventions to reduce daytime sleeping specifically. In the study by Ancoli-Israel and coworkers [25], bright light therapy and daytime sleep restriction were compared. In this study, participants did not show an overall reduction in the amount of sleep during the daytime hours, although there were some improvements in nighttime sleep and circadian activity rhythms among participants who received exposure to bright light during the day. Alessi and coworkers [32] used a comprehensive 24-hour intervention to regularize sleep-wake patterns among nursing home residents with baseline nighttime sleep the intervention trial. This intervention resulted in a substantial reduction in daytime sleeping. Residents in the intervention group decreased daytime sleeping from 32% at baseline to 21% at follow-up with no change in usual-care control participants. This intervention, however, led to only modest changes in nighttime sleep quality.

Summary

Sleep disturbances in nursing home patients are common, and often are a consequence of multiple factors including primary sleep disorders, medical and psychiatric illnesses, concomitant drug use, circadian rhythm changes, and environmental factors. Sleep difficulties in nursing home patients may increase the risk of falls, affect the ability to concentrate and recall, and decrease the overall quality of life. It is important to recognize that sleep difficulties are not an inevitable part of aging or of residing in an institutionalized setting. Sleep and circadian rhythm disorders can and should be treated in this population to avoid the burdensome health

<table>
<tr><td>

Box 1:   Tips for healthier sleep in nursing homes

Improve environment
Keep environment dark at night
Keep environment bright during the day
Keep the environment quiet at night
Match roommates (eg, night owls with night owls)

Adjust behavior
Timing of medication (eg, sedatives given at night, stimulants during the day)
Avoid caffeine
Limit time in bed during the day
Increase activity and socialization

</td></tr>
</table>

problems that they might cause or accentuate. To enhance the quality of life in institutionalized elderly, doctors and nurses providing health care in nursing homes need to be able to recognize the symptomatology, prevalence, and possible etiologies of the sleep disturbances in this population and the appropriate treatments and environmental changes that can be applied to facilitate better sleep (Box 1).

References

[1] Vitiello MV, Prinz PN, Williams DE, et al. Sleep disturbances in patients with mild-stage Alzheimer's disease. J Gerontol 1990;45:M131–8.

[2] Gaugler JE, Edwards AB, Femia EE, et al. Predictors of institutionalization of cognitively impaired elders: family help and the timing of placement. J Gerontol B Psychol Sci Soc Sci 2000;55:247–55.

[3] Vitiello MV, Borson S. Sleep disturbances in patients with Alzheimer's disease. CNS Drugs 2001;15:777–96.

[4] Donaldson C, Tarrier N, Burns A. Determinants of carer stress in Alzheimer's disease. Int J Geriatr Psychiatry 1998;13:248–56.

[5] Ancoli-Israel S, Jones DW, McGuinn P, et al. Sleep disorders. In: Morris J, Lipshitz J, Murphy K, et al, editors. Quality care for the nursing home. St Louis: Mosby Lifeline; 1997. p. 64–73.

[6] Alessi CA, Schnelle JF. Approach to sleep disorders in the nursing home setting. Sleep Med Rev 2000;4:45–56.

[7] Monane M, Glynn RJ, Avorn J. The impact of sedative-hypnotic use on sleep symptoms in elderly nursing home residents. Clin Pharmacol Ther 1996;59:83–92.

[8] Jacobs D, Ancoli-Israel S, Parker L, et al. Twenty-four hour sleep-wake patterns in a nursing home population. Psychol Aging 1989;4:352–6.

[9] Ancoli-Israel S, Parker L, Sinaee R, et al. Sleep fragmentation in patients from a nursing home. J Gerontol 1989;44:M18–21.

[10] Schnelle JF, Ouslander JG, Simmons SF, et al. Nighttime sleep and bed mobility among incontinent nursing home residents. J Am Geriatr Soc 1993;41:903–9.

[11] Schnelle JF, Cruise PA, Alessi CA, et al. Sleep hygiene in physically dependent nursing home residents. Sleep 1998;21:515–23.

[12] Martin JL, Webber AP, Alam T, et al. Daytime sleeping, sleep disturbance and circadian rhythms in nursing home residents. Am J Geriatr Psychiatry 2006;14(2):121–9.

[13] Clapin-French E. Sleep patterns of aged persons in long-term care facilities. J Adv Nurs 1986; 11:57–66.

[14] Ancoli-Israel S, Parker L, Sinaee R, et al. Sleep in a nursing home population [abstract]. Sleep Res 1987;16:298.

[15] Ancoli-Israel S, Klauber MR, Jones DW, et al. Variations in circadian rhythms of activity, sleep and light exposure related to dementia in nursing home patients. Sleep 1997;20:18–23.

[16] Shochat T, Martin J, Marler M, et al. Illumination levels in nursing home patients: effects on sleep and activity rhythms. J Sleep Res 2000;9:373–80.

[17] Schnelle JF, Ouslander JG, Simmons SF, et al. The nighttime environment, incontinence care, and sleep disruption in nursing homes. J Am Geriatr Soc 1993;41:910–4.

[18] Manabe K, Matsui T, Yamaya M, et al. Sleep patterns and mortality among elderly patients in a geriatric hospital. Gerontology 2000;46: 318–22.

[19] Brassington GS, King AC, Bliwise DL. Sleep problems as a risk factor for falls in a sample of community-dwelling adults aged 64–99 years. J Am Geriatr Soc 2000;48:1234–40.

[20] Avidan AY, Fries BE, James MC, et al. Insomnia and hypnotic use, recorded in the minimum data set, as predictors of falls and hip fractures in Michigan nursing homes. J Am Geriatr Soc 2005;53:955–62.

[21] Middelkoop HA, Kerkhof GA, Smilde-van den Doel DA, et al. Sleep and ageing: the effect of institutionalization on subjective and objective characteristics of sleep. Age Ageing 1994; 23:411–7.

[22] Lenzer J. FDA warns about using antipsychotic drugs for dementia. BMJ 2005;330:922.

[23] NIH State of the Science Conference Statement on Insomnia. Manifestations and Management of Chronic Insomnia in Adults June 13–15, 2005. Sleep 2005;28:1049–58.

[24] Ancoli-Israel S, Gehrman PR, Martin JL, et al. Increased light exposure consolidates sleep and strengthens circadian rhythms in severe Alzheimer's disease patients. Behavioral Sleep Medicine 2003;1:22–36.

[25] Ancoli-Israel S, Martin JL, Kripke DF, et al. Effect of light treatment on sleep and circadian

rhythms in demented nursing home patients. J Am Geriatr Soc 2002;50:282–9.

[26] Ancoli-Israel S, Poceta JS, Stepnowsky C, et al. Identification and treatment of sleep problems in the elderly. Sleep Med Rev 1997;1:3–17.

[27] Alessi CA, Yoon EJ, Schnelle JF, et al. A randomized trial of a combined physical activity and environmental intervention in nursing home residents: do sleep and agitation improve? J Am Geriatr Soc 1999;47:784–91.

[28] Fetveit A, Bjorvatn B. The effects of bright-light therapy on actigraphical measured sleep last for several weeks post-treatment: a study in a nursing home population. J Sleep Res 2004;13:153–8.

[29] Naylor E, Penev PD, Orbeta L, et al. Daily social and physical activity increases slow-wave sleep and daytime neuropsychological performance in the elderly. Sleep 2000;23:87–95.

[30] Alessi CA, Schnelle JF, MacRae PG, et al. Does physical activity improve sleep in impaired nursing home residents? J Am Geriatr Soc 1995; 43:1098–102.

[31] Schnelle JF, Alessi CA, Al-Samarrai NR, et al. The nursing home at night: effects of an intervention on noise, light and sleep. J Am Geriatr Soc 1999; 47:430–8.

[32] Alessi CA, Martin JL, Webber AP, et al. Randomized, controlled trial of a nonpharmacological intervention to improve abnormal sleep/wake patterns in nursing home residents. J Am Geriatr Soc 2005;53:803–10.

[33] Ouslander JG, Connell BR, Bliwise DL, et al. A nonpharmacological intervention to improve sleep in nursing home patients: results of a controlled clinical trial. J Am Geriatr Soc 2006; 54:38–47.

[34] Richards KC, Beck C, O'Sullivan PS, et al. Effect of individualized social activity on sleep in nursing home residents with dementia. J Am Geriatr Soc 2005;53:1510–7.

[35] Chen ML, Lin LC, Wu SC, et al. The effectiveness of acupressure in improving the quality of sleep of institutionalized residents. J Gerontol A Biol Sci Med Sci 1999;54:M389–94.

[36] Young T, Palta M, Dempsey J, et al. The occurrence of sleep disordered breathing among middle-aged adults. N Engl J Med 1993;328: 1230–5.

[37] Ancoli-Israel S, Kripke DF, Klauber MR, et al. Sleep disordered breathing in community-dwelling elderly. Sleep 1991;14:486–95.

[38] Ancoli-Israel S, Klauber MR, Butters N, et al. Dementia in institutionalized elderly: relation to sleep apnea. J Am Geriatr Soc 1991;39:258–63.

[39] Gehrman PR, Martin JL, Shochat T, et al. Sleep disordered breathing and agitation in institutionalized adults with Alzheimer's disease. Am J Geriatr Psychiatry 2003;11:426–33.

[40] Martin JL, Mory AK, Alessi CA. Nighttime oxygen desaturation and symptoms of sleep-disordered breathing in long-stay nursing home residents. J Gerontol A Biol Sci Med Sci 2005;60:104–8.

[41] Nieto FJ, Young T, Lind B, et al. Association of sleep-disordered breathing, sleep apnea, and hypertension in a large community-based study. JAMA 2000;283:1829–36.

[42] Newman AB, Nieto FJ, Guidry U, et al. Relation of sleep-disordered breathing to cardiovascular disease risk factors: the Sleep Heart Health Study. Am J Epidemiol 2001;154:50–9.

[43] Ancoli-Israel S, DuHamel ER, Stepnowsky C, et al. The relationship between congestive heart failure, sleep disordered breathing and mortality in older men. Chest 2003;124:1400–5.

[44] Ancoli-Israel S, Kripke DF, Klauber MR, et al. Morbidity, mortality and sleep disordered breathing in community dwelling elderly. Sleep 1996;19:277–82.

[45] Ancoli-Israel S, Klauber MR, Fell RL, et al. Sleep disordered breathing: preliminary natural history and mortality results. In: Seifert RA, Carlson J, editors. International perspective on applied psychophysiology. New York: Plenum Publishing; 1994. p. 103–11.

[46] van Someren E, Kessler A, Mirmiran M, et al. Indirect bright light improves circadian rest-activity rhythm disturbances in demented patients. Biol Psychiat 1997;41:955–63.

SLEEP
MEDICINE
CLINICS

ELSEVIER
SAUNDERS

Sleep Med Clin 1 (2006) 299–303

Index

Note: Page numbers of article titles are in **boldface** type.

A

Acid reflux, sleep disturbances in older adults related to, 238

Aging, alterations in Circadian rhythms with, **187–196**
- Circadian amplitude, 189
- Circadian clock, 188
  - responsiveness of to photic and nonphotic stimuli, 188–189
- Circadian phase, 189–190
- decreased exposure to synchronizing agents, 190–192
- entrainment of, 190
- manipulation of, therapeutic implications, 192
- neurobiology of, 187–188

normal, sleep and cognition in, **207–220**

normal, sleep in, **171–176**
- causes of disturbed sleep in, 174–175
- Circadian rhythms in, 173
- napping and excessive daytime sleepiness in, 173–174

Alcohol dependence, sleep disturbances in older adults due to, 235–236

Alternative therapies, non-hormonal, impact on sleep in midlife women, 202

Alzheimer's disease, sleep disturbances in patients with, 274–277
- Circadian rhythm disturbances in, 276
- sleep architecture in, 275–276
- sleep-disordered breathing in, 276
- treatment of, 276–277

Amyotrophic lateral sclerosis, sleep disturbances in elderly patients with, 284

Anxiety disorders, sleep disturbances in older adults due to, 234–235

Arthritis, sleep disturbances in older adults related to, 237

B

Behavioral treatments, for sleep disturbances in nursing homes, 295–296

Bereavement, sleep disturbances in older adults due to stresses of, 234

Bipolar affective disorder, sleep disturbances in older adults due to, 234

Breathing disorders, sleep-related, in the elderly, **247–262**
- clinical assessment and management, 255–257
  - presentation and diagnosis, 255–256
  - treatment, 256–257
- clinical features, 248–249
- epidemiology, 249–250
  - prevalence and incidence, 249–250
  - risk factors, 250
- in nursing home patients, 296
- morbidity and mortality associated with, 250–255
  - cardiovascular consequences, 250–252
  - cognitive impairment and dementia, 253–254
  - falls and fractures, 254–255
  - metabolic consequences, 252–253
  - mortality, 254
- physiologic features, 248

C

Caffeine, sleep disturbances in older adults due to, 236

Cancer, sleep disturbances in older adults related to, 239

Cardiovascular consequences, of sleep-disordered breathing in the elderly, 250–252

Caregiving, sleep disturbances in older adults due to demands of, 234

1556-407X/06/$ – see front matter © 2006 Elsevier Inc. All rights reserved.
sleep.theclinics.com

doi:10.1016/S1556-407X(06)00049-X

Moving?

Make sure your subscription moves with you!

To notify us of your new address, find your **Clinics Account Number** (located on your mailing label above your name), and contact customer service at:

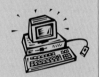

E-mail: elspcs@elsevier.com

800-654-2452 (subscribers in the U.S. & Canada)
407-345-4000 (subscribers outside of the U.S. & Canada)

Fax number: 407-363-9661

Elsevier Periodicals Customer Service
6277 Sea Harbor Drive
Orlando, FL 32887-4800

*To ensure uninterrupted delivery of your subscription, please notify us at least 4 weeks in advance of move.

ELSEVIER